Clinical Cardiology
An Illustrated Text

Published by Chapman & Hall, 2–6 Boundary Row, London SE1 8HN, UK

Chapman & Hall, 2–6 Boundary Row, London SE1 8HN, UK

Chapman & Hall GmbH, Pappelallee 3, 69469 Weinheim, Germany

Chapman & Hall USA, 115 Fifth Avenue, New York, NY 10003, USA

Chapman & Hall Japan, ITP-Japan, Kyowa Building, 3F, 2-2-1 Hirakawacho, Chiyoda-ku, Tokyo 102, Japan

Chapman & Hall Australia, 102 Dodds Street, South Melbourne, Victoria 3205, Australia

Chapman & Hall India, R. Seshadri, 32 Second Main Road, CIT East, Madras 600 035, India

First edition 1988
First revised edition 1990
Second revised edition 1998

© 1988, 1990, 1998 Current Medical Literature Ltd

Typeset in Goudy
Printed in the UK by Bath Press Colourbooks

ISBN 0 412 78310 X

A catalogue record for this book is available from the British Library

Clinical Cardiology
An Illustrated Text

George C. Sutton

MD, FRCP, FACC

*Consultant Cardiologist, Hillingdon Hospital, Uxbridge
and Senior Lecturer in Cardiology, National Heart and Lung Institute
Imperial College School of Medicine, London, UK*

Kanu Chatterjee

MB, FRCP (Lond), FRCP (Edin), FCCP, FACC, MACP

*Professor of Medicine and Lucie Stern Professor of Cardiology
University of California, San Francisco, USA*

Forewords by

Philip A. Poole-Wilson MD, FRCP, FACC, FESC
*Professor of Cardiology, National Heart and Lung Institute, Imperial College School of Medicine
London, UK*

William W. Parmley MD, FACC
*Professor of Medicine, Vilensky Professor of Cardiology, Division of Cardiology, University of California,
San Francisco, USA*

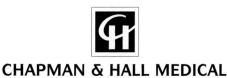

CHAPMAN & HALL MEDICAL
London · Weinheim · New York · Tokyo · Melbourne · Madras

Major Series Contributors

Professor M. Davies
St George's Hospital Medical School, London, UK

Dr Y. Ho
National Heart and Lung Institute, Imperial College School of Medicine, London, UK

Mr G. Leech
St George's Hospital Medical School, London, UK

Dr J. Mann
St George's Hospital Medical School, London, UK

Dr P. Nihoyannopoulos
National Heart and Lung Institute, Imperial College School of Medicine, London, UK

Dr D. Pennell
National Heart and Lung Institute, Imperial College School of Medicine, London, UK

Dr M. Raphael
Middlesex Hospital, London, UK

Professor J. Swales
University of Leicester School of Medicine, Leicester, UK

Acknowledgements

Appreciation is extended to Kim Fox, who co-edited *A Colour Atlas of Heart Disease* (1990) with Dr Sutton. Some of the material included in this book also appeared in that title.

The authors are grateful to John Swales, Professor of Medicine, University of Leicester, for the chapter on Hypertension; many of the illustrations used in this chapter were generously made available by Dr E.H. Mackay of Leicester General Hospital.

The authors gratefully acknowledge the contributions of Robert Anderson, John Bayliss, John Cleland, John Davies, David Hackett, Stuart Hunter, Ian Kerr, Fergus McCartney, Simon Rees, Michael Rigby, and Richard Underwood.

Thanks also go to Dr Elyse Foster, Dr Rita Redberg, and Dr Eli Botvinick, Moffitt-Long Hospital, University of California, San Francisco, USA, for providing many of the illustrations.

Clinical Cardiology
An Illustrated Text

Contents

Forewords		vi
Preface		vii
Chapter 1	***Ischemic Heart Disease***	
	Stable Angina	3
	Variant Angina	34
	Unstable Angina	40
	Acute Myocardial Infarction	47
Chapter 2	***Heart Failure***	93
Chapter 3	***Hypertension***	129
Chapter 4	***Valve Disease***	
	Mitral Stenosis	169
	Mitral Regurgitation	188
	Aortic Stenosis	206
	Aortic Regurgitation	230
	Tricuspid Valve Disease	251
Chapter 5	***Congenital Heart Disease***	
	Atrial Septal Defect	269
	Ventricular Septal Defect	283
	Persistent Ductus Arteriosus	296
	Pulmonary Stenosis	306
	Fallot's Tetralogy	314
	Coarctation of the Aorta	321
Chapter 6	***The Cardiomyopathies***	
	Dilated Cardiomyopathy	331
	Hypertrophic Cardiomyopathy	342
	Restrictive Cardiomyopathy	359
Chapter 7	***Miscellaneous Cardiac Conditions***	
	Cardiac Tumors	373
	Pulmonary Embolic and Pulmonary Vascular Disease	389
	Pericardial Disease	409
Index		421

Forewords

This book is different, very different. The reasons arise from fundamental questions with regard to medical education and the approach to health delivery and patient care. At the present time in many countries, the cost of modern medicine has exceeded the resources which those countries choose to allocate to healthcare. This financial deficit is particularly evident in specialties, such as cardiology, where frequent use is made of high technology. At the same time, there has been much enthusiasm for evidence-based medicine, control of allocation of resources, and measures which, when applied to the population as a whole, should bring about a fall in the incidence and prevalence of selected medical conditions.

This book is a majestic riposte and provides an alternative approach which might, by contrast, be called patient-based medicine – that is, clinical medicine where prominence is given to establishing a correct diagnosis and tailoring treatment to the individual patient. The book has a uniform style because, unlike many others, it has only two authors. The two are well known clinical cardiologists who were brought up in a school of cardiology in the United Kingdom which placed great emphasis on the elucidation of a proper history, a detailed clinical examination, and the use of selected investigations. The book provides clear evidence that such skills will not and should not be lost.

The book uses illustrations, diagrams, and drawings to allow the reader to understand with little difficulty many conditions which otherwise appear complex. Much attention has been paid to the detail of presentation. The way in which this is done is based on modern ideas concerning the optimum organization of a page for learning and teaching. The combination of high quality presentation and the emphasis on clinical cardiology makes this book different from all other current textbooks. Books are usually written to be read and may be long and tedious. Only a few give pleasure when just held or on turning the pages. The reader is then drawn in by curiosity and spurred on by the possibility of secret revelations hidden on other pages. This is just such a book. It is a book which will give endless pleasure to the clinical cardiologist.

Philip A. Poole-Wilson MD, FRCP, FACC, FESC
Professor of Cardiology, National Heart and Lung Institute, Imperial College School of Medicine
London, UK
Past President, European Society of Cardiology

In industrialized countries, heart disease remains a major cause of mortality. There are so many textbooks, monographs, etc. published on heart disease that one might legitimately ask, why do we need another book on heart disease? I believe the answer is related to the unique nature of this illustrated text by Drs Sutton and Chatterjee.

Cardiology has become a very visual specialty. From electrocardiograms to echocardiography, angiography, chest X-rays, radionuclide imaging, computed tomography, and magnetic resonance imaging and spectroscopy, we are constantly reviewing 'pictures' in the evaluation and management of patients. Truly, 'a picture is worth a thousand words'. Readers of this new account on clinical cardiology will be pleased with the high quality illustrations which accompany a very clinically oriented text comprising the full spectrum of cardiac diseases. The authors have an international reputation as teachers of clinical cardiology, so it is no surprise that they have written a clear, concise text, which complements the value of the images.

I believe that this work will be an extremely useful addition to a cardiology library. It will be especially helpful to students, house officers, and fellows to use as a quick source of reference for any given cardiac problem. The combination of pictures and text will provide a more lasting remembrance of a disease than the numerous words to be found in standard textbooks. I recommend it not only to the novice but also as an important reference book for the most seasoned cardiologist.

William W. Parmley MD, FACC
Professor of Medicine, Vilensky Professor of Cardiology, Division of Cardiology
University of California, San Francisco, USA
Editor-in-Chief, Journal of the American College of Cardiology
Past President, American College of Cardiology

Preface

The purpose of this work is to present cardiology in a way which makes clinical diagnosis and management easy to understand by undergraduates and postgraduates alike. It is neither a textbook of cardiology nor an atlas. The text, which is the most important aspect, comprises a concise account of the main clinical, investigatory, and management features of the principal cardiological conditions which affect adults. We believe that knowledge of the pathology and deranged physiology of these conditions will enable the reader to understand the clinical presentation, the investigatory features, and their role in management, as well as the actual management of the individual patient.

The contents are copiously illustrated, providing an important resource for the teacher of cardiology. It is not a text written around a collection of illustrations, but a text of clinical cardiology which is appropriately illustrated.

The following account represents the synthesis of many years devoted to the care of patients with heart disease, and our teaching of medical students and physicians. It would never have been completed without the support, patience, and understanding of our wives. We would like to express our sincere thanks to Jane and Docey.

George C. Sutton MD, FRCP, FACC
Consultant Cardiologist, Hillingdon Hospital, Uxbridge
and Senior Lecturer in Cardiology, National Heart and Lung Institute
Imperial College School of Medicine, London, UK

Kanu Chatterjee MB, FRCP (Lond), FRCP (Edin), FCCP, FACC, MACP
Professor of Medicine and Lucie Stern Professor of Cardiology
University of California, San Francisco, USA

CHAPTER 1
Ischemic Heart Disease

STABLE ANGINA

VARIANT ANGINA

UNSTABLE ANGINA

ACUTE MYOCARDIAL INFARCTION

Abbreviations

A	Aneurysm	LLATL	Left lateral
AMVL	Anterior mitral valve leaflet	LV	Left ventricle
ANT	Anterior	LVEF	Left ventricular ejection fraction
Ao	Aorta	MV	Mitral valve
AoV	Aortic valve	MVL	Mitral valve leaflet
AP	Antero-posterior	N	Negative contrast effect
ED	End-diastole	PMVL	Posterior mitral valve leaflet
Eff	Effusion	PVW	Posterior ventricular wall
ES	End-systole	RA	Right atrium
IVS	Interventricular septum	RAO	Right anterior oblique
LA	Left atrium	RV	Right ventricle
LAD	Left anterior descending	TV	Tricuspid valve
LAO	Left anterior oblique	VSD	Ventricular septal defect
LAT	Lateral		

General Pathology

Ischemic heart disease almost always results from atherosclerosis of the coronary arteries [1]. Although atheroma may occur to a variable extent in the coronary arterial tree, the histologic pattern is consistent. Over 75% of the atherosclerotic lesions are eccentric [2]. Concentric lesions involving the whole circumference of the coronary artery occur less frequently. An advanced atheromatous plaque consists of a thickened intima with intramural deposition of lipids (primarily cholesterol and cholesteryl esters) in and around cells of the arterial wall. There is also cellular proliferation, fibrosis, and calcification. Sometimes advanced plaques are separated from the lumen by a thin layer of fibrous tissue. Early atherosclerotic lesions are characterized by the appearance of cholesterol-laden macrophages that accumulate in the subintimal space immediately below the endothelial cells lining the artery (fatty streaks). Concentric coronary artery lesions tend to produce fixed luminal obstruction. In the presence of eccentric lesions, the smooth muscles in the uninvolved segment of the arterial wall remain responsive to vasoactive stimuli; thus, dynamic changes in the luminal diameter can occur.

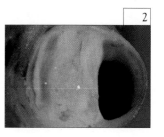

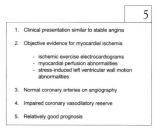

Myocardial ischemia and necrosis may occur very infrequently in the absence of obstructive atherosclerotic coronary artery disease. Coronary artery spasm, coronary emboli, anomalous origin of the coronary artery, coronary arteritis, Kawasaki's disease [3], collagen vascular disease, cardiomyopathies, and cocaine abuse are clinical examples in which myocardial ischemia with its consequences can occur in the absence of atherosclerotic coronary artery disease.

Although coronary atherosclerosis is the common pathologic substrate of ischemic heart disease, considerable differences can be identified in the pathophysiologic mechanisms of the different clinical syndromes. The important clinical syndromes are stable angina, variant angina (also known as Prinzmetal or vasospastic angina), unstable angina, and acute myocardial infarction. These will be described in the subsections that follow. Variant angina, unstable angina, and acute myocardial infarction constitute the acute cardiac ischemic syndromes.

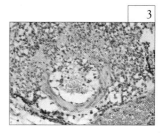

STABLE ANGINA

Definition

Chest pain (or dyspnea) occurs usually at a repetitive and predictable level of exercise. It can be precipitated by emotional stress. The heart rate–systolic blood pressure product (an index of myocardial oxygen demand) at the onset of angina or ischemic ST-segment changes in the exercise electrocardiogram (angina or ischemic threshold) usually does not vary.

Pathophysiology

In the vast majority of patients, obstructive atherosclerotic coronary artery lesions are present, limiting the required increase in coronary blood flow to meet the increased metabolic demand during physical activity or emotional stress. Although initially coronary blood flow increases as the heart rate–blood pressure product increases, at the onset of myocardial ischemia flow becomes limited relative to the demand for increase in myocardial oxygen requirement during physical activity. Thus, excessive increase in myocardial oxygen demand is the dominant mechanism for the imbalance of myocardial oxygen demand and supply which produces myocardial ischemia and results in the symptoms of stable angina [4].

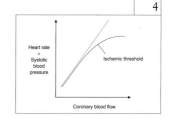

Some patients with exertional stable angina have been shown to have anatomically normal coronary arteries, yet demonstrate stress-induced myocardial ischemia. This relatively uncommon condition is termed syndrome X. Impaired coronary vasodilatory reserve may be the mechanism [5].

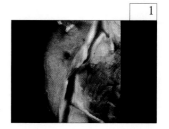

1. Clinical presentation similar to stable angina
2. Objective evidence for myocardial ischemia
   - ischemic exercise electrocardiograms
   - myocardial perfusion abnormalities
   - stress-induced left ventricular wall motion abnormalities
3. Normal coronary arteries on angiography
4. Impaired coronary vasodilatory reserve
5. Relatively good prognosis

Presentation

Symptoms

In stable angina, chest pain typically occurs at a predictable level of physical exercise or during emotional stress. Cold weather, heavy meals (postprandial angina), or the recumbent position may precipitate angina in some patients. Usually, but not invariably, the greater the degree of coronary artery narrowing, the lesser the level of activity or stress required to precipitate angina. Typically, the chest pain is relieved with cessation of activity or stress. Relief of the discomfort with nitroglycerin is suggestive but not diagnostic of pain due to myocardial ischemia. The duration of chest pain in stable angina rarely exceeds 15 minutes. The location of chest pain is usually retrosternal or precordial but ischemic pain may occasionally start in the epigastric or infrascapular regions. The radiation of pain may extend to the neck, lower jaw, epigastrium, back, or arms. The character of the pain is usually 'deep and dull'. Instead of pain, patients may describe heaviness, tightness, pressure, or an indigestion-like sensation [6]. A minority of patients complain predominantly of dyspnea with little or no chest discomfort. Momentary sensations or prolonged duration (hours) make the diagnosis of angina unlikely. The term 'important' angina may be used for those patients whose normal life-style is significantly affected.

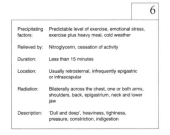

Discomfort similar to that of myocardial ischemia may occur in non-cardiac conditions such as esophageal pathology [7], and gall bladder, peptic ulcer, and pancreatic disease. The pain of costo-chondritis (Tietze's syndrome) may be similar to that of angina. In particular, the pain accompanying esophageal spasm may be relieved by nitroglycerin and have an identical radiation to that of myocardial ischemia.

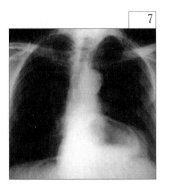

Signs
In the majority of patients with stable angina, particularly those without prior myocardial infarction, abnormal physical findings are not detected. However, if the patient is examined during the episode of angina, a palpable double apical impulse, and/or audible atrial (fourth) or third heart sounds, reversed splitting of the second heart sound, and the murmurs of mitral regurgitation may be detected. If these abnormal findings are transient, the diagnosis of myocardial ischemia is very likely.

Investigations

Radiology
Most patients with stable angina, in the absence of left ventricular dysfunction, have a normal plain chest radiograph.

Electrocardiography
The resting ECG may often be normal. However, it may show evidence of an old myocardial infarction, ST-T abnormalities, and intra-ventricular conduction defects (e.g. left bundle branch block).

Exercise Stress Testing
Treadmill exercise or bicycle ergometry with concurrent recording of the ECG is useful for the diagnosis of myocardial ischemia, particularly in patients with established or suspected stable angina. The most specific change is downsloping ST-segment depression, particularly in association with the development of chest pain [8]. Usually 1 mm ST-segment depression is suggestive of myocardial ischemia. Upsloping ST-segment changes, increased voltage of the QRS complex, T-wave inversion, and pseudonormalization of the T-waves have less diagnostic value. Failure of the systolic blood pressure to rise or an actual fall, an inadequate rise in heart rate (chronotropic incompetence), and prolonged recovery time of exercise-induced myocardial ischemia may indicate severe coronary artery disease including left main coronary artery stenosis. However, the onset of ischemia in the early stages of exercise (within stage 2, Bruce protocol) is probably the most sensitive indicator of severe myocardial ischemia. ST-segment elevation during exercise indicates transmural ischemia due to severe proximal coronary artery stenosis in patients with stable angina. Exercise-induced ST-segment elevation may also be observed in patients with variant angina or in patients with recent anterior myocardial infarction [9]. Occasionally arrhythmias develop in association with ischemic ST-segment

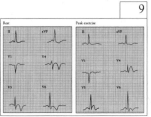

changes [10]. The presence of an abnormal resting ECG, particularly left bundle branch block, makes interpretation of ST-segment changes unrewarding.

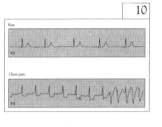

Ambulatory ECG Recording
Continuous ambulatory ECG recording provides information both about rhythm abnormalities and about myocardial ischemia in patients with ischemic heart disease. The technique is useful in patients with episodic chest pain thought to be due to myocardial ischemia (see sections on Variant Angina and Unstable Angina). Striking ST-segment shift may occur during episodes of chest pain, but it may also occur in patients with ischemic heart disease without chest pain ('silent' ischemia) [11]. The frequency of silent ischemic episodes is much higher than those associated with chest pain. Silent ischemia can be precipitated by an increase in myocardial oxygen demand, such as an increase in heart rate, or by a spontaneous reduction in coronary blood flow due to an increase in coronary vascular tone. The prognostic significance of silent ischemia in various clinical syndromes of ischemic heart disease remains controversial. The management of patients with or without silent ischemia remains the same. Some patients with episodic chest pain may be shown by ambulatory ECG monitoring to have transient, unsuspected arrhythmias responsible for chest pain.

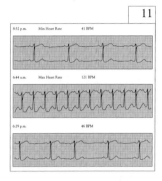

Nuclear Techniques
Various nuclear imaging tests provide information regarding myocardial perfusion and function which complement the anatomic information obtained by coronary arteriography. Thallium-201 imaging is most frequently employed to assess myocardial perfusion. The thallium-201 isotope is actively extracted by myocardial cells in proportion to coronary blood flow and myocardial perfusion. Thallium images therefore provide a map of myocardial perfusion with defects representing areas of impaired perfusion due to ischemic or fibrotic myocardium. The isotope is injected intravenously at peak stress with imaging being performed immediately afterwards and again after rest. Areas of infarction demonstrate fixed defects, but ischemic myocardium has impaired uptake initially and improved uptake following redistribution [12,13]. The introduction of tomographic techniques to enhance the thallium perfusion image has improved the sensitivity and specificity of nuclear perfusion imaging techniques in the diagnosis of myocardial ischemia.

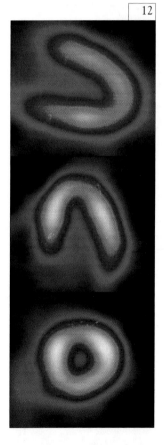

The usual technique of redistribution imaging at four hours after initial post-stress imaging may not always reveal redistribution in the ischemic myocardial segments, which may thus appear as fixed defects. Reinjection of thallium-201 after redistribution imaging at four hours often enhances thallium uptake by the ischemic myocardium by increasing isotope concentration in the blood [14]. Delayed imaging at 24 hours may also demonstrate greater thallium-201 uptake by the ischemic myocardial segments compared with the redistribution imaging at four hours [15]. These newer techniques, along with use of single photon emission computed tomography (SPECT), appear to have higher positive and negative predictive values, compared with standard thallium-201 planar imaging techniques, in the diagnosis of the presence of ischemic myocardial segments. Newer radionuclide tracers such as technetium-99m isonitrile (^{99m}Tc MIBI) have been used for the diagnosis of ischemia [16].

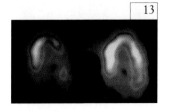

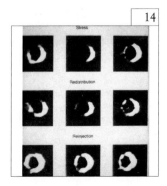

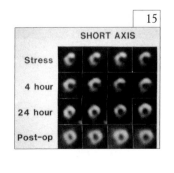

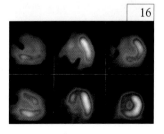

Pharmacologic stress induction using dipyridamole [17], adenosine [18] (both potent coronary vasodilators), or intravenous dobutamine [19] can be used to enhance or substitute for exercise in the detection of myocardial ischemia by thallium scanning. In clinical practice, perfusion imaging using pharmacologic stress is most frequently employed when exercise stress testing cannot be performed or is contraindicated (lower extremity peripheral vascular disease or musculo-skeletal disease).

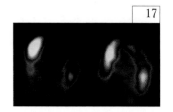

Perfusion imaging is most useful when the ECG is abnormal at rest and cannot be used to show ST-segment shift reflecting myocardial ischemia. The sensitivity and specificity of perfusion imaging for the diagnosis of ischemia and the detection of coronary artery disease are higher than those of stress electrocardiography [20]. Perfusion imaging is superior in determining the extent of myocardial ischemia and to identify coronary artery disease patients with a poor prognosis [21]. Results of revascularization procedures (coronary angioplasty or surgery) can also be evaluated by perfusion imaging [22].

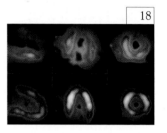

Radionuclide ventriculography using technetium-99m to label the intra-cardiac blood pool can assess the presence, extent, and functional consequences of myocardial ischemia. Imaging is performed either during the first passage of the bolus through the central circulation or when it has reached equilibrium [23]. Left and right ventricular volumes, global ejection fraction (systolic function), and the filling rate (diastolic function) can be measured. Regional wall motion can also be assessed, and helpful methods of displaying both the extent and the timing of contraction are the Fourier amplitude and phase images [24,25]. The phase image is particularly helpful in defining areas of dyskinesis suggesting a localized left ventricular aneurysm. Imaging during exercise or pharmacologic stress may reveal global or regional ventricular functional abnormalities reflecting stress-induced myocardial ischemia [26,27]. The degree of functional impairment, especially ejection fraction, is a powerful prognostic indicator.

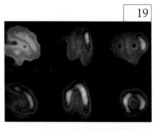

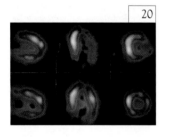
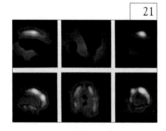
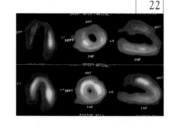
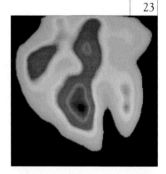

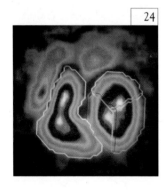
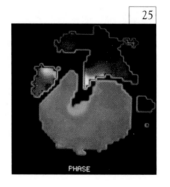
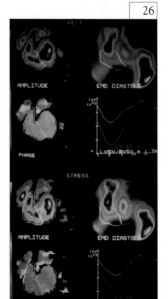
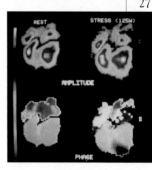

Concurrent assessment of myocardial perfusion by thallium-201 scintigraphy allows the diagnosis of the presence and extent of 'hibernating' myocardium. Hibernating myocardium is defined as a poorly functioning myocardial segment which recovers after revascularization. Such areas of myocardium are probably chronically underperfused with matched downgrading of contraction. Hibernating myocardium almost always results from severe coronary artery stenosis. If successful angioplasty or coronary artery bypass surgery improves perfusion of hibernating myocardium, a significant improvement in regional and global ejection fraction may result [28].

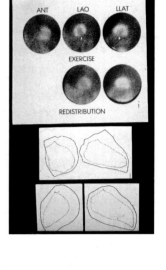

Positron emission tomography (PET) has the capability to evaluate regional myocardial blood flow and metabolism [29]. PET scans using perfusion markers such as nitrogen-13 ammonia ($^{13}NH_3$) and rubidium-82 can detect myocardial ischemia and hence the presence of obstructive coronary artery disease. The relative advantages of very expensive PET imaging over presently available, much less expensive, other nuclear imaging techniques have not been established.

Magnetic Resonance Imaging (MRI) and Computed Tomography (CT)
Gated MR images can reveal abnormalities of ventricular function and regional wall motion abnormalities in patients with chronic ischemic heart disease [30,31]. ECG gated CT has the potential to detect ischemic myocardial segments by identifying lack of systolic thickening. CT imaging may be helpful in detecting coronary artery calcification, which usually suggests significant coronary atherosclerotic disease [32].

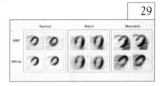

The relative merits of MRI or CT compared with other imaging techniques for the diagnosis and management of ischemic heart disease have not been established in clinical practice.

Echocardiography
In patients with stable angina without prior myocardial infarction, echocardiograms at rest may not reveal any abnormality. Where there has been prior infarction, regional wall motion abnormalities, generalized dilatation of the left ventricle with reduced systolic function [33], or a localized left ventricular aneurysm may be detected [34].

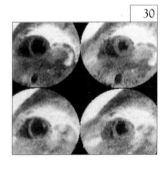

Stress echocardiography (during exercise or dobutamine infusion [35]) may reveal regional wall motion abnormalities, lack of systolic thickening of myocardial segments, transient reduction of global ejection fraction, and impaired diastolic function, all of which suggest myocardial ischemia and the presence of coronary artery disease.

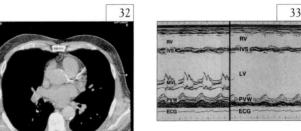

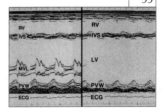

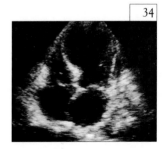

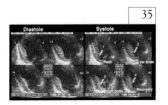

Cardiac Catheterization and Angiography

In patients with stable angina without prior myocardial infarction, the resting hemodynamic measurements, left ventricular ejection fraction, and regional wall motion are all usually normal. In patients with prior myocardial infarction and chronic left ventricular dysfunction, the resting hemodynamics are frequently abnormal, particularly in terms of an elevated left ventricular end-diastolic pressure. Angiography may show a reduced ejection fraction, segmental wall motion abnormalities, and diastolic dysfunction.

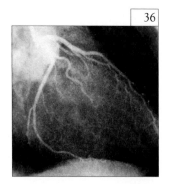

In order to demonstrate the exact pattern of coronary artery narrowing, coronary arteriography is required, both in patients with chronic ischemic heart disease and with acute ischemic syndromes [36–42]. In patients with stable angina, both eccentric and concentric coronary artery lesions can be detected [37,39]. The surface of the lesions is usually smooth. Complicated lesions or diffuse lesions are less frequently encountered in patients with stable angina.

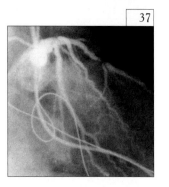

Coronary arteriography is also required for the diagnosis of non-atherosclerotic coronary artery disease or coronary artery anomalies when they are the anatomic substrate for angina. Coronary arteries, by definition, are normal in patients with syndrome X.

Principles of Management

General measures consist of weight reduction (if overweight), cessation of cigarette smoking, control of hypertension and diabetes, and regular exercise [43]. The reduction of blood cholesterol with the use of lipid-lowering agents, particularly with statins (HMG coenzyme reductase inhibitors), has been shown to be of benefit both in primary prevention (decreasing cardiovascular morbidity and mortality, and total mortality) and in patients with established coronary artery disease who have raised cholesterol levels.

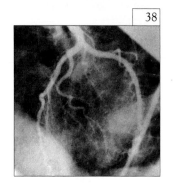

The use of sublingual nitroglycerin or a nitroglycerin spray should be encouraged not only for the immediate relief of angina but also prophylactically before engaging in the physical activity that is likely to precipitate angina. For maintenance therapy, relatively long-acting nitroglycerin or nitrates, beta-adrenergic blocking agents, and calcium channel blocking agents (long-acting vasoselective dihydropyridines, slow-release dihydropyridines, or slow-release non-dihydropyridines) should be used either alone or

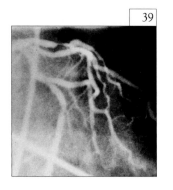

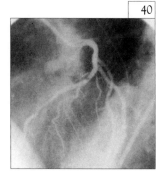

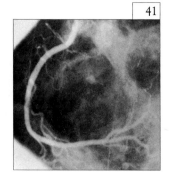

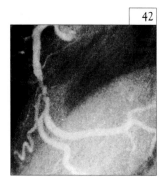

43

1. Establish the diagnosis – history and exercise ECG; other investigations when indicated

2. Modify risk factors – reduce weight, stop smoking, control hypertension, diabetes

3. Regular exercise if not contraindicated

4. Lipid-lowering agents for hypercholesterolemic patients (particularly with statins)

5. Nitroglycerin for immediate relief of angina and as a prophylactic agent

6. Beta-adrenergic antagonists, calcium channel blocking agents, and long-acting nitrates for maintenance therapy

7. Revascularization in patients refractory to medical therapy

8. Intramyocardial laser revascularization, extended external counterpulsation in selected patients with refractory angina

in combination to control angina. Although there is little evidence that combination therapy is more effective than, for instance, beta-blockers alone, most physicians tend to prescribe combination therapy for patients with important angina. In those patients who remain significantly symptomatic despite medical therapy, coronary arteriography should be performed with a view to a revascularization procedure by coronary angioplasty or by coronary artery bypass surgery [44,45]. Coronary arterial stents in conjunction with angioplasty are being used increasingly. The indications for stenting include complex arterial lesions, completely obstructed arteries, and restenosis following a previously, apparently successful, angioplasty [46]. Patients with stable angina who can neither tolerate nor accept medical therapy are also candidates for a revascularization procedure. From a prognostic point of view, those patients with left main coronary artery stenosis (and stable angina) or those with severe disease affecting all three main coronary arteries and reduced left ventricular ejection fraction should also be considered for revascularization surgery. Some patients with refractory angina and not candidates for conventional revascularization procedures may benefit from intramyocardial laser recanalization or extended external counterpulsation therapy.

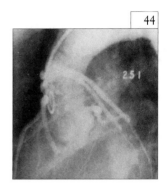

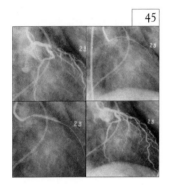

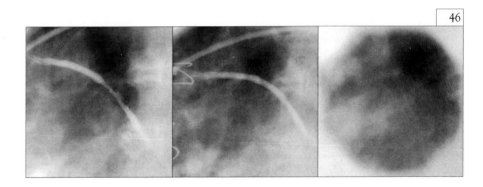

1   Longitudinal slice of coronary artery showing at least 80% narrowing of the lumen by atherosclerotic plaques.

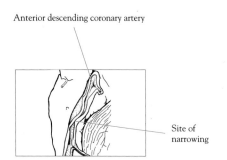

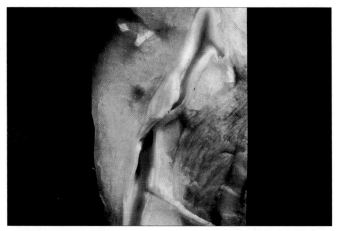

2   Narrowed coronary artery due to atherosclerosis. The plaque is situated eccentrically, allowing the retention of an arc of normal vessel wall. The plaque itself has a central core of lipid, with the rest of the plaque being made up of white collagen tissue.

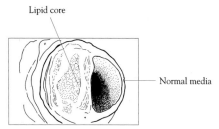

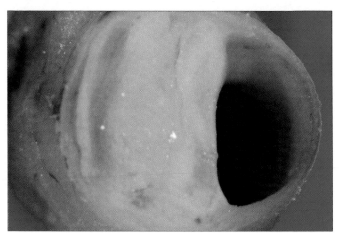

3   Cross-section through a coronary artery with massive inflammatory infiltration of the wall in Kawasaki's disease.

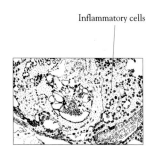

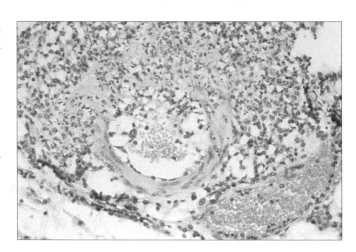

4   Normally, coronary blood flow increases proportionately as the myocardial oxygen requirements (heart rate × systolic blood pressure) increase. In the presence of obstructive coronary artery disease, luminal obstruction limits the appropriate increase in coronary blood flow for the magnitude of increase of myocardial oxygen demand, producing an imbalance between myocardial oxygen demand and supply, the principal mechanism for myocardial ischemia in patients with stable angina during exercise.

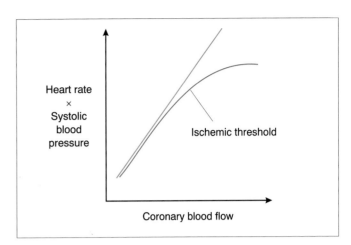

5   Features of syndrome X.

1. Clinical presentation similar to stable angina

2. Objective evidence for myocardial ischemia

    - ischemic exercise electrocardiograms
    - myocardial perfusion abnormalities
    - stress-induced left ventricular wall motion abnormalities

3. Normal coronary arteries on angiography

4. Impaired coronary vasodilatory reserve

5. Relatively good prognosis

6   The diagnostic features of effort angina.

Precipitating factors:	Predictable level of exercise, emotional stress, exercise plus heavy meal, cold weather
Relieved by:	Nitroglycerin, cessation of activity
Duration:	Less than 15 minutes
Location:	Usually retrosternal, infrequently epigastric or infrascapular
Radiation:	Bilaterally across the chest, one or both arms, shoulders, back, epigastrium, neck, and lower jaw
Description:	'Dull and deep', heaviness, tightness, pressure, constriction, indigestion

7   A chest X-ray of a patient with a hiatus hernia which may produce chest discomfort similar to angina.

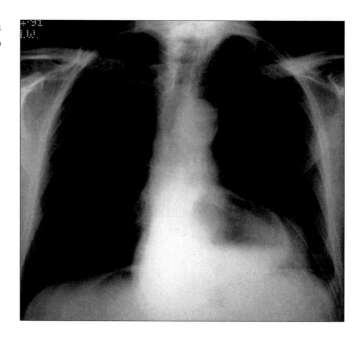

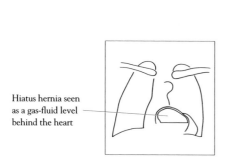

Hiatus hernia seen as a gas-fluid level behind the heart

8

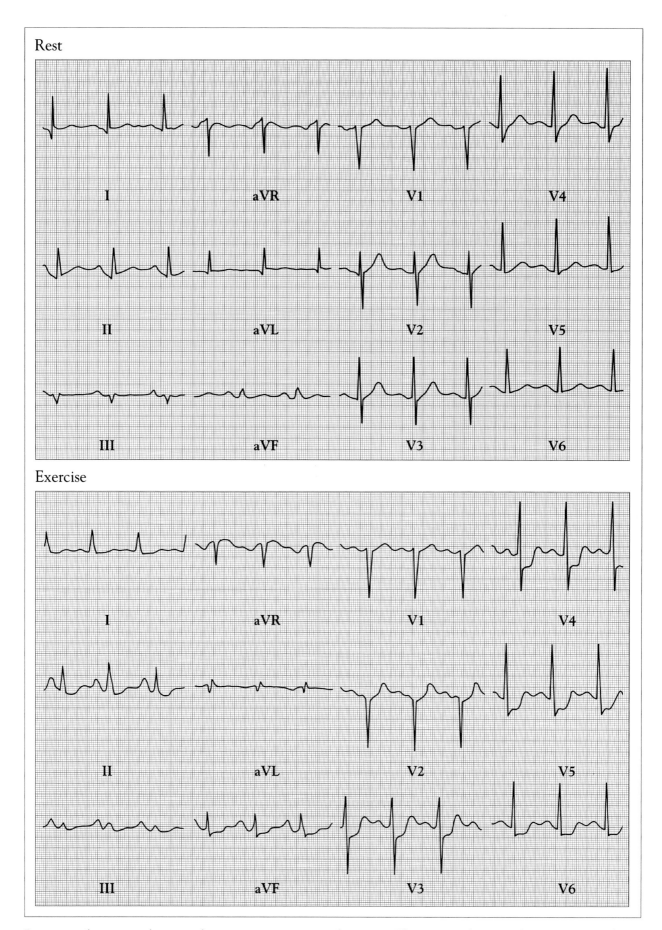

Resting and exercise electrocardiograms in a patient with angina. The resting electrocardiogram is normal. On exercise there is both horizontal and downsloping ST-segment depression in the anterior chest leads associated with the development of chest pain.

9

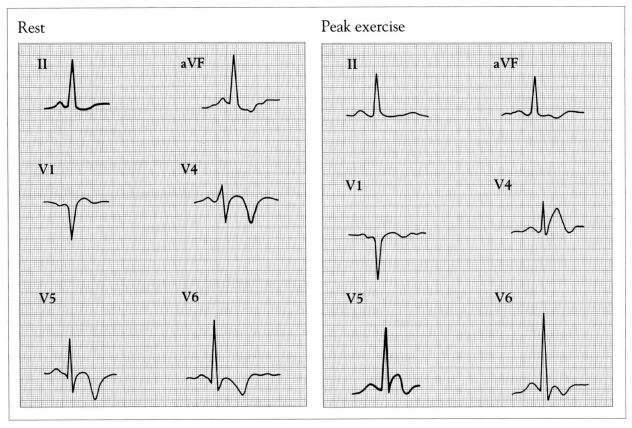

Elevation of ST segments during exercise in leads V1, V4, V5, and V6 in a patient with stable angina with a history of a recent anterior myocardial infarction. Resting electrocardiogram shows symmetrical T-wave inversions in the same leads. Coronary arteriography revealed subtotal occlusion of the left anterior descending coronary artery.

10

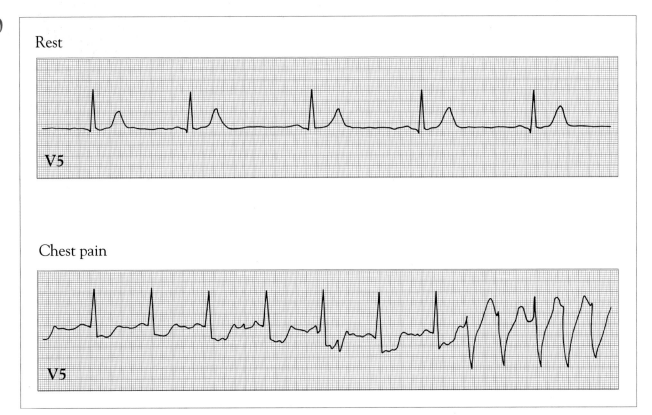

Electrocardiogram recorded during 24-hour ambulatory monitoring showing ST-segment depression and the development of ventricular tachycardia during chest pain.

11

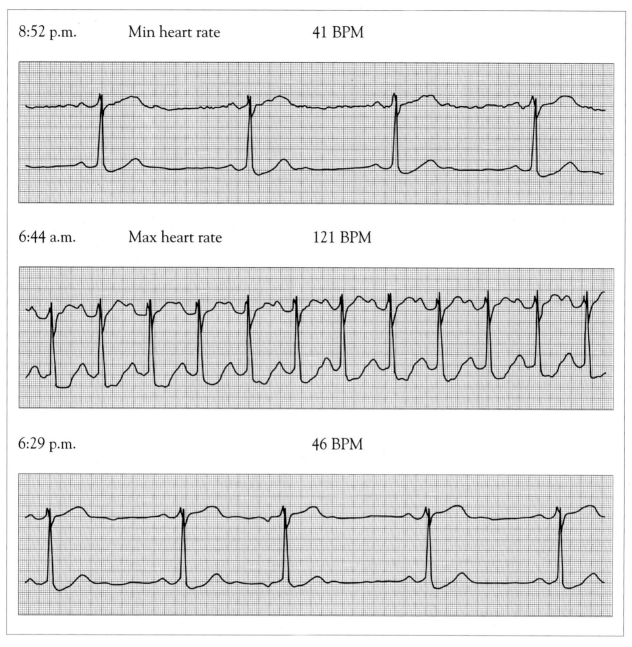

8:52 p.m.   Min heart rate   41 BPM

6:44 a.m.   Max heart rate   121 BPM

6:29 p.m.   46 BPM

Ambulatory electrocardiograms in a patient with stable angina. The upper and lower panels show sinus brady-cardia with minor ST-segment depression. In the middle panel, marked ST-segment depression occurred with increased heart rate but without chest pain, indicating 'silent' myocardial ischemia.

12 Normal emission tomograms after stress in (a) vertical long-axis, (b) horizontal long-axis, and (c) short-axis planes. There is uniform uptake of thallium-201 throughout the myocardium.

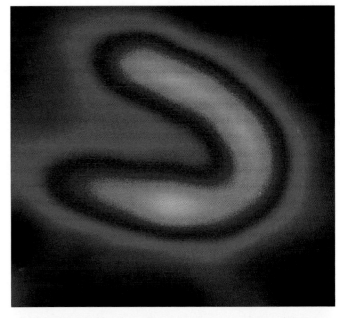

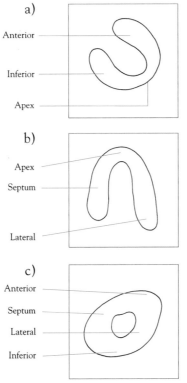

a)

Anterior

Inferior

Apex

b)

Apex

Septum

Lateral

c)

Anterior

Septum

Lateral

Inferior

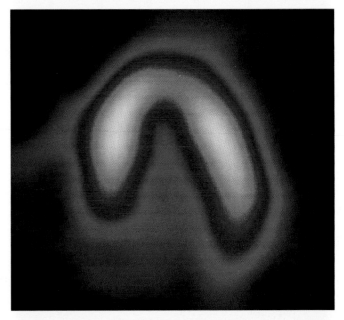

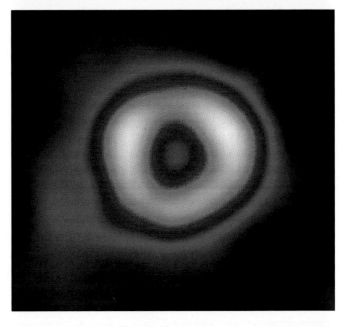

13

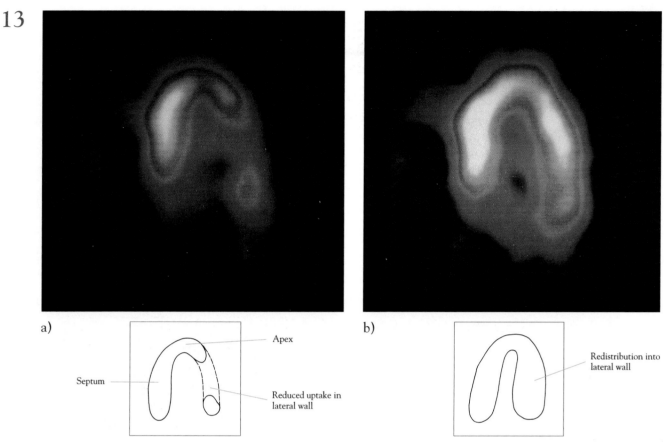

a)

Apex

Septum

Reduced uptake in lateral wall

b)

Redistribution into lateral wall

Stress (a) and redistribution (b) horizontal long-axis tomograms showing reversible lateral wall ischemia in a patient with left circumflex coronary artery disease.

14

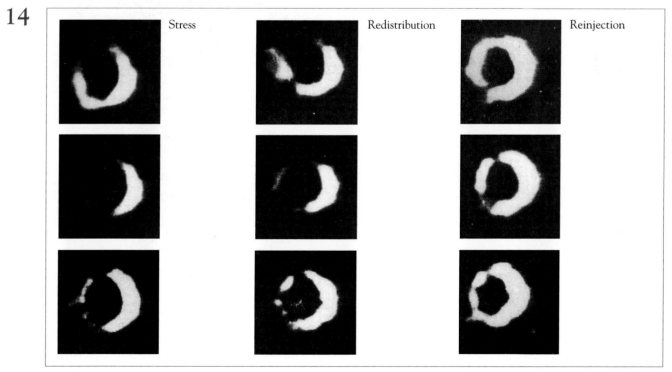

Stress Redistribution Reinjection

Thallium-201 myocardial perfusion images in a patient with stable angina after stress, after redistribution prior to reinjection, and after reinjection of thallium-201. Stress images showed reduced perfusion in the anteroseptal region. Redistribution images prior to reinjection showed virtually no change (fixed defects), which usually indicates the presence of scar tissue. Images after reinjection of thallium showed almost normal uptake of the same regions, indicating the presence of considerable residual myocardium in the apparently fixed defect.

15 Stress, four-hour, 24-hour, and postoperative short-axis thallium-201 myocardial perfusion tomograms in a patient with stable angina. Stress images demonstrated perfusion defects in the lateral wall of the left ventricle which persisted in the four-hour redistribution images. Redistribution images at 24 hours, however, revealed almost normal uptake of the same regions, indicating the presence of viable ischemic myocardium. Following successful coronary artery bypass surgery, normal perfusion of the left ventricular lateral wall is evident.

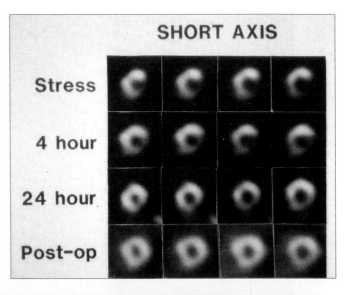

16

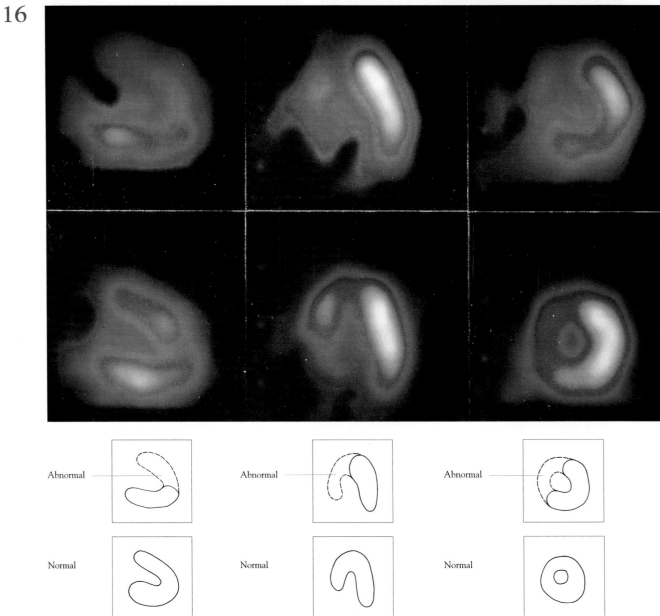

MIBI SPECT imaging after stress and at rest showing reversible anteroseptal myocardial ischemia.

17

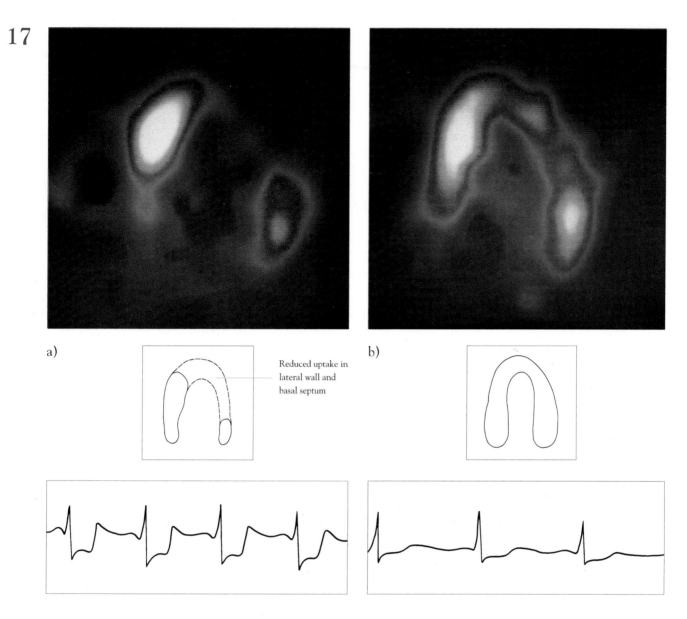

a)

Reduced uptake in
lateral wall and
basal septum

b)

Stress (a) and redistribution (b) horizontal long-axis tomograms (top) with ECG (bottom) showing reversible ischemia of the lateral wall and basal septum. In this case, the abnormality was produced by intravenous infusion of dipyridamole and no exercise was necessary.

18 Thallium tomography with adenosine stress. The upper row shows thallium tomograms acquired after the infusion of adenosine for six minutes in a patient with a left main stem coronary artery lesion. There is greatly reduced tracer uptake in the anterior wall, apex, and lateral wall which shows complete redistribution in the rest images in the lower row after three hours.

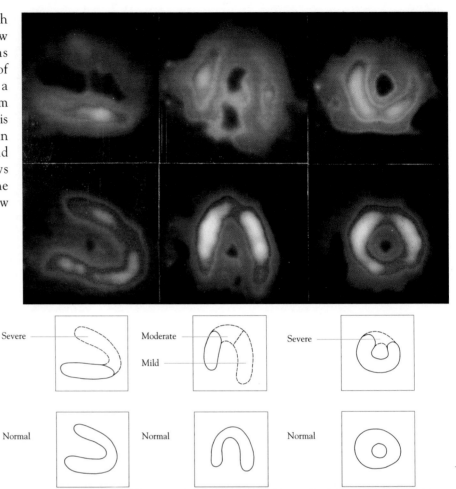

19 Thallium myocardial tomography after dobutamine stress. The upper row shows reduced perfusion in the anterior wall, apex, and inferior wall in a patient with left anterior descending and right coronary artery disease. The redistribution images in the lower row show improvement in all areas except the basal inferior wall, which is infarcted.

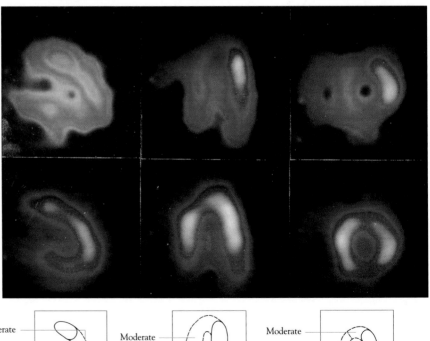

20 Thallium tomography in a patient with angina. Thallium tomography revealed the presence of a lateral wall perfusion abnormality after stress which showed full redistribution, confirming the presence of a left circumflex lesion. In this patient, exercise ECG was normal.

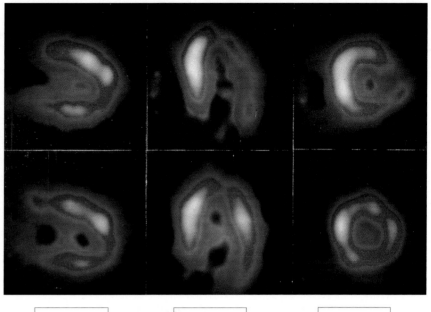

21 Thallium tomography in a patient with severe coronary artery disease. The stress images (upper row) show reduced tracer uptake throughout the heart, except for a small portion of the anterior wall. There is full redistribution after three hours (lower row), showing that all the myocardium is viable. Both the extent and the severity of the stress hypoperfusion indicate a high risk of future cardiac events.

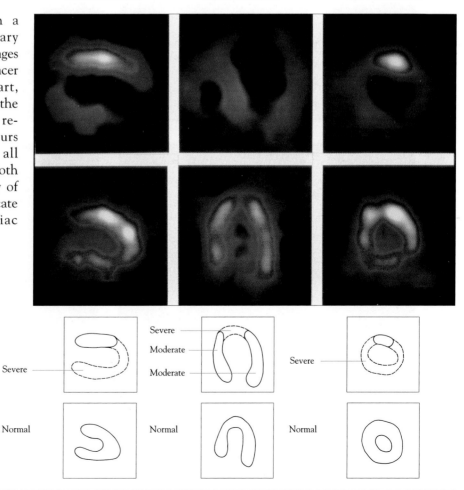

22

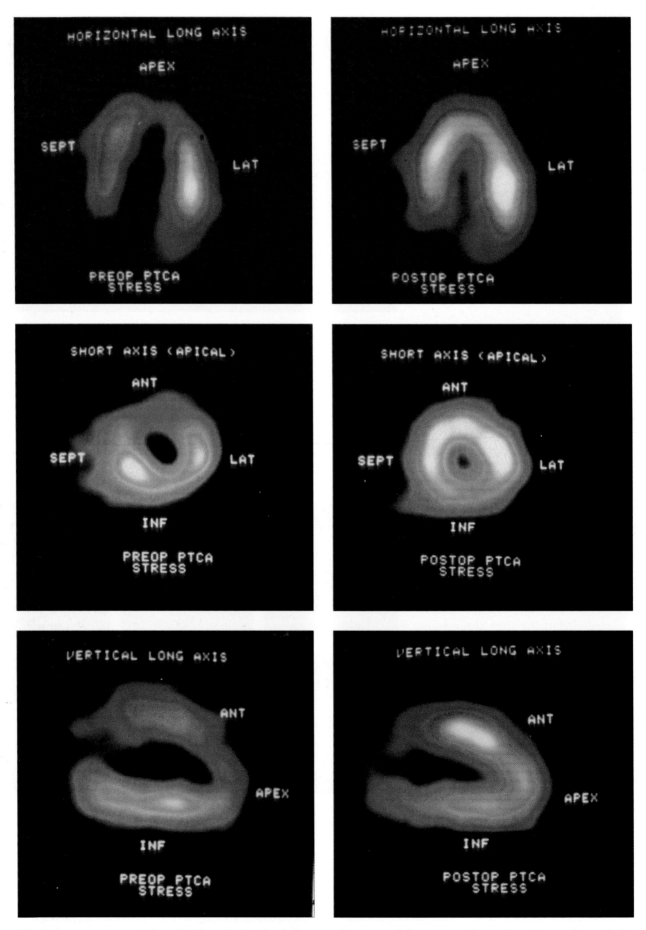

Thallium tomograms before (left) and after (right) angioplasty to a left anterior descending lesion beyond the first septal branches. The small distal anterior area of ischemia is abolished.

23 Normal left anterior oblique end-diastolic image from an equilibrium radionuclide ventriculogram.

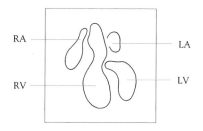

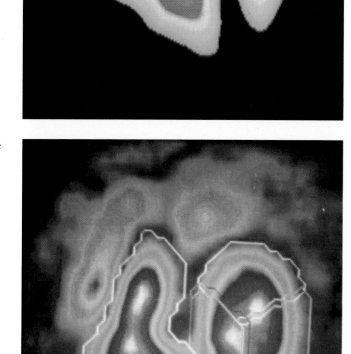

24 Normal amplitude image showing high amplitude of all parts of the left ventricle.

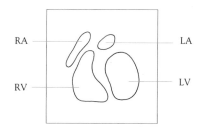

25 Normal phase image showing synchronous contraction of all parts of both ventricles in green. The atria and great vessels are 180° out of phase and are seen in red.

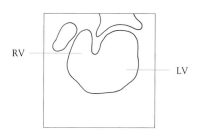

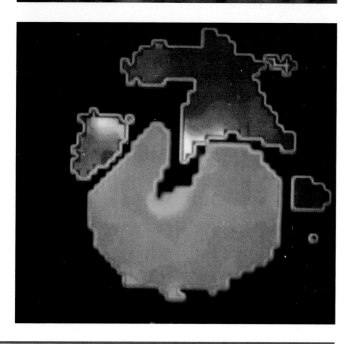

26

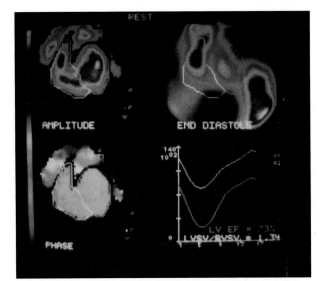
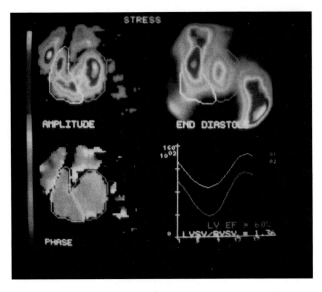

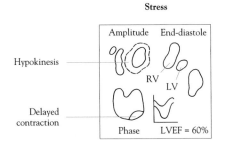

Stress

Rest (left) and stress (right) radionuclide ventriculograms with phase and amplitude images in a patient with coronary heart disease. The LVEF is normal at rest (73%) with normal regional wall motion shown on the amplitude and phase images. During stress, the LVEF falls (60%), and the amplitude and phase images show septal hypokinesis with delayed contraction.

27 Rest (left) and stress (right) amplitude and phase images. Regional wall motion is normal at rest, but delayed apical contraction develops during stress.

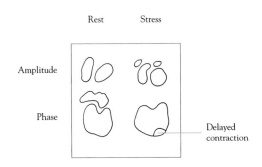

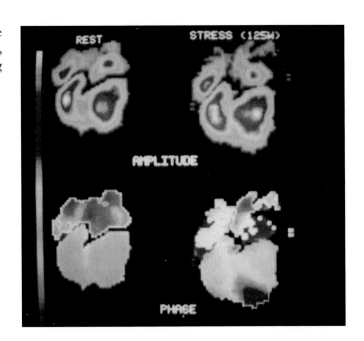

28 (a) Planar thallium-201 myocardial perfusion images in anterior (ANT), left anterior oblique (LAO), and lateral (LLAT) projections during exercise and redistribution show reversible perfusion defects of the left ventricular inferior wall (arrows), suggesting ischemia. (b) Superimposed left ventricular end-diastolic and end-systolic outlines in left anterior oblique and right anterior oblique projections obtained during preoperative contrast ventriculography show reduced systolic motion of the inferior wall of the left ventricle, suggesting 'hibernating' myocardium. (c) Following coronary artery bypass surgery, systolic motion of the inferior wall of the left ventricle markedly improved.

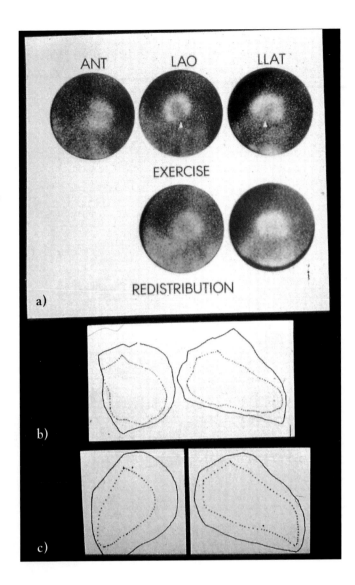

29

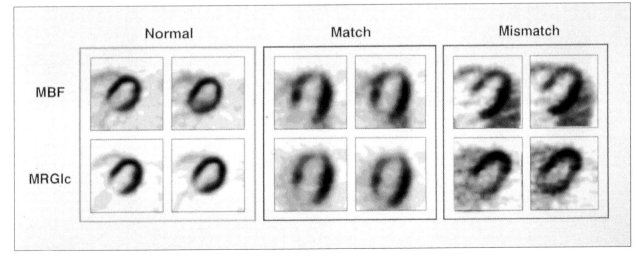

Two contiguous transaxial images of the left ventricular myocardium obtained by positron emission tomography in three patients. The blood flow images (MBF) obtained with nitrogen-13 ammonia ($^{13}NH_3$) are compared with glucose uptake images (MRGlc)obtained with fluorine-18 deoxyglucose (FDG). Normal $^{13}NH_3$ uptake indicates preserved perfusion. FDG uptake in the same segments suggests metabolically active myocardium. Decreased $^{13}NH_3$ and FDG uptake (Match) indicates scar tissue. Decreased $^{13}NH_3$ uptake and increased FDG uptake (Mismatch) indicates 'hibernating' myocardium.

30 Magnetic resonance imaging of left ventricular wall motion in a patient with coronary artery disease. The upper row shows a diastolic image (left) and a systolic image (right) from a cardiac cine study showing normal contraction throughout the myocardium. The lower row shows the same plane after the administration of dipyridamole. There is no systolic wall thickening in the antero-septal region.

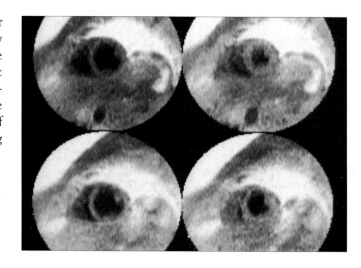

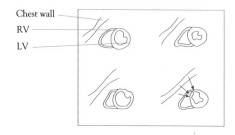

31

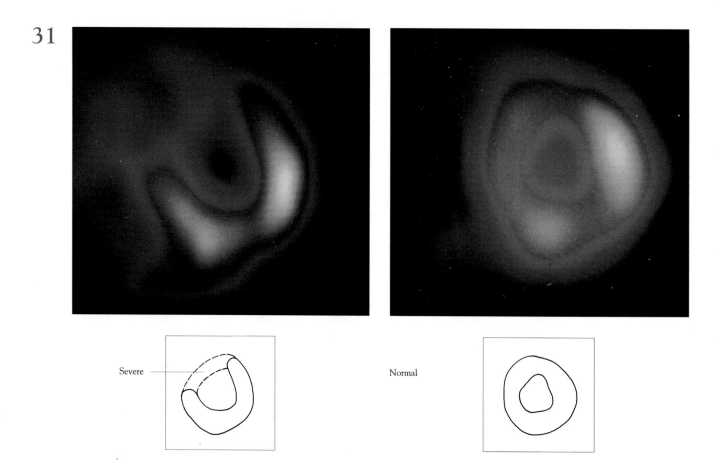

The corresponding thallium tomogram of the same patient shows the presence of an antero-septal perfusion defect with full redistribution after three hours. The patient has anterior descending coronary artery disease.

32 Ultrafast CT image of coronary calcification. In this transaxial plane the calcium deposited in the coronary arteries can be seen in the wall of the aorta, the left main stem, the left anterior descending coronary artery, and the first diagonal branch.

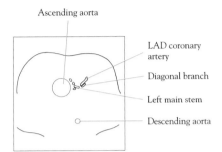

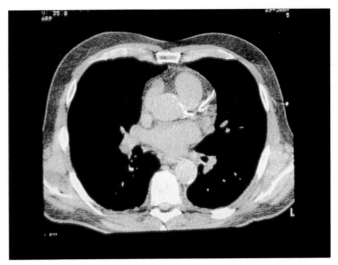

33

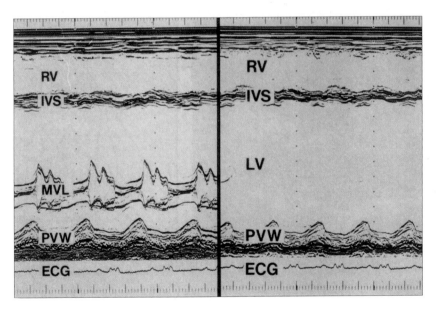

M-mode recordings from a patient with heart failure secondary to ischemic heart disease. The left-hand panel shows that the mitral valve opening excursion is small due to low flow and this, combined with the enlarged ventricle, leads to abnormally large separation between the interventricular septum and the mitral E-point (maximal anterior motion in early diastole). The right-hand panel shows the left ventricle to be very large and systolic function poor. The infarcted interventricular septum shows increased echo intensity with little movement or systolic thickening.

34

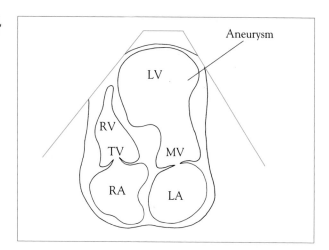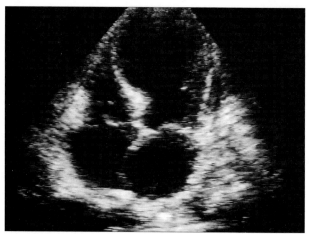

Apical four-chamber view showing a large apical left ventricular aneurysm. The apical region has a bulbous shape, is thin-walled, and expands rather than contracts during systole.

35

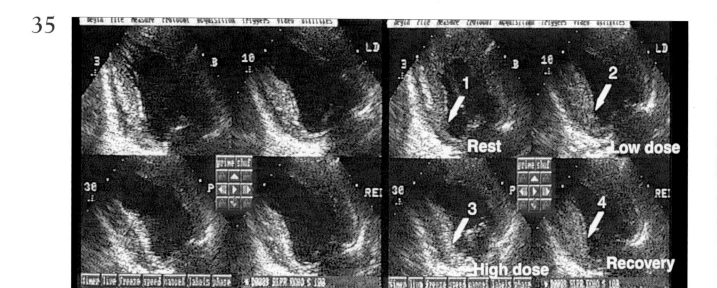

Groups of four still-frame two-dimensional images taken at end-diastole (left) and end-systole (right) during a dobutamine stress test. The upper left image of each group shows the baseline condition. During low-dose dobutamine infusion (upper right images), there is an increased systolic motion of the infero-basal segment (arrowed). At higher dose rate (lower left), the same segment shows lack of thickening and decreased systolic wall motion, indicating the presence of ischemic myocardium as a result of obstructive right coronary artery disease. The bottom right images show the post-infusion recovery to baseline.

36 Normal left coronary arteriogram in the right anterior oblique (RAO) view.

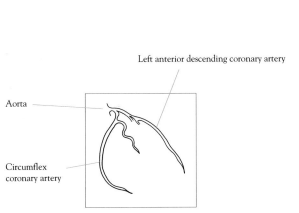

Aorta

Left anterior descending coronary artery

Circumflex coronary artery

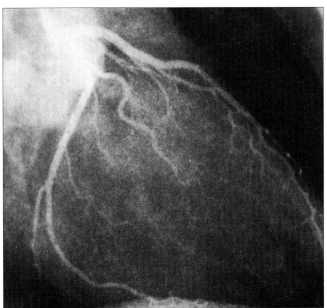

37 Left coronary artery injection in the right anterior oblique (RAO) projection. A severe concentric stenotic lesion in the anterior descending branch of the left coronary artery has been demonstrated (arrow).

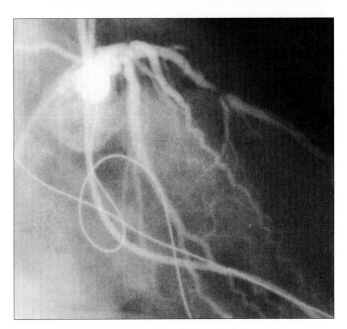

38 Angiogram in the left anterior oblique (LAO) projection showing a normal left coronary artery.

Left anterior descending coronary artery

Diagonal branch of left anterior descending coronary artery

Circumflex coronary artery

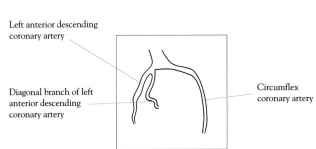

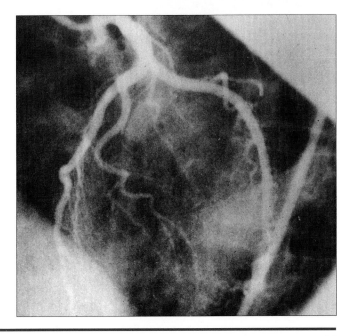

39 Angiogram showing an eccentric smooth surfaced atherosclerotic plaque (arrow) of the anterior descending coronary artery.

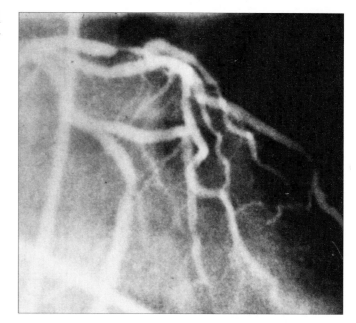

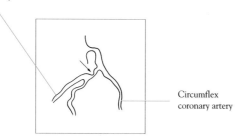

40 Left anterior oblique angiogram showing atherosclerotic narrowing of the anterior descending coronary artery (arrow).

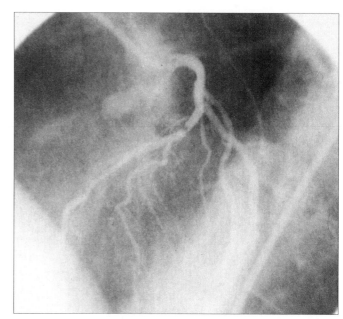

Left anterior descending coronary artery

Circumflex coronary artery

41 Angiogram in the left anterior oblique (LAO) projection showing a normal right coronary artery.

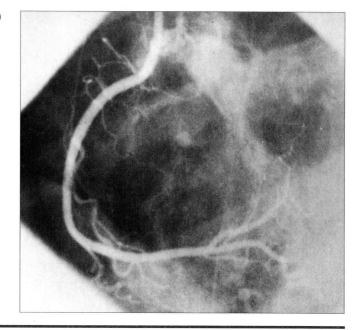

Right coronary artery

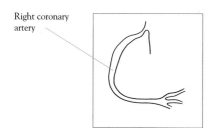

42   Right coronary artery in the left anterior oblique (LAO) projection. The right coronary artery is dominant and shows a localized, severe, irregular stricture as it descends down the right heart border (arrow).

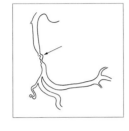

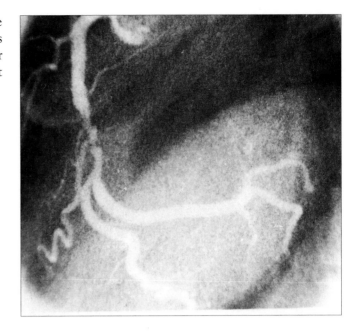

ISCHEMIC HEART DISEASE   **STABLE ANGINA / Principles of Management**

43   Principles of management of stable angina.

1. Establish the diagnosis – history and exercise ECG; other investigations when indicated

2. Modify risk factors – reduce weight, stop smoking, control hypertension, diabetes

3. Regular exercise if not contraindicated

4. Lipid-lowering agents for hypercholesterolemic patients (particularly with statins)

5. Nitroglycerin for immediate relief of angina and as a prophylactic agent

6. Beta-adrenergic antagonists, calcium channel blocking agents, and long-acting nitrates for maintenance therapy

7. Revascularization in patients refractory to medical therapy

8. Intramyocardial laser revascularization, extended counterpulsation in selected patients with refractory angina

44   Vein bypass graft surgery. A root aortogram reveals four patent vein grafts going to the right, anterior descending, diagonal, and circumflex arteries.

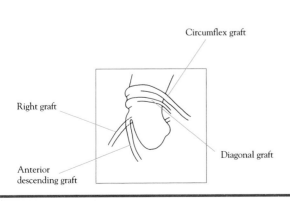

Circumflex graft

Right graft

Diagonal graft

Anterior descending graft

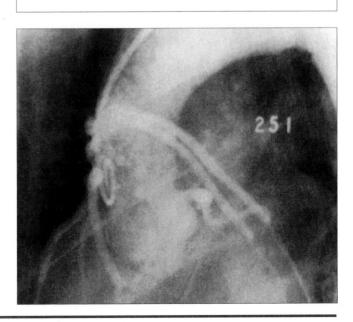

45

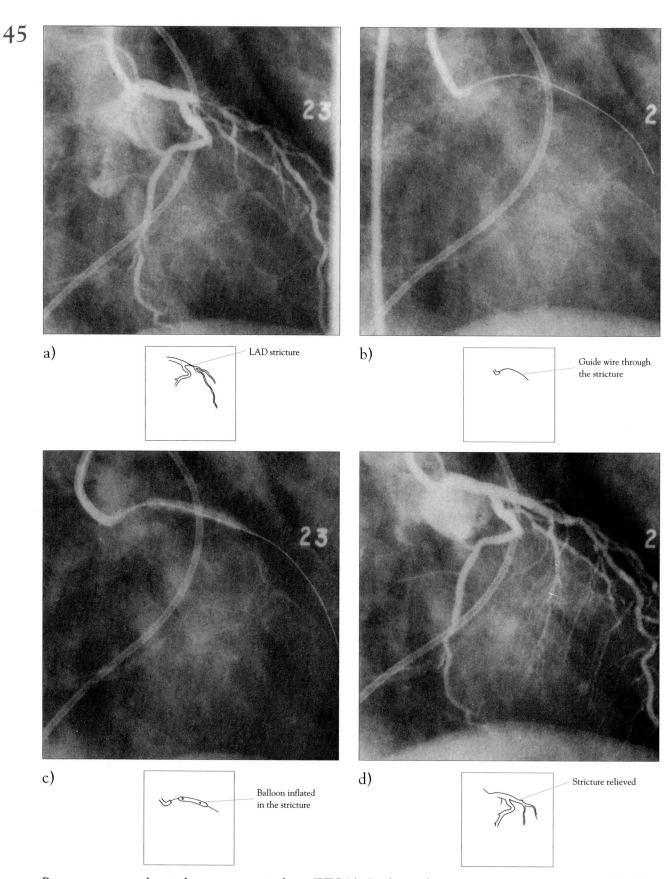

a)   LAD stricture

b)   Guide wire through
                                                      the stricture

c)   Balloon inflated
                                                      in the stricture

d)   Stricture relieved

Percutaneous transluminal coronary angioplasty (PTCA). In this technique, coronary strictures are dilated by high pressure balloons positioned within the lumen by percutaneous catheters. (a) Selective left coronary angiography shows a severe stricture in the anterior descending branch of the left coronary artery. (b) A fine guide wire is passed through the special preshaped guide catheter into the anterior descending coronary artery and across the stricture. (c) The high pressure balloon is inflated with dilute contrast medium. (d) After inflation, contrast injection shows that the stenosis is markedly reduced.

46 Stent insertion. (a) Stricture in a graft. (b) After balloon angioplasty and stent insertion the stricture is no longer visible. (c) Stent in position; a coned view shows how difficult it is to see the stent during deployment.

a)

Vein graft stricture

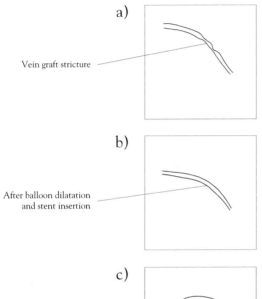

b)

After balloon dilatation
and stent insertion

c)

Stent in position

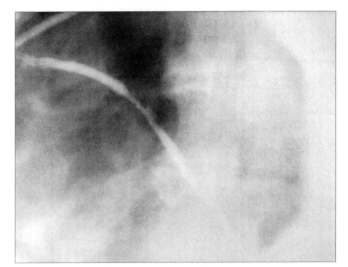

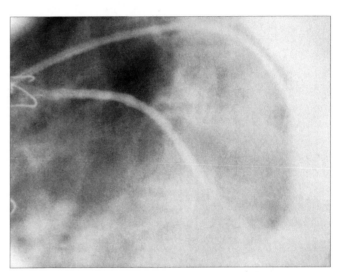

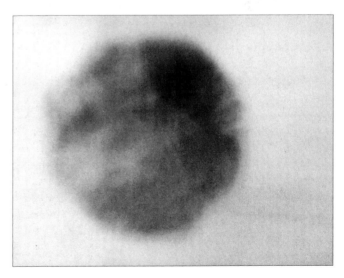

VARIANT ANGINA

Definition

Variant angina (Prinzmetal or vasospastic angina) is defined as chest pain due to myocardial ischemia occurring spontaneously at rest, usually without a history of exertional angina. A characteristic feature of variant angina is ST-segment elevation in the electrocardiogram occurring during the episode of pain, reverting to normal with the regression of pain.

Pathophysiology

It has been well documented that myocardial ischemia and spontaneous angina arise as a result of focal spasm of the epicardial coronary artery and, consequently, a primary reduction of coronary blood flow. An increase in myocardial oxygen requirement may or may not accompany the reduction in coronary blood flow due to coronary artery vasospasm. In about 90% of patients, some degree of coronary atherosclerosis at the site of spasm is present, although the degree of luminal obstruction due to atherosclerosis may be hemodynamically insignificant. Angiographically normal coronary arteries are detected in approximately 10% of patients. Coronary artery spasm is usually localized, although diffuse narrowing of the coronary arteries may be observed in some patients with variant angina. The cause of coronary artery spasm is likely to be multifactorial. Increased vagal tone, with or without withdrawal of sympathetic tone, has been postulated. Endothelial dysfunction with decreased endothelium-derived relaxing factor (EDRF), imbalance between alpha- and beta-adrenergic-receptor activity, lack of the vasodilator prostacyclin, increase in the vasoconstrictor thromboxane, and enhanced activity of serotonin receptors have all been proposed as the potential mechanism of vasospasm [1]. No single mechanism, however, has been identified as the cause of coronary vasospasm in all patients with variant angina. The clinical relevance of this lack of understanding of the mechanism of coronary artery spasm is that it is necessary to use non-specific coronary vasodilators for the relief of coronary vasospasm.

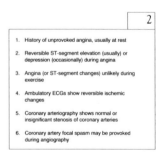

Presentation

Symptoms

Recurrent episodes of rest angina without provocation comprise the most common symptom [2]. A history of effort angina is usually absent, although in the occasional patient angina may occur at a very high level of exercise. Angina occurs more frequently during the early hours of the morning; some patients experience angina soon after getting up. In many patients a history of angina occurring repetitively at the same time of day is obtained, although such a history is not a prerequisite for a diagnosis of variant angina. A history of migraine and Raynaud's phenomenon is common in patients with variant angina. The duration of angina may be more prolonged than that of effort angina. The pain almost invariably responds to nitroglycerin. Dyspnea, due to a transient increase in pulmonary capillary wedge pressure, and syncope, due to ventricular tachycardia or atrioventricular block, may accompany angina in the occasional patient.

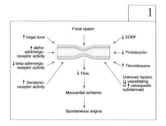

1. History of unprovoked angina, usually at rest
2. Reversible ST-segment elevation (usually) or depression (occasionally) during angina
3. Angina (or ST-segment changes) unlikely during exercise
4. Ambulatory ECGs show reversible ischemic changes
5. Coronary arteriography shows normal or insignificant stenosis of coronary arteries
6. Coronary artery focal spasm may be provoked during angiography

Signs

Abnormal physical findings are usually not detected except during the episodes of angina, when atrial and ventricular gallops and a murmur suggestive of transient mitral regurgitation may be observed.

Investigations

Electrocardiography

The ECGs taken during episodes of angina reveal reversible ischemic changes. ST-segment elevation indicating transmural ischemia is particularly characteristic [3]. However, ST-segment depression suggesting subendocardial ischemia may also occur in

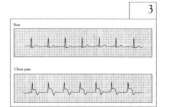

the same patient during other episodes of angina [4]. In the vast majority of patients, the episodes of ischemia resolve spontaneously without developing evidence of myocardial infarction. In less than 10% of patients, Q-wave myocardial infarction develops.

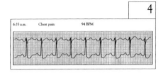

Recording of the electrocardiogram during an episode of angina is the most important and informative investigation in the diagnosis of variant angina. If such an opportunity is not available, ambulatory electrocardiographic monitoring may reveal spontaneous episodes of ischemia with ST-segment depression or elevation. Many of these episodes may not be accompanied by chest pain [5].

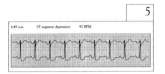

Echocardiography, Nuclear Techniques, Magnetic Resonance Imaging (MRI), and Computed Tomography (CT)

The echocardiogram may reveal reversible regional wall motion abnormalities when obtained during ischemia [6]. Nuclear imaging, MRI, and CT studies are not usually performed during pain but modern isotope perfusion tracers can be injected during pain, and imaging performed up to four hours later when the patient's condition has stabilized. Due to the lack of redistribution with these tracers, the perfusion at the time of pain is 'frozen' for the later imaging [7].

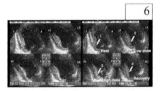

Cardiac Catheterization and Angiography

Coronary arteriography is indicated when the diagnosis of variant angina is strongly suspected. Demonstration of normal coronary arteries or hemodynamically insignificant coronary artery lesions virtually confirms the diagnosis. In some patients, provocative tests with the intravenous administration of ergonovine or methacholine or hyperventilation are employed to induce coronary artery spasm [8]. If focal coronary spasm occurs in response to provocation, together with the development of angina and ECG changes of ischemia, the diagnosis of variant angina is very likely. In the presence of hemodynamically significant atherosclerotic lesions, provocative tests should not be performed.

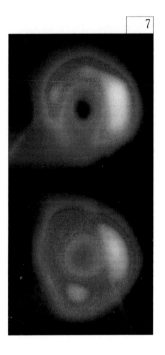

Principles of Management

In patients with normal coronary arteries or with hemodynamically minor coronary artery lesions, calcium channel blockers and nitrates may be effective for the prevention of coronary spasm [9]. In refractory patients, the addition of amiodarone to calcium channel blockers and nitrates may be effective in controlling angina.

In patients with significant fixed coronary artery stenosis, revascularization surgery may be required in addition to pharmacotherapy.

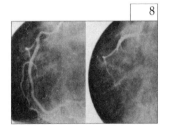

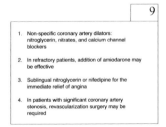

1. Non-specific coronary artery dilators: nitroglycerin, nitrates, and calcium channel blockers

2. In refractory patients, addition of amiodarone may be effective

3. Sublingual nitroglycerin or nifedipine for the immediate relief of angina

4. In patients with significant coronary artery stenosis, revascularization surgery may be required

1
Potential mechanisms of variant angina. Focal spasm of a segment of an epicardial coronary artery decreases coronary blood flow producing spontaneous episodes of myocardial ischemia and angina.

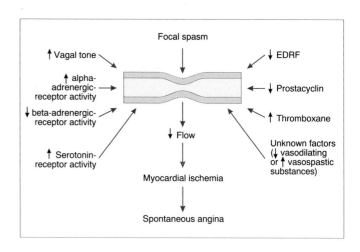

2
Diagnostic approach to variant angina.

1. History of unprovoked angina, usually at rest

2. Reversible ST-segment elevation (usually) or depression (occasionally) during angina

3. Angina (or ST-segment changes) unlikely during exercise

4. Ambulatory ECGs show reversible ischemic changes

5. Coronary arteriography shows normal or insignificant stenosis of coronary arteries

6. Coronary artery focal spasm may be provoked during angiography

3

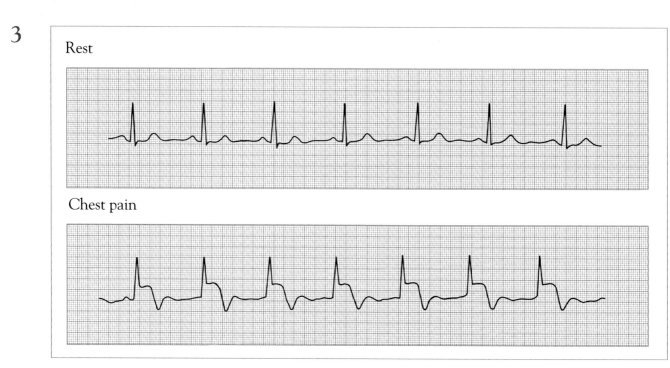

ECGs obtained during spontaneous angina showing ST-segment elevation indicating transmural ischemia. It also shows A-V dissociation. With relief of angina, ST-segment changes normalize.

4

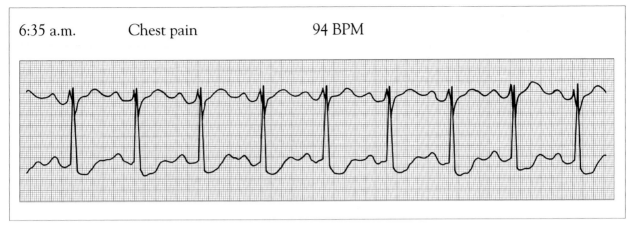

6:35 a.m.	Chest pain	94 BPM

Spontaneous ST-segment depression suggesting subendocardial ischemia in a patient with variant angina. The episodes of ST-segment depression were associated with chest pain.

5

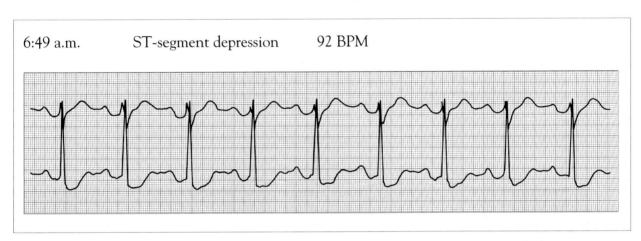

6:49 a.m.	ST-segment depression	92 BPM

Ambulatory ECG showing ST-segment depression which occurred without provocation in the same patient with variant angina as in [4]. This episode of ST-segment depression was not accompanied by chest pain, indicating spontaneous silent myocardial ischemia.

6

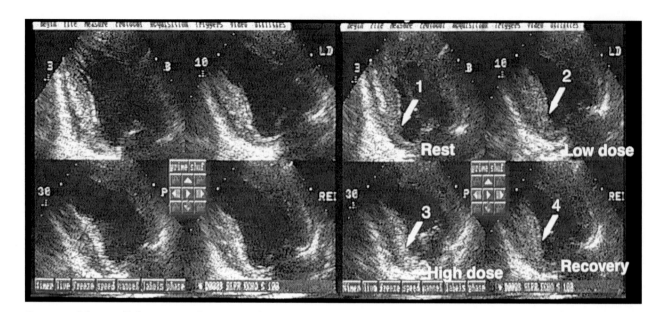

Groups of four still-frame two-dimensional images taken at end-diastole (left) and end-systole (right) during a dobutamine stress test. The upper left image of each group shows the baseline condition. During low-dose dobutamine infusion (upper right images), there is an increased systolic motion of the infero-basal segment (arrowed). At higher dose rate (lower left), the same segment shows lack of thickening and decreased systolic wall motion, indicating the presence of ischemic myocardium as a result of obstructive right coronary artery disease. The bottom right images show the post-infusion recovery to baseline.

7

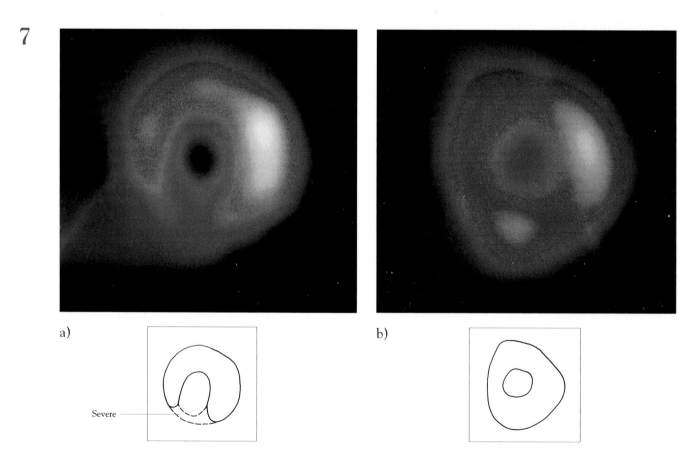

Reversible thallium-201 perfusion defect [(a) in pain, (b) pain-free] during an episode of spontaneous angina in a patient with variant angina. The perfusion abnormality is in the infero-septal region in the distribution of the right coronary artery.

8

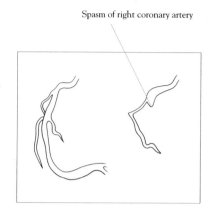

Spasm of right coronary artery

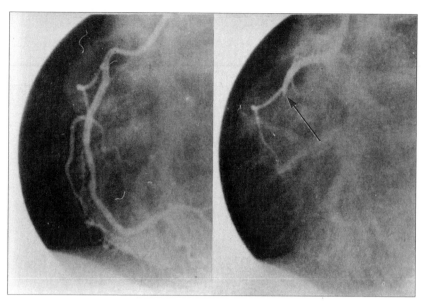

Coronary artery spasm. The angiogram on the left (left anterior oblique projection) shows normal blood flow in the right coronary artery. The angiogram on the right shows coronary artery spasm (arrow) completely occluding the right coronary artery.

ISCHEMIC HEART DISEASE   VARIANT ANGINA / Principles of Management

9   Principles of management of variant angina.

1. Non-specific coronary artery dilators: nitroglycerin, nitrates, and calcium channel blockers

2. In refractory patients, addition of amiodarone may be effective

3. Sublingual nitroglycerin or nifedipine for the immediate relief of angina

4. In patients with significant coronary artery stenosis, revascularization surgery may be required

UNSTABLE ANGINA

Definition

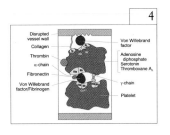

Angina occurring at rest, the new onset of angina in relation to exertion, and a recent deterioration in a previously stable pattern of angina constitute the usually accepted definitions of unstable angina. It is likely that not all three definitions have a common pathophysiologic explanation.

Pathophysiology

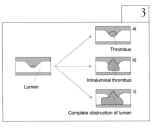

In unstable angina, a decrease in coronary blood flow induces myocardial ischemia in the vast majority of patients. Excessive increase in myocardial oxygen demand as the mechanism for myocardial ischemia at rest is infrequent.

The decrease in coronary blood flow appears to result from the formation of labile thrombi in association with an atheromatous plaque. Fissuring or ulceration of a usually soft lipid-rich eccentric plaque initiates platelet aggregation and adhesion, and formation of thrombus over the disrupted plaque [1]. The intra-intimal [2] and mural thrombi produce variable degrees of luminal narrowing and reduction of coronary blood flow. Spontaneous resolution of the thrombus restores normal coronary blood flow, relieving myocardial ischemia and, hence, angina. However, the presence of a disrupted plaque and residual thrombus, containing thrombin and other thrombogenic factors, encourages recurrent thrombus formation, further luminal narrowing, and, hence, recurrent episodes of ischemia and rest angina [3]. In addition to anatomic luminal obstruction by labile thrombi, dynamic luminal narrowing can also occur concurrently due to increased coronary arterial tone around the disrupted plaque, mediated by elaborated vasoactive substances such as thromboxane and serotonin. Deficiency in the endogenous thrombolytic mechanism or activation of endogenous thrombotic systems and proinflammatory state may contribute to the pathogenesis of unstable angina [4].

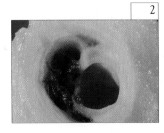

Although coronary atherosclerosis is invariably present, hemodynamically relatively minor stenoses (50% or less) are present in many patients.

Presentation

Symptoms
A history of single or multiple episodes of angina at rest is characteristic of unstable angina. A change in character, intensity, duration, and precipitating factors for angina in patients with a history of stable angina of long duration or the recent onset of exertional angina should also raise the possibility of unstable angina. Some patients experience dyspnea accompanying the angina. Dizziness due to transient ventricular tachycardia or atrioventricular block during the episodes of spontaneous ischemia is an infrequent presenting symptom. Frank syncope is rare.

Signs
In patients without prior myocardial infarction and in the absence of ongoing myocardial ischemia, abnormal cardiac findings are usually absent. Clinical findings suggestive of myocardial ischemia, such as atrial or ventricular gallops, can be detected during an episode of angina.

Investigations

Radiology
The plain chest X-ray does not reveal any abnormal findings, except in patients with prior myocardial infarction and chronic ischemic damage, in whom cardiomegaly and signs of pulmonary venous congestion may be present.

Electrocardiography

ECGs during angina demonstrate evidence of ischemia, such as reversible ST-segment changes, T-wave inversion, and pseudonormalization of T-waves in the majority of patients [5]. In a small proportion of patients, the ECGs remain normal during episodes of angina. A normal ECG initially is associated with a favorable prognosis; abnormal initial ECGs indicate a worse prognosis. Furthermore, in patients with abnormal ECGs, the frequency of angiographically detected mural coronary artery thrombi is much higher. Continuous electrocardiographic monitoring may reveal episodes of transient ST-T abnormalities without chest pain. The prognosis of such patients with respect to the development of myocardial infarction or death is worse.

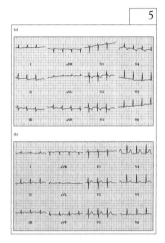

Echocardiography

Echocardiograms obtained during ischemia provoked by exercise or infusion of an inotrope may reveal the consequences of ischemia such as abnormalities of myocardial systolic and diastolic function. When the patient is stable, stress echocardiography can detect the consequences of myocardial ischemia (regional wall motion abnormalities) and the extent of myocardium at ischemic risk.

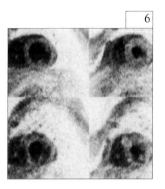

Nuclear Techniques, Magnetic Resonance Imaging (MRI), and Computed Tomography (CT)

Nuclear imaging with ^{99m}Tc agents can be performed in unstable angina, either by injecting during pain and imaging up to four hours later, or by using a mobile gamma camera on the coronary care unit. MRI and CT are not usually performed during episodes of ischemia. However, they may be used to evaluate left ventricular function after stabilization [6].

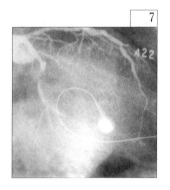

Cardiac Catheterization and Angiography

Coronary arteriography in patients with angina at rest usually reveals eccentric atherosclerotic lesions with an irregular ragged surface [7]. However, concentric lesions, eccentric lesions with a smooth surface, and diffuse lesions are also identified in a smaller percentage of patients. Coronary arteriography performed shortly after the development of pain may show thrombus at the site of the plaque or distal to it, particularly in patients with abnormal ECGs at the time of the onset of pain [8]. Angioscopic studies pre- and intraoperatively have also revealed coronary arterial mural thrombi in the majority of patients with unstable angina.

In patients without angina at rest (deterioration of stable angina or newly recognized stable angina) the coronary artery lesions are similar to those with stable angina.

Hemodynamic abnormalities resulting from myocardial ischemia may be present during catheterization if the procedure is performed during an episode of ischemia. Otherwise, the hemodynamics may be normal or similar to those of long-standing myocardial damage.

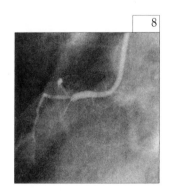

Contrast left ventriculography may not reveal any abnormality in patients without myocardial ischemia at the time of investigation. In patients with prior myocardial infarction or chronic myocardial damage, abnormalities of global and regional myocardial systolic and diastolic function can be detected. It should be recognized that cardiac catheterization is not necessary for the routine evaluation of a patient with unstable angina.

Principles of Management

The medical treatment of unstable angina is currently in a state of flux. Patients with a history of recurrent episodes of rest angina and abnormal ECGs should be monitored in the cardiac care unit [9]. Initial therapy should include aspirin (shown to affect prognosis favorably), nitroglycerin, and nitrates. Patients already on aspirin or with a history of recurrent episodes of rest angina may receive a continuous intravenous infusion of heparin. Anti-thrombotic and anti-platelet aggregation agents, such as low-molecular weight heparins and glycoprotein IIb/IIIa receptor antagonists, respectively, are currently the subject of clinical research. The addition of beta-adrenergic blocking agents should be considered for those who continue to experience angina. In some patients refractory to nitrates and beta-blockers, addition of slow-release or long-acting vasoselective dihydropyridines or slow-release non-dihydropyridines may control angina. With such medical therapy, most patients become free of angina. Subsequently, however, such patients are likely to have stable angina and may need coronary arteriography and revascularization. Intervention in the acute phase of unstable angina is undesirable, although those patients whose pain is refractory to medical therapy may require angioplasty or coronary artery bypass surgery. Angioplasty during the acute phase is associated with a high incidence of abrupt reocclusion. The incidence of myocardial infarction and death is higher after angioplasty than after coronary artery bypass surgery in patients with unstable angina.

9

1. Patients with a history of recurrent episodes of rest angina should be monitored in the cardiac care unit

2. Aspirin in patients not already receiving this medication and GP IIb/IIIa antagonists in selected patients

3. Intravenous nitroglycerin followed by non-parenteral nitrates

4. Intravenous continuous heparin infusion or low-molecular weight heparins in selected patients with recurrent episodes of angina at rest

5. Addition of beta-blockers in patients symptomatic despite nitroglycerine

6. Addition of slow release or long-acting dihydropyridines or slow release non-dihydro-pyridines to nitrates and beta-blockers in refractory patients

7. Revascularization therapy in patients refractory to medical therapy

1   (Left) Diagrammatic representation of a lipid-rich stable eccentric plaque causing luminal obstruction as seen in stable angina. (Right) Diagrammatic representation of the longitudinal section of a segment of a coronary artery containing a disrupted eccentric atheromatous plaque with an intraintimal and intraluminal thrombus causing luminal obstruction.

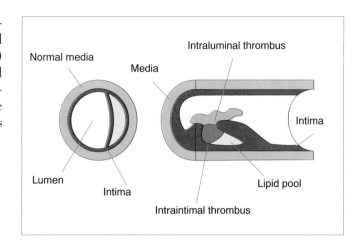

2   Transverse section of a coronary artery. The plaque cap has a fissure which has allowed blood into the lipid core, allowing the formation of a massive thrombus within the plaque itself.

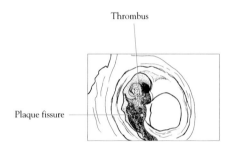

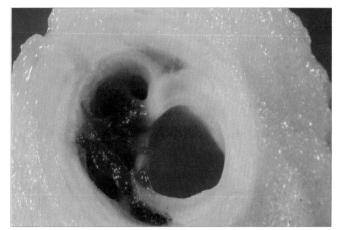

3   Diagrammatic illustrations of the potential outcomes of plaque development and fissure. (a) Healed fissures with buried incorporated thrombus may cause enlargement and progression of the plaque. (b) Fissuring leading to formation of labile intraintimal and intraluminal thrombi may cause recurrent luminal obstruction and reduction in coronary blood flow producing unstable angina syndrome. (c) When large occlusive thrombus develops following fissuring of the plaque, total interruption of blood flow may cause acute myocardial infarction.

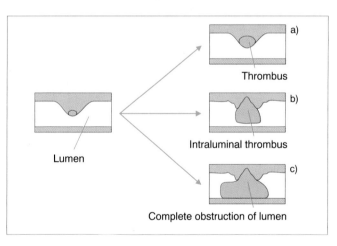

4   Schematic illustration of the interactions of platelet membrane receptors (glycoproteins Ia/Ib, IIb/IIIa), adhesive macromolecules, and the disrupted vessel wall. The different pathways of platelet activation are dependent on collagen, thrombin, adenosine diphosphate, and serotonin and thromboxane A_2.

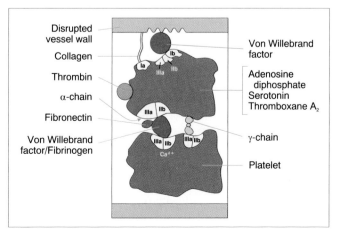

5

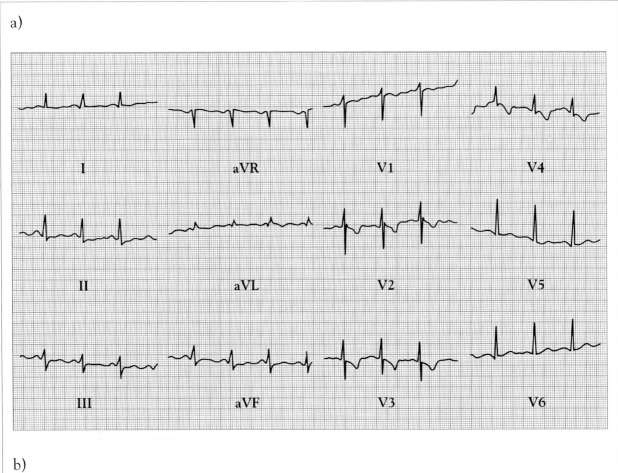

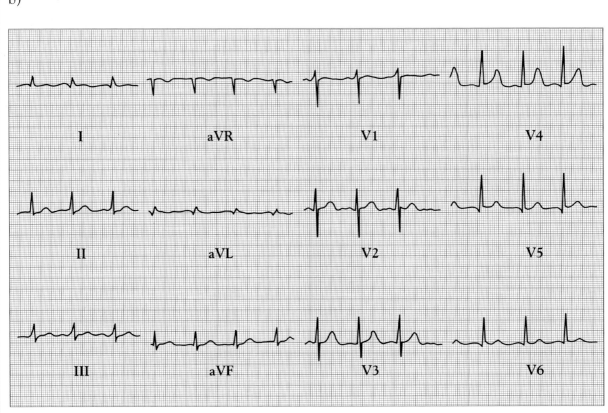

Resting electrocardiograms taken during chest pain in a patient with ischemic heart disease showing ST-T wave abnormalities in the anterior chest leads (a). After the pain has subsided, the ST-segment changes return to normal (b).

6   Magnetic resonance imaging showing regional wall motion abnormality in a patient with angina. The upper row shows the diastolic (left) and systolic (right) images in the absence of angina. The lower panel shows wall motion abnormality involving the infero-septal region of the left ventricle (arrowed) during angina induced by dobutamine.

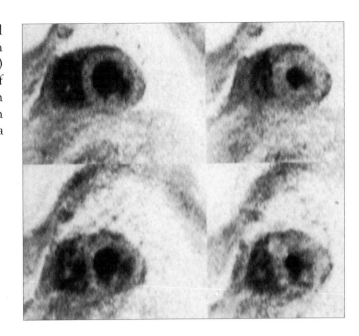

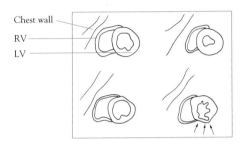

7   Coronary arteriography demonstrating a complex lesion with ragged irregular surface.

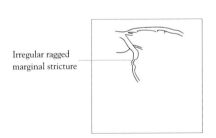

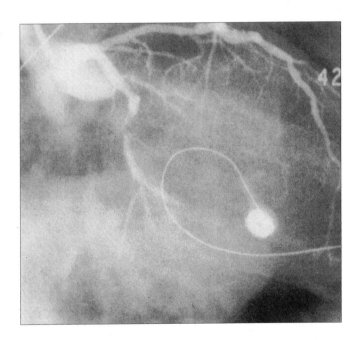

8   Coronary arteriogram during acute ischemic pain. Right coronary injection shows a sharp cut-off of the contrast column, typical of an acute occlusion. The occlusion is clearly soft thrombus and the angioplasty wire has passed easily into it.

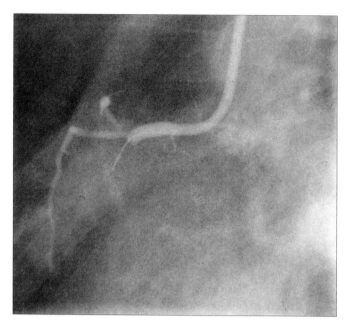

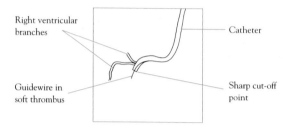

9   Principles of management of unstable angina.

1. Patients with a history of recurrent episodes of rest angina should be monitored in the cardiac care unit

2. Aspirin in patients not already receiving this medication and GP IIb/IIIa antagonists in selected patients

3. Intravenous nitroglycerin followed by non-parenteral nitrates

4. Intravenous continuous heparin infusion or low-molecular weight heparins in selected patients with recurrent episodes of angina at rest

5. Addition of beta-blockers in patients symptomatic despite nitroglycerin

6. Addition of slow-release or long-acting dihydro-pyridines or slow-release non-dihydropyridines to nitrates and beta-blockers in refractory patients

7. Revascularization therapy in patients refractory to medical therapy

ACUTE MYOCARDIAL INFARCTION

Definition

Acute myocardial necrosis with loss of myocardial function.

Pathophysiology

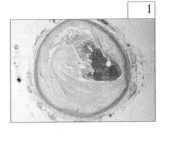

Acute interruption of blood flow producing prolonged myocardial ischemia is the most frequent cause of myocardial infarction. Clinical myocardial infarction almost always results from occlusion of an atherosclerotic epicardial coronary artery by thrombus. In over 90% of patients, the occlusive thrombus forms at the site of, or close to, an atheromatous plaque [1]. Increase in circumferential stress within the artery may initiate rupture or ulceration of the plaque resulting in the extrusion of the contents of the plaque (collagen, lipids, and other thrombogenic material) into the vessel lumen [2] (also see [2] in Unstable Angina), inducing platelet aggregation and adhesion. The formation of intra-intimal, intraluminal, and propagating thrombus prevents antegrade blood flow. Whereas transmural myocardial infarction is almost always associated with the development of a thrombus which completely occludes the vessel [3], non-Q-wave myocardial infarction is usually associated with a non-occlusive labile thrombus at the site of a fissured plaque [4]. Vasoconstrictive substances (e.g. thromboxane) may also contribute to the reduction of coronary blood flow. Decreased blood flow and stasis promote thrombosis. Transient impairment of the endogenous thrombolytic mechanism and enhancement of the thrombotic mechanism have also been documented in acute myocardial infarction.

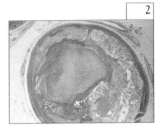

Acute myocardial infarction without reperfusion produces coagulation necrosis, which can be transmural or non-transmural [5]. With reperfusion, hemorrhagic infarction can occur [6]. However, commonly, contraction band necrosis is found [7].

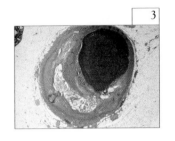

During the acute phase of myocardial infarction, mitral regurgitation may result from ischemic dysfunction or rupture [8] of the papillary muscle. Acute papillary muscle rupture produces severe mitral regurgitation, whereas papillary muscle dysfunction is associated with chronic mild to moderate mitral regurgitation [9]. Rupture of the ventricular septum usually results in left-to-right shunt [10]. Rupture of the free wall results in fatal cardiac tamponade [11,12]. A relatively large transmural myocardial infarction often leads to the development of a left ventricular aneurysm [13].

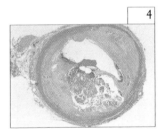

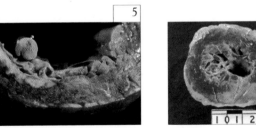

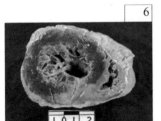

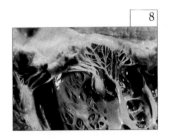

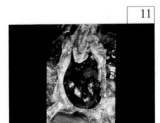

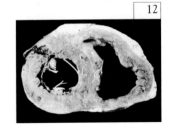

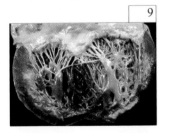

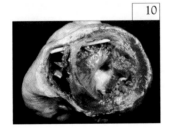

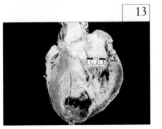

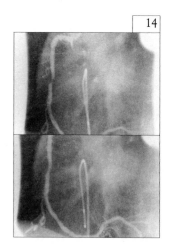

Occasionally, myocardial infarction occurs in the absence of obstructive atherosclerotic coronary artery disease. Coronary embolism, coronary vasospasm [14], anomalous origin of a coronary artery, coronary arteritis, coronary artery aneurysm (including Kawasaki's disease), pseudo-xanthoma elasticum, and metabolic disorders such as mucopoly-saccharoidosis and Fabry's disease are rare causes of acute myocardial infarction. Myocardial necrosis can occur in patients with valvular heart disease, particularly in patients with aortic stenosis or regurgitation and also in patients with hypertrophic cardiomyopathy.

Presentation

Symptoms

Patients usually present with prolonged chest pain. The location, radiation, and character of the pain are very similar to those of angina. However, the pain of myocardial infarction is usually more severe and longer in duration. Associated symptoms such as sweating, nausea, vomiting, dizziness, and dyspnea are more common in patients with myocardial infarction than with angina. Chest pain may be similar to that of acute myocardial infarction in patients with a thoracic aortic dissection, pericarditis, pneumothorax, and upper abdominal disease. Pain may be absent in some patients with acute myocardial infarction. Patients who present with severe dyspnea due to acute pulmonary edema, with stroke at the onset of infarction, or with syncope may not complain of chest pain. Patients who die suddenly and are immediately resuscitated usually have not had a myocardial infarct, and have no recollection of chest pain. In approximately 10% of patients, myocardial infarction occurs without any symptoms and the diagnosis is made by the characteristic electrocardiographic changes.

Signs

Even in patients with an uncomplicated acute myocardial infarct, evidence of impaired left ventricular function can be detected. A double apical impulse and an atrial sound (due to augmented atrial contraction) indicate an elevated left ventricular diastolic pressure. Sometimes a sustained outward movement of the apical impulse occurs, indicating decreased left ventricular ejection fraction. Patients in pulmonary edema may have basal crepitations. Hypoperfusion is recognized by the presence of cool extremities, reduced urine output, and mental obtundation. Cardiogenic shock is diagnosed when hypotension (systolic blood pressure less than 90 mmHg) accompanies evidence of hypoperfusion such as a urine output of less than 20 ml/hour, confusion, and a cold clammy skin. Right ventricular infarction is suspected when there is an elevated jugular venous pressure with Kussmaul's sign and a right ventricular third heart sound in the absence of pulmonary edema.

Acute rupture of the infarct is a serious, often fatal complication. If an infarct which involves the papillary muscle ruptures, there is usually pulmonary edema with a low output state and cardiogenic shock. A pansystolic or early systolic murmur of mitral regurgitation indicates papillary muscle dysfunction or rupture, respectively. In patients with an infarct resulting in rupture of the ventricular septum, a pansystolic murmur, often accompanied by a thrill, is present along the lower left sternal border. It is, however, difficult to differentiate between mitral regurgitation and ventricular septal rupture based on the physical findings alone. Ventricular free wall rupture produces tamponade causing rapid demise of the patient and antemortem diagnosis is rarely possible.

Pericarditis associated with a transmural myocardial infarct (episternopericarditis) is common, and diagnosed by pericardial pain with a transient pericardial rub. Pericarditis, with or without effusion, is also a feature of Dressler's syndrome (post-myocardial infarction syndrome), which usually occurs late after myocardial infarction. Pericardial pain, fever, pleuritic chest pain, arthralgia, pulmonary infiltrates, and an obvious pericardial rub are the usual findings of Dressler's syndrome.

In patients who develop a left ventricular aneurysm with the passage of time, a double, sustained apical impulse and an atrial sound may be the only abnormal physical findings.

Investigations

Radiology

Even in patients with uncomplicated transmural myocardial infarction, the plain chest X-ray, obtained soon after the onset of infarction, may show radiologic evidence of pulmonary venous congestion such as upper lobe blood diversion, Kerley B-lines, and perihilar haziness. These findings may persist for several hours after the pulmonary capillary wedge pressure has returned to normal. Evidence of florid pulmonary edema (alveolar edema, 'bat-wing' appearance) is present in patients who develop acute pulmonary edema due to extensive myocardial infarction, papillary muscle infarction, or ventricular septal rupture [15–17]. Cardiomegaly is usually absent except in patients with prior myocardial damage or a pre-existing left ventricular aneurysm. In patients with a ruptured ventricular septum, the pattern of pulmonary vessels may suggest both a left-to-right shunt with pulmonary arterial engorgement and pulmonary venous congestion. Pulmonary plethora, typical of a left-to-right shunt, will only become obvious with the passage of time.

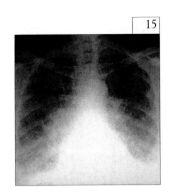

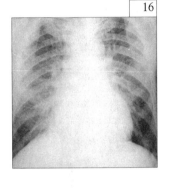

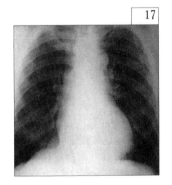

Electrocardiography

At the onset of myocardial infarction, only ST-segment elevation is present in the electrocardiographic leads representing the site of infarction [18]. In those leads remote from the site of infarction, reciprocal ST-segment depression may be present [18]. Soon after the onset of infarction, the presence of Q-waves or loss of R-waves denotes myocardial necrosis [19]. With the further passage of time, ST segments become isoelectric and T-wave inversion appears. Persistent ST-segment elevation with Q-waves suggests a chronic left ventricular aneurysm.

The location of the infarct can be roughly determined from the electrocardiogram; thus, an acute anterior infarct shows Q-waves and ST-segment elevations in the anterior precordial leads (V1 to V4) with similar changes in leads I, aVL, and V5 to V6 [20]. An inferior infarct shows similar changes in the inferior leads (I, II, aVF) [21]. A true posterior infarction shows dominant R-wave in leads V1 and V2, reflecting the absence of posterior forces [22].

Patients with ventricular septal rupture following myocardial infarction show ECG findings of either inferior or anterior infarction, as ventricular septal rupture occurs with almost equal frequency in inferior and anterior infarction [23]. Patients with papillary muscle infarction or ischemia usually show evidence of inferior infarction, as this complication is more frequent in inferior infarction.

When the infarct is non-transmural (non-Q-wave infarct), Q-waves or loss of R-waves are not seen but ST-segment depression and T-wave inversion are present, which may resolve with time [24,25].

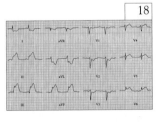 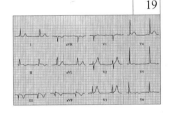 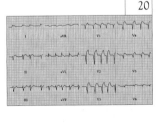 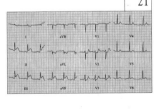

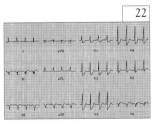 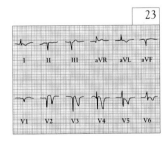 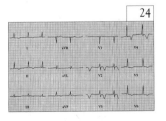 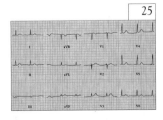

Right ventricular infarction may show characteristic ECG changes. ECG changes of inferior or infero-posterior infarction are accompanied by ST-segment elevations in the anterior precordial leads, usually V1 and V2, and also in the right precordial leads V3R to V7R. The magnitude of the Q-wave in lead III is usually greater than that in aVF [26].

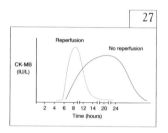

In ventricular free wall rupture, the ECGs may demonstrate evidence of Q-wave infarction or only ischemic ST-T changes. Sudden slowing of the sinus rate followed by a junctional or idioventricular rhythm with diminution of QRS amplitude may indicate acute or subacute rupture. The sudden appearance of tall peaking of precordial T-waves in a patient with previous ST-segment depression or T-wave inversion may also indicate hemopericardium.

Laboratory Studies

Estimation of serum enzymes is necessary to confirm acute myocardial necrosis. Elevation of the MB fraction of creatine kinase (CK) is almost diagnostic. Elevations of the MM fraction of CK, LDH isoenzymes, SHBD, and myoglobin are less sensitive. However, the increased ratio of MM3/MM1 or LDH1/LDH2 appear to be equally as sensitive as CK-MB for the diagnosis of acute myocardial necrosis. The early appearance and early peaking of cardiac enzymes have been thought to indicate recanalization of the infarct-related artery and myocardial reperfusion [27]. Troponin-T and cardiospecific troponin-I measurements have high sensitivity and specificity in the diagnosis of acute myocardial necrosis.

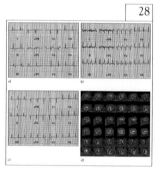

Exercise ECG Post-Myocardial Infarction

Exercise ECG testing in patients following uncomplicated myocardial infarction may show both the development of chest pain on exercise and ECG changes typical of myocardial ischemia [28]. The absence of pain or ECG changes of ischemia is associated with a good prognosis.

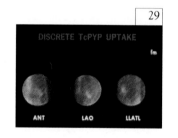

Nuclear Techniques

Although thallium perfusion imaging has been used in the diagnosis of acute myocardial infarction, it cannot distinguish between recent and old myocardial infarction.

Infarct-avid scintigraphy, using technetium-99m stannous pyrophosphate or technetium-99m imidodiphosphonate, for the diagnosis of acute myocardial necrosis, can be useful in some clinical circumstances. The distribution of radioactivity may be either discrete, which is specific for myocardial damage, or diffuse, which is related to blood pool radioactivity [29]. Although technetium-99m pyrophosphate imaging has a high degree of diagnostic sensitivity for transmural myocardial infarction (particularly anterior infarction), it is seldom used in routine diagnosis. However, it may be useful in the diagnosis of perioperative myocardial infarction following coronary artery bypass surgery, as electrocardiograms and enzymatic changes are less reliable. It is also useful in the localization of infarction in patients with intraventricular conduction defects such as left bundle branch block. Right ventricular, true posterior, and lateral myocardial infarcts are also better identified and localized by technetium-99m pyrophosphate imaging [30].

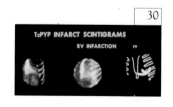

Assessment of left ventricular regional and global, systolic and diastolic function by radionuclide ventriculography, using technetium-99m to label the intracardiac blood pool, provides useful diagnostic and prognostic information in patients with acute myocardial infarction. Imaging is performed either during the first passage of the bolus through the central circulation or when it has reached equilibrium. Left ventricular volumes, ejection fraction, and parameters of diastolic function, such as filling rates, can be measured. Amplitude and phase images are useful in determining the location of an infarct. The timing of regional myocardial motion is useful in defining areas of dyskinesis [31,32].

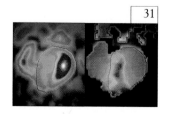
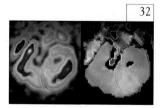

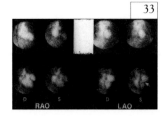

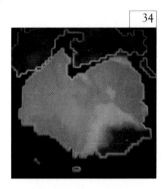

Radionuclide ventriculography used to determine left ventricular ejection fraction may be helpful in assessing the long-term prognosis of patients with acute myocardial infarction. The one-year mortality probability is less than 10% when the ejection fraction is greater than 45%, whereas it is close to 50% when the ejection fraction is 25% or less. A true left ventricular aneurysm with dyskinetic wall motion, as well as a pseudoaneurysm with a narrow neck connecting the aneurysmal cavity to the fundus, can be easily diagnosed by radionuclide ventriculography [33]. Phase imaging during radionuclide ventriculography can also demonstrate a left ventricular aneurysm [34].

A right ventricular ejection fraction of less than 40%, with a regional wall motion abnormality, virtually confirms the diagnosis of right ventricular infarction. The left ventricular ejection fraction may remain normal in these patients [35].

Serial left ventricular radionuclide ventriculography may be useful for the assessment of the extent of 'stunned' myocardium after successful reperfusion therapy [36].

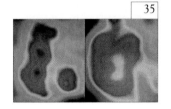

Echocardiography

Regional wall motion abnormalities revealing hypokinesis, akinesis, or dyskinesis and thinning of the affected myocardial segments are the most important echocardiographic findings in acute myocardial infarction [37,38]. In ischemia without infarction, similar regional systolic wall motion abnormalities can be recognized but myocardial thinning is usually absent. Wall motion abnormalities involving the base of the inferior or the diaphragmatic wall suggest inferior infarction, while abnormalities of the septum, apex, and anteroseptal regions indicate anterior myocardial infarction. The diagnosis of right ventricular infarction may be suggested if right ventricular volumes are increased [39]. Regional wall motion abnormalities of the right ventricle are often difficult to recognize, even by two-dimensional echocardiography.

A number of complications of acute myocardial infarction can be diagnosed by Doppler echocardiography. Mitral regurgitation due to papillary muscle dysfunction can be detected [40a & b]. Severe mitral regurgitation, resulting from a papillary muscle infarct with or without rupture, can be detected by transthoracic, transesophageal, and Doppler echocardiography [41a & b]. Rupture of the ventricular septum may be demonstrated by a combination of imaging, color, and continuous-wave Doppler [42a, b & c].

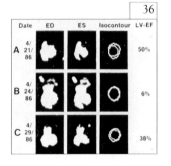

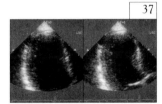

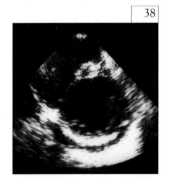

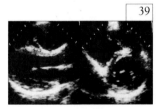

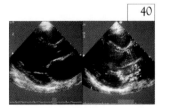

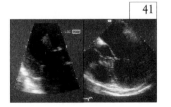

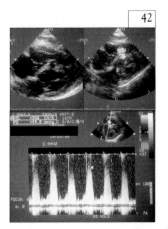

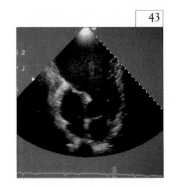

43

Left ventricular aneurysm following acute myocardial infarction is recognized by the presence of dyskinetic, thin myocardial segments. An antero-apical aneurysm incorporating the distal part of the septum is the most common [43]. Pseudoaneurysms which result from subacute rupture of the ventricular free wall are characterized by the presence of a narrow neck connecting the cavity of the aneurysm to the cavity of the ventricle [44]. The free walls of the pseudoaneurysm are formed by the pericardium, and these anatomic features can be identified by two-dimensional echocardiography.

Left ventricular thrombi occur frequently in antero-apical infarcts and only occasionally in inferior infarcts. Thrombi are recognized by the presence of highly reflective or luminescent intracavitary masses. These masses may be mobile, protruding into the cavity, or sessile with a laminated appearance [45a & b].

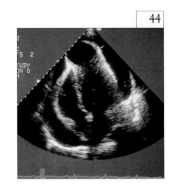

44

Magnetic Resonance Imaging and Computed Tomography

Magnetic resonance imaging can reveal the extent of myocardial loss after an acute myocardial infarction [46] and complications of infarctions, such as left ventricular aneurysm [47,48] and mural thrombus [49], in much the same way but often with better resolution than two-dimensional echocardiography.

Cine and gated computed tomography, like magnetic resonance imaging, can demonstrate areas of myocardial thinning and regional wall motion abnormalities in acute myocardial infarction. Computed tomography is also capable of diagnosing complications of acute myocardial infarction such as mitral regurgitation, ventricular septal defect, and mural thrombi [50]. In clinical practice, however, neither magnetic resonance imaging nor computed tomography is often needed for the diagnosis and management of patients with acute myocardial infarction.

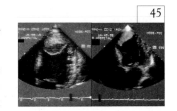

45

Cardiac Catheterization and Angiography

Right heart catheterization with the use of balloon flotation (Swan–Ganz) catheters is usually required to measure the hemodynamic disturbance during the management of severe heart failure, low output state, and cardiogenic shock complicating acute myocardial infarction [51]. A marked elevation of pulmonary capillary wedge pressure with reduced cardiac output is the characteristic hemodynamic abnormality of severe acute heart failure. In cardiogenic shock, the wedge pressure is elevated, the cardiac

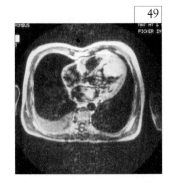

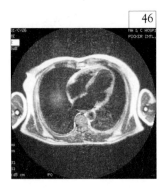

46

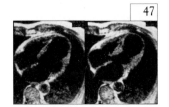

47

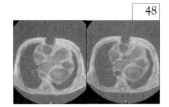

48

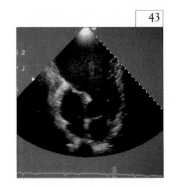

49

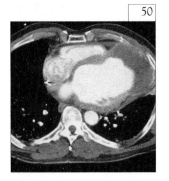

50

51

Subset	Pulmonary capillary wedge pressure	Right atrial pressure	Cardiac output
Uncomplicated	Normal	Normal	Normal
Heart failure	Elevated	Normal	Normal
Cardiogenic shock	Elevated	Normal or elevated	Low
Right ventricular infarction	Normal	Elevated	Low or normal
Hypovolemic shock	Low	Low	Low

output low, while the right atrial pressure is either normal or elevated. Disproportionate elevation of right atrial pressure compared with the pulmonary capillary wedge pressure is the hemodynamic abnormality of right ventricular infarction [52]. In hypovolemic shock both right atrial and pulmonary capillary wedge pressures are lower than normal, the cardiac output is reduced, and there is arterial hypotension.

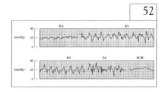

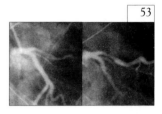

Coronary arteriography in acute myocardial infarction usually reveals total occlusion of the infarct-related vessel as well as other abnormalities in other vessels. When coronary arteriography is performed after thrombolytic therapy, the infarct-related artery shows varying degrees of residual stenosis [53], mural thrombi, and complex atherosclerotic lesions. In the absence of recanalization, the total occlusion of the infarct-related artery with a thrombus is easily recognized [54].

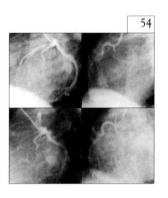

In patients with rupture of the ventricular septum, a step up in oxygen saturation in the pulmonary arterial blood confirms the presence of a left-to-right shunt [55]. A contrast left ventriculogram shows opacification of the right ventricle due to the ventricular septal defect [56].

An early peaked giant 'v' or regurgitant wave in the pulmonary capillary wedge pressure tracing and a reflected 'v' wave in the pulmonary artery pressure tracing usually indicates acute or subacute severe mitral regurgitation seen in patients with a papillary muscle infarct [57]. Contrast left ventriculography reveals almost instantaneous left atrial opacification due to severe mitral regurgitation [58]. With the advent of Doppler and two-dimensional echocardiography, contrast ventriculography is seldom required for the diagnosis of the complications of acute myocardial infarction or assessment of left ventricular function.

Principles of Management

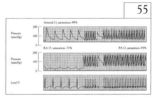

Pain relief with appropriate analgesics is usually required. Thrombolysis with streptokinase, anisoylated plasminogen streptokinase activator complex (APSAC), or recombinant tissue plasminogen activator (rtPA) has been shown to reduce mortality in patients with myocardial infarction irrespective of age, sex, or location of infarct. Aspirin has also been shown to reduce mortality. If thrombolysis achieves successful recanalization of an infarct-related occluded artery, pain is relieved and left ventricular function improved, thereby improving long-term prognosis. There may be hematologic contra-indications to thrombolysis, when aspirin can be substituted.

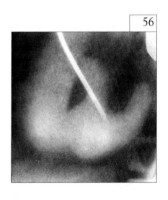

Other drugs which may be used at the time of uncomplicated myocardial infarction and shortly afterwards include beta-adrenergic blocking agents, angiotensin converting enzyme (ACE) inhibitors, and lipid-lowering agents, all of which have been shown to decrease mortality [59]. ACE inhibitors, either administered early or relatively late after onset of symptoms, reduce mortality, particularly in patients with reduced left ventricular ejection fraction and those with overt heart failure [60]. They also preserve left ventricular function in certain patients with myocardial infarction and have the potential to decrease recurrent infarction and unstable angina. Intravenous magnesium over 24 hours has been shown to decrease ventricular arrhythmias. Anticoagulation is used in patients with documented mural thrombus. Attempts should be made to modify the risk factors for the

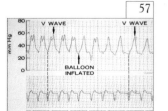

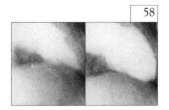

PHARMACOLOGIC RISK MODIFICATION
IN ISCHEMIC HEART DISEASE

Intervention	Approximate % risk reduction of death and/or non-fatal myocardial infarction
Beta-blockers	13 – 23%
ACE inhibitors	19 – 37%
Lipid-lowering agents	30 – 42%

progression of coronary heart disease [61]. Lipid-lowering agents have been shown to improve prognosis in those patients with hypercholesterolemia.

Post-Infarction Angina

Patients may have either silent or overt (painful) myocardial ischemia following myocardial infarction. The prognosis for such patients is worse than those who have no ischemia. Post-infarction angina may be improved with intravenous heparin, nitrates, calcium channel blockers, and beta-adrenergic blockers. If angina persists, coronary arteriography, with a view to revascularization by angioplasty or surgery, is required.

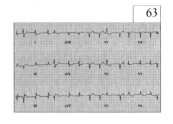

Dysrhythmias

Dysrhythmias of all kinds are common following acute myocardial infarction [62]. Ectopic beats, particularly of ventricular origin [63], are almost invariably present. Unless ventricular ectopics are frequent (>5/min), they do not require treatment. Ventricular fibrillation [64] is treated by cardioversion followed by intravenous lidocaine. Non-sustained ventricular tachycardia should be treated with intravenous lidocaine. Procainamide and amiodarone may be required in refractory monomorphic ventricular tachycardia [65] and ischemic polymorphous ventricular tachycardia [66,67].

Atrioventricular block of various types is common in acute infarction, particularly in patients with inferior wall myocardial infarction [68,69].

Slow heart rates causing symptoms may respond to atropine, while symptomatic atrioventricular block (particularly in association with anterior infarction) requires temporary transvenous pacing. Atrioventricular dissociation with accelerated idioventricular rhythm does not require pacing [70]. Prophylactic temporary pacing is required in patients who develop bifascicular [71] or trifascicular conduction defects complicating myocardial infarction. Sustained atrial fibrillation [72] and flutter are relatively uncommon tachyarrhythmias in acute infarction. Atrial tachyarrhythmias, including atrial fibrillation, require digitalization following cardioversion in the presence of hemodynamic compromise.

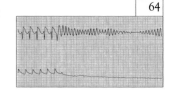

Pulmonary Edema

Prompt oxygenation is necessary, including intubation when there is severe hypoxia. Intravenous morphine or diamorphine, diuretics, or nitrates have all been shown to be of benefit. Echo-Doppler studies should be carried out to check that a surgically correctable mechanical complication, such as rupture of the ventricular septum or a papillary muscle, is not present. Hemodynamic assessment of left and right heart pressures and cardiac output may facilitate management with vasodilator or positive inotropic drugs.

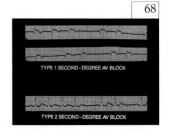

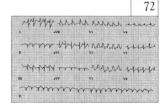

In patients refractory to such treatment, coronary arteriography with a view to primary angioplasty may be of benefit. Intra-aortic balloon counterpulsation may be used as supportive treatment [73].

Cardiogenic Shock

Systemic arterial hypotension (systolic blood pressure <90 mmHg) and diminished organ perfusion (peripheral vasoconstriction, oliguria, and mental obtundation) constitute the syndrome of cardiogenic shock. The mortality associated with cardiogenic shock is extremely high, irrespective of treatment. Primary angioplasty of the infarct-related artery might be feasible and has been shown to improve prognosis of both cardiogenic shock and pulmonary edema. Hemodynamic monitoring is required to direct logical treatment with vasodilators, inotropic agents, or intra-aortic balloon counterpulsation [74]. If acute cardiac transplantation is a possibility, left ventricular assist devices may be employed as a preliminary, temporary measure.

Mechanical Complications

There is a high mortality from either significant rupture of the ventricular septum or rupture (partial or complete) of a papillary muscle with resultant severe mitral regurgitation. Intra-aortic balloon counterpulsation [75] may be used as a 'holding' procedure until it is technically possible to correct these lesions by surgery. Vasodilator and inotropic agents may also help temporarily.

Right Ventricular Infarction

In hypotensive patients with a low right atrial pressure, intravenous fluid therapy is worthwhile. If the pressure is already raised and the cardiac output low, inotropic agents might help. Primary angioplasty might help the critically ill patient. Atrioventricular block is relatively common and best treated with sequential atrioventricular pacing [76].

Non-Q-Wave (Subendocardial) Myocardial Infarction

As the pathophysiology is closer to unstable angina than transmural (Q-wave) infarction, thrombolytic agents have not been effective. With respect to the development of subsequent myocardial infarction or angina, the prognosis is worse than for Q-wave infarction. Evaluation and therapy are similar to those of unstable angina. Non-dihydropyridine calcium entry blocking agents may decrease reinfarction and post-infarction angina.

Pericarditis

No specific treatment is required apart from analgesics. Aspirin may be particularly useful, as well as other non-steroidal anti-inflammatory agents. Steroids should be reserved for those with severe refractory pericardial pain, as they have been shown to induce a higher incidence of recurrent pericarditis. Colchicine may benefit some patients with recurrent pericarditis.

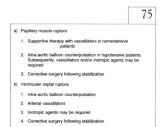

73

1. Supplemental oxygen (60 – 100%) by face mask; intubation in patients remaining hypoxic
2. Intravenous morphine, diamorphine
3. Intravenous frusemide
4. Sublingual nitroglycerin followed by intravenous nitroglycerin
5. Echo-Doppler to exclude the presence of mechanical defects
6. Hemodynamic monitoring for maintenance vasodilator and/or inotropic therapy
7. Consider coronary arteriography and primary angioplasty if no response to treatment as above

74

1. Coronary angiography with a view to primary angioplasty of the infarct-related artery
2. Vasopressors to maintain arterial pressure
3. Intra-aortic balloon counterpulsation therapy as soon as feasible
4. Supportive pharmacotherapy according to hemodynamics
5. Treat pulmonary edema
6. Echo-Doppler to exclude mechanical defects
7. Left ventricular assist devices as a bridge to cardiac transplant in refractory patients

75

a) Papillary muscle rupture
  1. Supportive therapy with vasodilators in normotensive patients
  2. Intra-aortic balloon counterpulsation in hypotensive patients. Subsequently, vasodilators and/or inotropic agents may be required
  3. Corrective surgery following stabilization
b) Ventricular septal rupture
  1. Intra-aortic balloon counterpulsation
  2. Arterial vasodilators
  3. Inotropic agents may be required
  4. Corrective surgery following stabilization

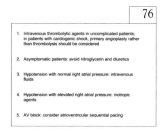

76

1. Intravenous thrombolytic agents in uncomplicated patients; in patients with cardiogenic shock, primary angioplasty rather than thrombolysis should be considered
2. Asymptomatic patients: avoid nitroglycerin and diuretics
3. Hypotension with normal right atrial pressure: intravenous fluids
4. Hypotension with elevated right atrial pressure: inotropic agents
5. AV block: consider atrioventricular sequential pacing

1   Thrombosed coronary artery in transverse section. The lumen is completely occluded by a mass of red thrombus. Above and to the left of the thrombus is a plaque of atheroma which contains lipid.

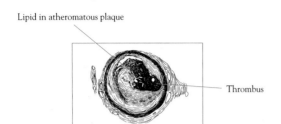

Lipid in atheromatous plaque

Thrombus

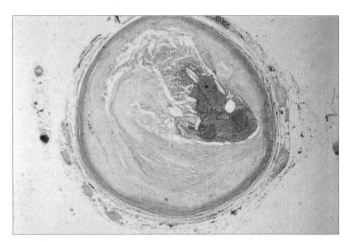

2   Transverse section of a coronary artery. The plaque cap has a fissure which has allowed blood into the lipid core, allowing the formation of a massive thrombus within the plaque itself.

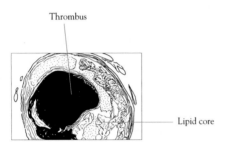

Thrombus

Lipid core

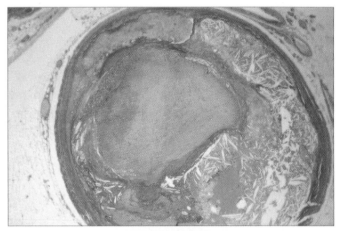

3   Histologic section of a coronary artery. The continuity between lipid in the core and thrombus completely occluding the lumen is due to rupture of the plaque cap.

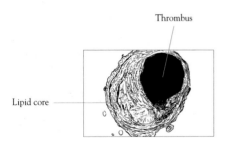

Thrombus

Lipid core

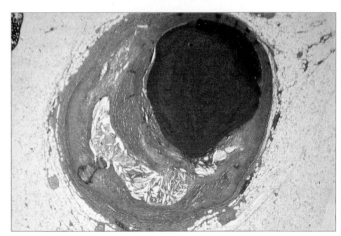

4   Cross-section through a coronary artery with an atherosclerotic plaque which has fissured, intraplaque hemorrhage, and mural thrombus.

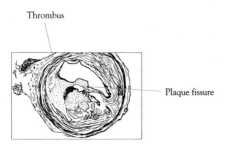

Thrombus

Plaque fissure

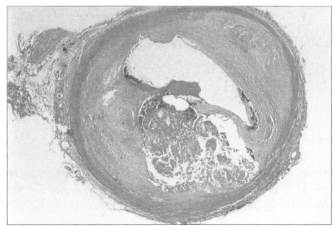

5 Four-day-old acute myocardial infarction, in which necrotic muscle is bright yellow. The infarction is non-transmural and involves the papillary muscle.

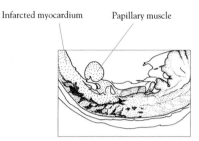

Infarcted myocardium   Papillary muscle

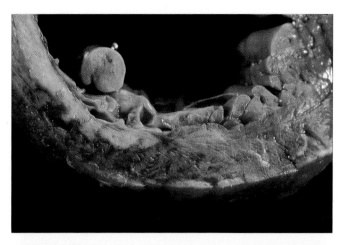

6 With reperfusion, the macroscopic appearances of an acute myocardial infarction change, and the myocardium becomes hemorrhagic.

Hemorrhagic infarction

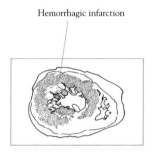

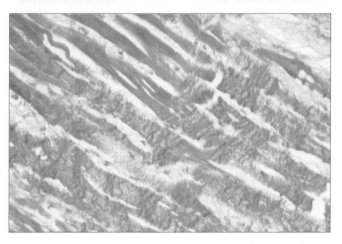

7 Histologic section of the myocardium in a patient with reperfusion injury. There is characteristic contraction band necrosis.

Contraction bands

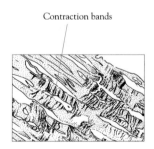

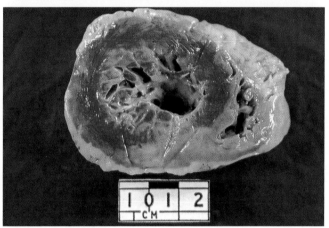

8 Acute myocardial infarction resulting in rupture of a papillary muscle.

Anterior cusp   Posterior cusp

Partially torn postero-medial papillary muscle

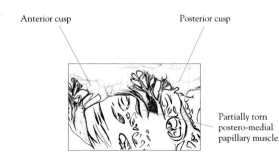

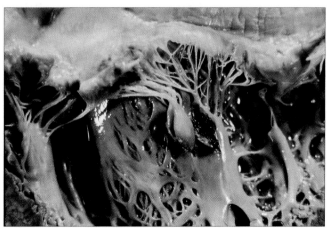

9   The left ventricle has been opened to show a papillary muscle infarct resulting in mitral regurgitation. The posterior papillary muscle is pale and shrunken due to infarction. The anterior papillary muscle (normal) is larger and darker. Subendocardial ischemic scarring is present in the left ventricle.

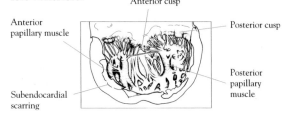

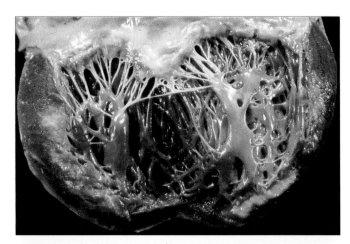

10   Acute myocardial infarction of the septum with rupture resulting in a ventricular septal defect (probe is shown passing through the defect).

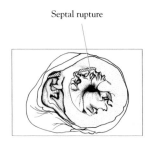

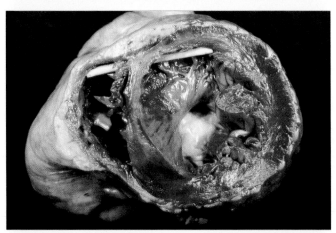

11   Pericardial sac filled with blood clot as a result of cardiac rupture due to myocardial infarction.

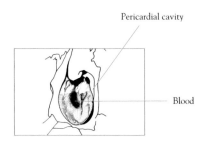

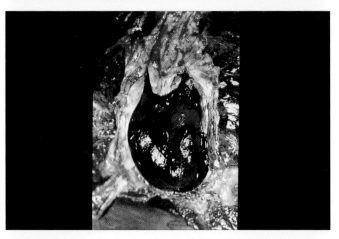

12   Rupture of the anterior wall of the left ventricle due to acute infarction.

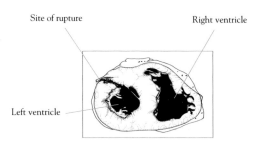

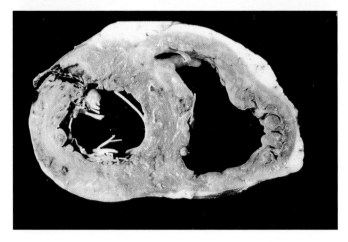

13 Localized left ventricular aneurysm due to old myocardial infarction. The aneurysm does not contain more than a fine deposit of thrombus and has a larger central cavity opening into the ventricle.

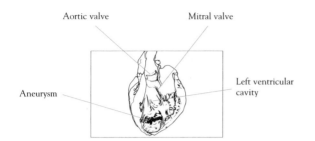

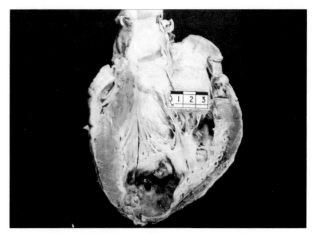

14

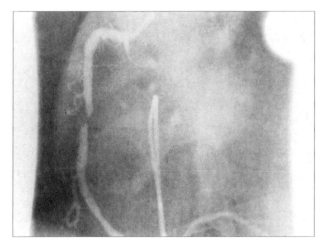

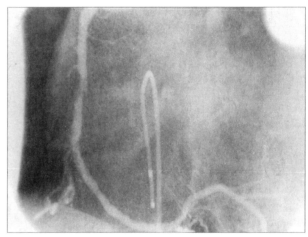

a)

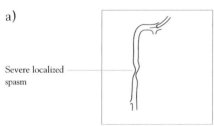

b)

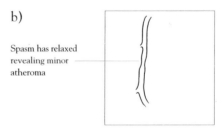

An example of coronary artery spasm, in the presence of minor atherosclerotic coronary artery disease. Angiogram of the right coronary artery in the right anterior oblique projection during spontaneous spasm (a), and following relaxation of spasm showing residual minor narrowing (b).

15 Chest X-ray showing pulmonary edema and bilateral pleural effusions following acute myocardial infarction.

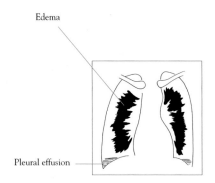

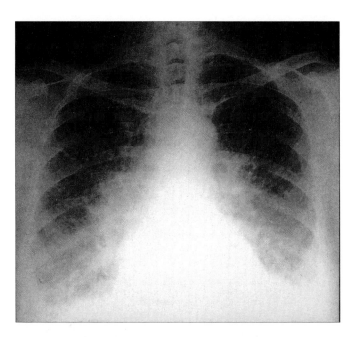

16 Chest X-ray showing cardiac enlargement with hilar edema and generalized increase in pulmonary vessel size due to left-to-right shunt through a ventricular septal defect complicating myocardial infarction.

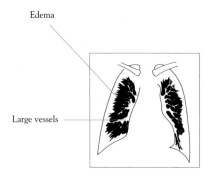

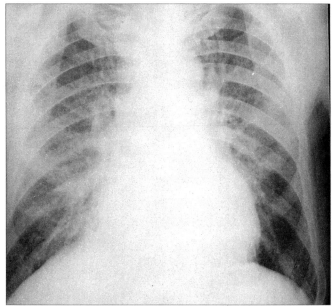

17 Chest X-ray of the same patient as in [16] showing normal pulmonary vascularity following surgical closure of the defect.

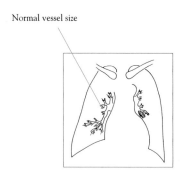

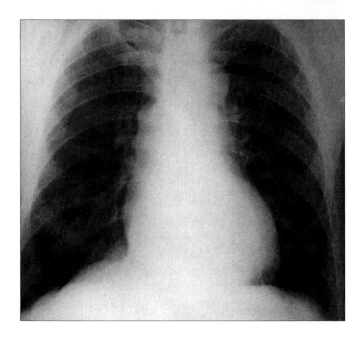

18

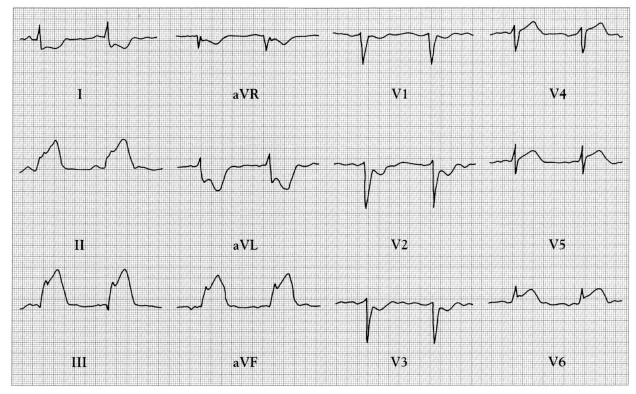

Electrocardiogram showing acute inferior myocardial infarction with ST-segment elevation in II, III and aVF. There is also ST-segment elevation in V5 and V6 and ST-segment depression in I, aVL, V2 and V3.

19

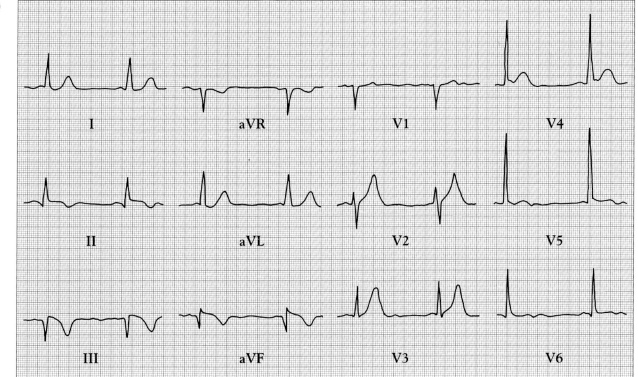

Electrocardiogram from the same patient as in [18] showing Q-waves and T-wave inversion in leads II, III and aVF.

20

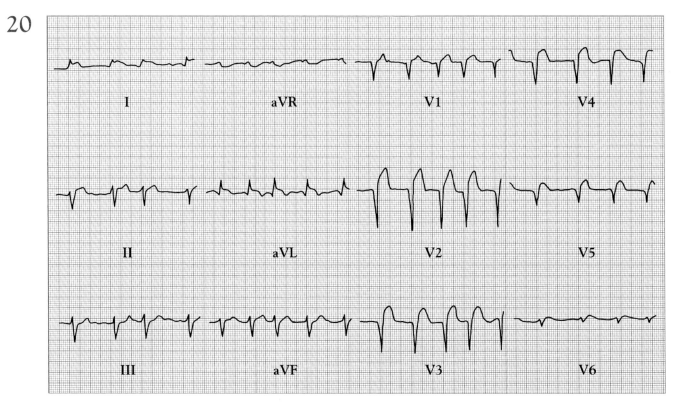

Electrocardiogram in a patient with acute antero-lateral myocardial infarction showing Q-waves and ST-segment elevation in V2–V5, I and aVF.

21

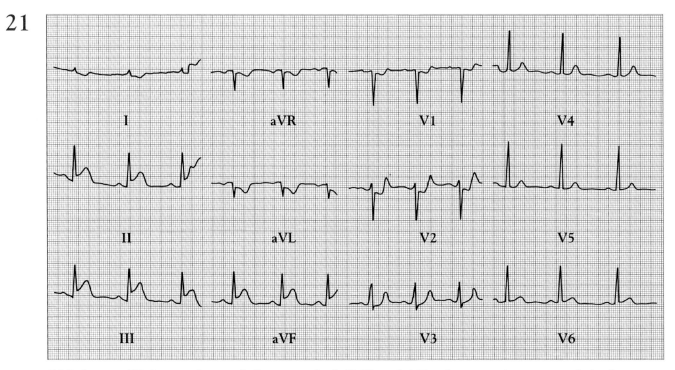

ECG showing ST changes along with Q-waves in leads II, III, and aVF, indicating inferior myocardial infarction.

22

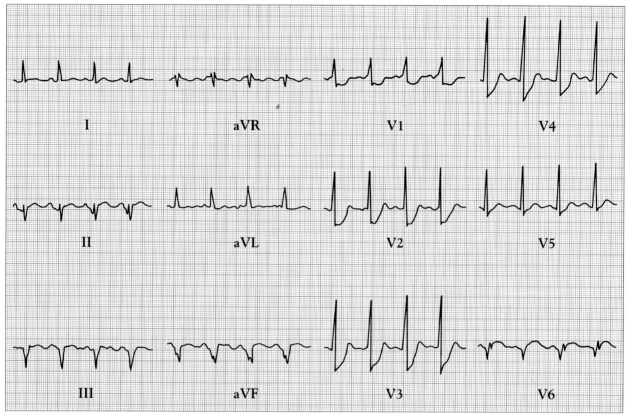

Electrocardiogram showing a true posterior myocardial infarction. There are Q-waves in II, aVF, and V6 with dominant R-waves in V1–V4 together with ST-segment depression in the anterior chest leads.

23 Electrocardiogram from a patient with a ruptured ventricular septum following myocardial infarction. There are Q-waves in leads V1–V3 indicating septal infarction.

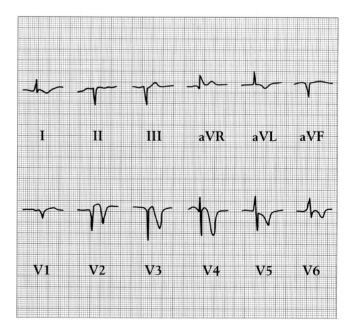

24

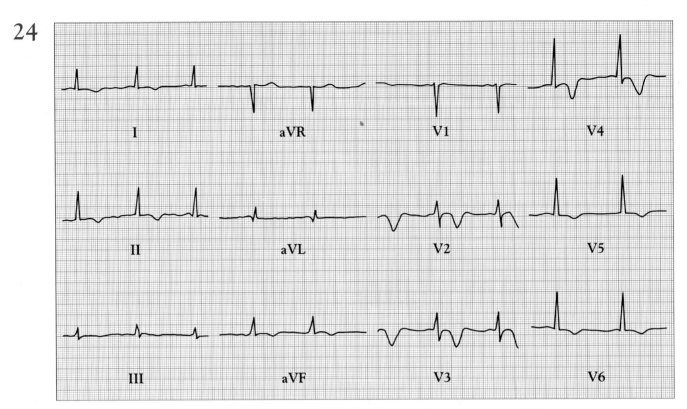

Electrocardiogram from a patient with a subendocardial infarction showing widespread T-wave inversion.

25

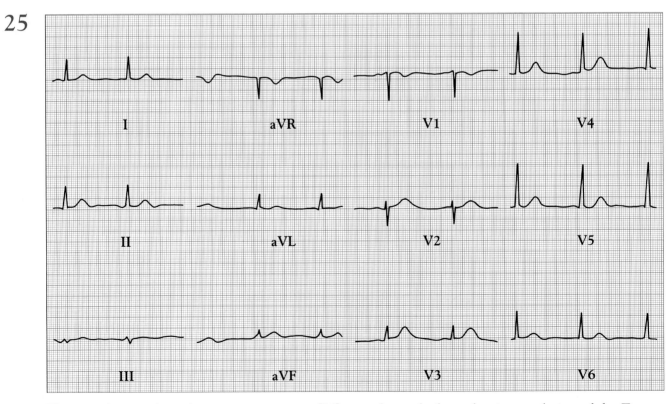

Electrocardiogram from the same patient as in [24] several months later showing resolution of the T-wave changes.

26

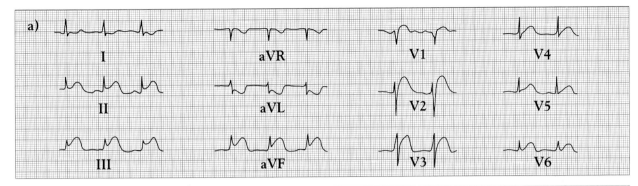

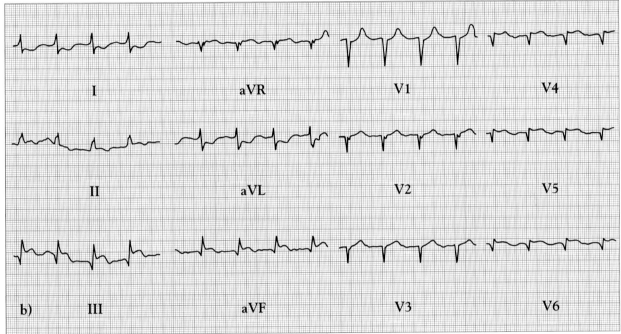

Electrocardiograms in two patients with acute right ventricular infarction. In (a), ST-segment elevation is present in leads II, III, and aVF as in inferior infarction. In addition, ST-segment elevation in the anterior precordial leads V1 to V3 suggests right ventricular infarction. In (b), ST-segment elevation in leads II, III, aVF, and in the right precordial leads V4-V6 suggests right ventricular infarction. The magnitude of the Q-wave in lead III is greater than the Q-wave in aVF. Q-waves are also present in the right precordial leads V3-V6. Also note the prolonged P-R interval indicating first degree A-V block.

27 Schematic illustration: CK-MB time–concentration curves in patients with reperfusion (blue line) and without reperfusion (red line). Sudden release of CK-MB and early peaking of the curve within 10–14 hours suggest recanalization of the infarct-related artery.

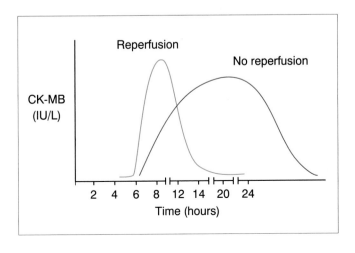

28

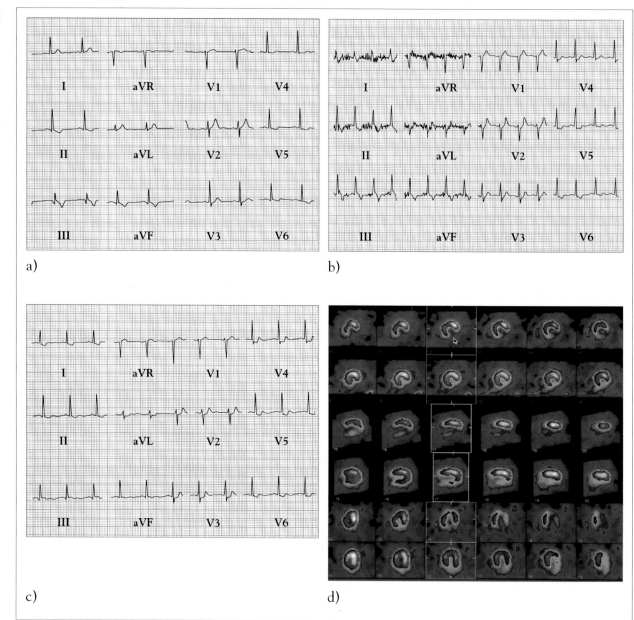

Stress electrocardiography and thallium perfusion scintigraphy in a patient with recent myocardial infarction. (a) The rest electrocardiogram indicates infero-lateral myocardial infarction. (b) During the early stages of exercise with only a modest increase in heart rate, upsloping ST depressions in leads V2-V3, and horizontal or down-sloping ST depressions in leads V4-V6, indicate myocardial ischemia in the left anterior descending coronary artery territory. (c) The recovery ECG continues to show ST-T abnormalities greater than at rest (a). (d) Thallium SPECT scintigraphy in various views demonstrates reversible thallium defects in the antero-septal regions of the left ventricle, indicating the presence of ischemic myocardial segments in the left anterior descending territory. Fixed thallium defects were present in the inferior wall in the territory of the right coronary artery.

29 ^{99m}Tc-pyrophosphate (TcPYP) images in anterior (ANT), left anterior oblique (LAO), and left lateral (LLATL) projections in a patient with a recent antero-lateral myocardial infarction showing pyrophosphate uptake in the antero-lateral wall of the left ventricle.

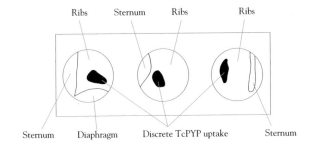

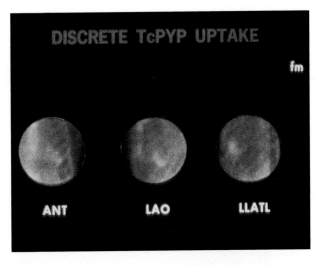

30 Right ventricular (RV) infarction diagnosed by ^{99m}Tc-pyrophosphate imaging. The presence of RV infarction is recognized by the horizontal extension of radioactivity from the inferior left ventricular (LV) wall to the sternum in the left anterior oblique projection. In RV infarction, LV inferior wall and inferior interventricular septum are almost always involved.

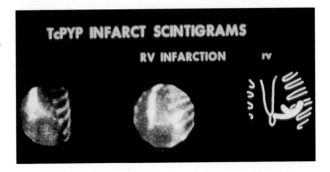

31

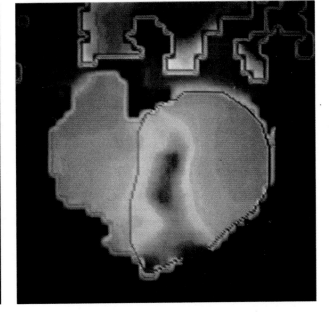

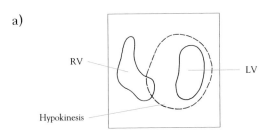

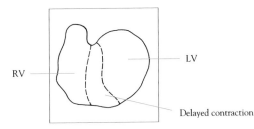

Amplitude (a) and phase (b) images in anteroseptal infarction. There are reduced values of amplitude and high phase in the region of the septum. This indicates hypokinesis and delayed contraction.

32

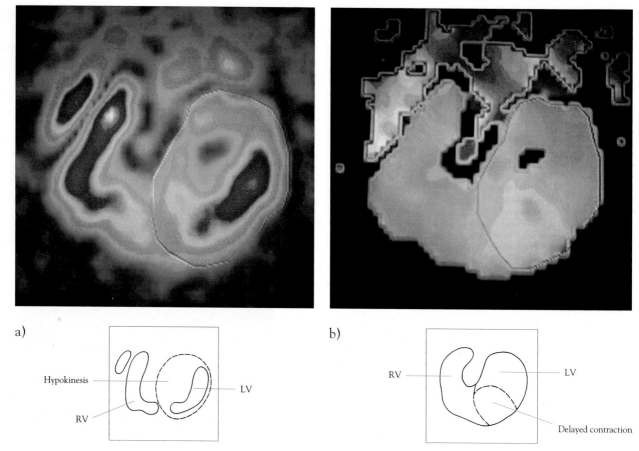

a)

Hypokinesis —— LV

RV ——

b)

RV —— LV

Delayed contraction

Amplitude (a) and phase (b) images in inferior infarction. The central amplitude defect and the delayed apical contraction are typical.

33

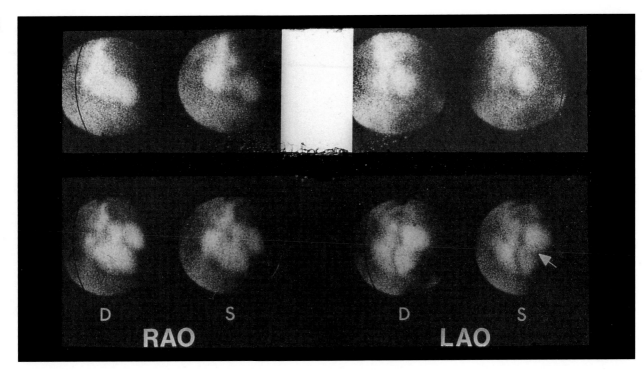

Radionuclide ventriculography (equilibrium gated blood pool scintigraphy) in right anterior oblique (RAO) and left anterior oblique (LAO) projections. Upper panels show true antero-apical aneurysm of the left ventricle with a broad neck. Lower panels show a false left ventricular aneurysm with a narrow neck (arrow).

34   Phase image in left ventricular aneurysm showing apical dyskinesis (red).

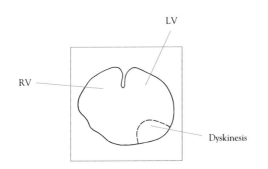

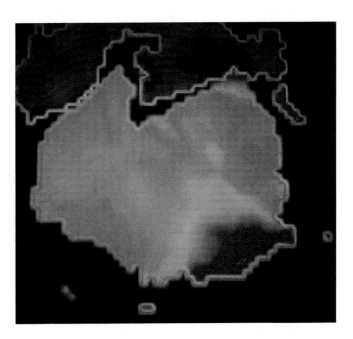

35

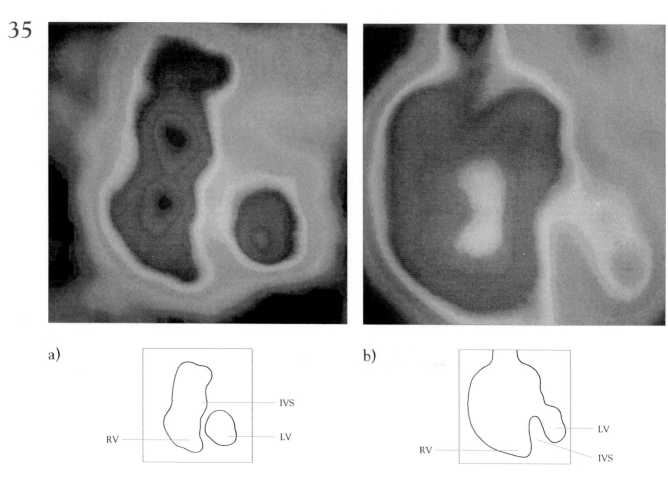

a)

RV

IVS

LV

b)

RV

LV

IVS

Radionuclide ventriculogram of a patient with right ventricular infarction showing a dilated poorly contracting right ventricle with reduced ejection fraction (b) compared with a normal subject (a). Left ventricular ejection fraction in this patient was normal.

36 Serial radionuclide gated equilibrium ventriculography in a patient with acute myocardial infarction, treated successfully with thrombolytic therapy. (A) The left ventricular ejection fraction (LVEF) was normal in this patient prior to the development of myocardial infarction. (B) LVEF fell markedly and remained low despite successful reperfusion of the ischemic myocardium by thrombolytic therapy. (C) Repeat radionuclide ventriculography five days later showed a significant increase of LVEF, suggesting the presence of 'stunned' myocardium following reperfusion.
ED=end-diastole; ES=end-systole;
Isocontour=automatic edge detection.

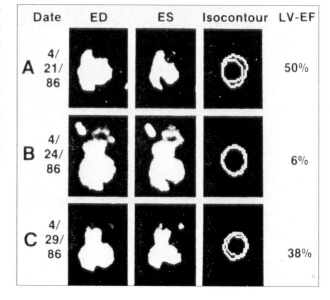

37

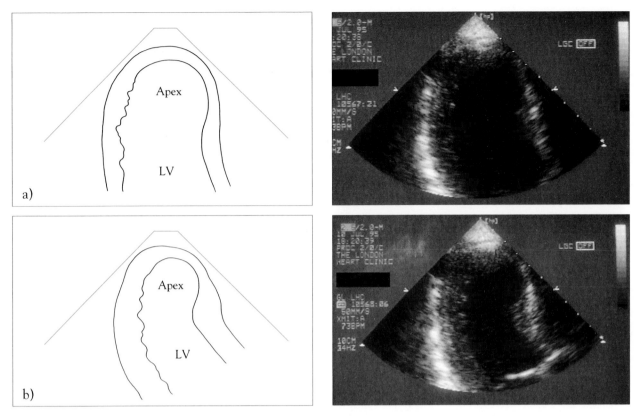

Apical long-axis views from a patient with an anterior/apical myocardial infarction at end-diastole (a) and end-systole (b). The apical portion of the anterior wall fails to thicken or contract.

38

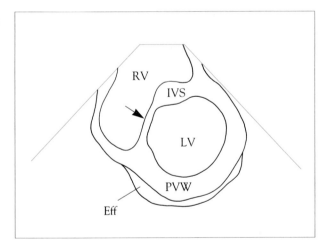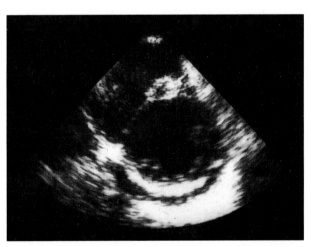

Parasternal short-axis view showing extreme thinning (arrow) of the interventricular septum resulting from myocardial infarction. There is a small pericardial effusion associated with post-infarction (Dressler's) syndrome.

39

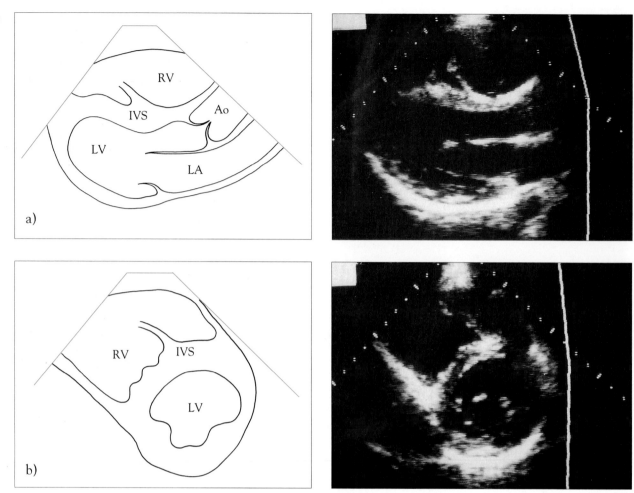

Parasternal long-axis (a) and parasternal short-axis (b) views from a patient with myocardial infarction involving the right ventricle. In the appropriate clinical setting, the finding of right ventricular enlargement with preserved left ventricular function can suggest this diagnosis.

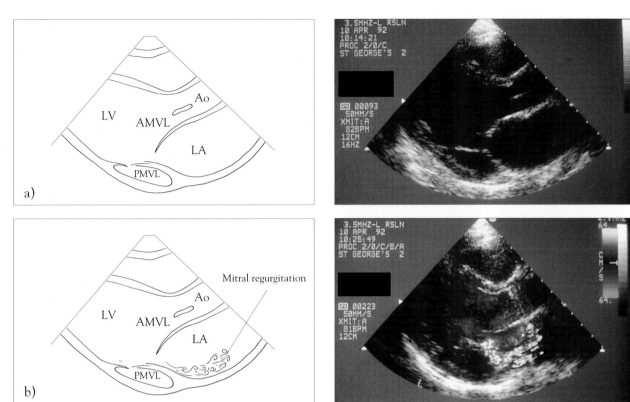

40

Parasternal long-axis view from a patient with infarction of the basal posterior wall involving one or both papillary muscles. (a) The result is to 'tether' the posterior mitral leaflet into the ventricle preventing it from aligning with the anterior leaflet. (b) Color-flow Doppler shows a posteriorly directed jet of mitral regurgitation.

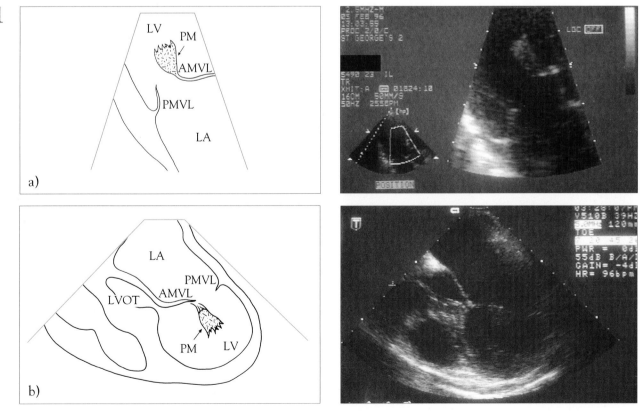

41

(a) Apical long-axis and (b) transesophageal study in a patient with a ruptured papillary muscle (PM) associated with inferior myocardial infarction. This is usually fatal but in this case a small, secondary chordal attachment to the ventricular wall prevented the ruptured muscle head from becoming totally 'flail' and limited the severity of the mitral regurgitation.

42

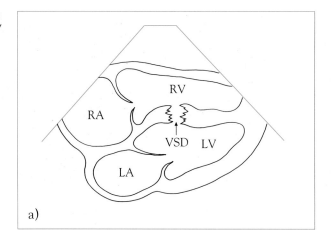

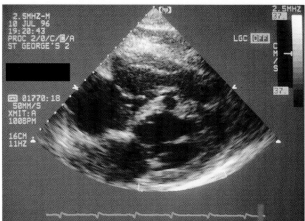

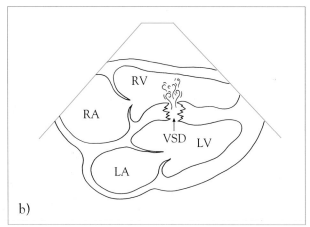

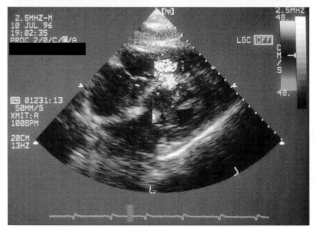

Sub-costal views from a patient with a ventricular septal rupture secondary to inferior myocardial infarction. (a) The standard image plane clearly shows a jagged tear in the interventricular septum (arrow). (b) Color-flow Doppler confirms the presence of left-to-right shunt. (c) Continuous-wave spectral Doppler allows the jet velocity to be measured, from which the (LV-RV) pressure gradient can be calculated using Bernoulli's equation. In this case, the gradient is 50 mmHg; since left ventricular pressure can be measured with a cuff sphygmomanometer, this allows right ventricular pressure to be calculated.

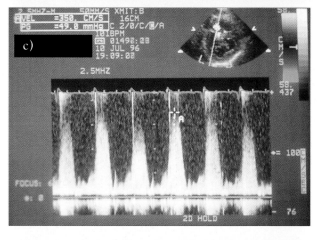

43

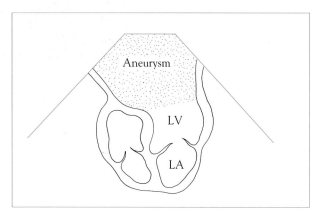

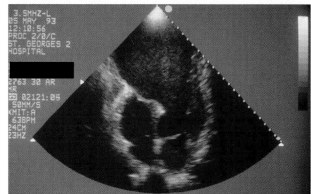

Apical four-chamber view showing an enormous apical left ventricular aneurysm. By reference to the scale of the other heart chambers, it is apparent that this is many times the volume of the normal ventricle. Static blood flow is evidenced by the dense 'spontaneous contrast' echoes.

44

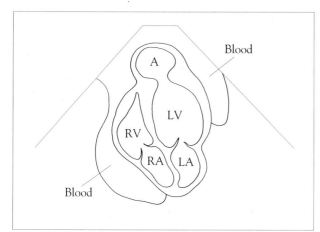
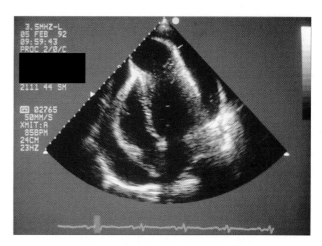

Apical four-chamber view showing a narrow-necked 'pseudoaneurysm' at the left ventricular apex. This is formed when near-rupture of the myocardium allows blood to accumulate between the myocardium and the visceral pericardium. In this example, some blood has also escaped into the pericardial sac.

45

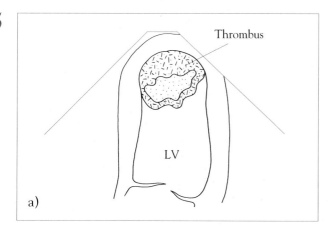
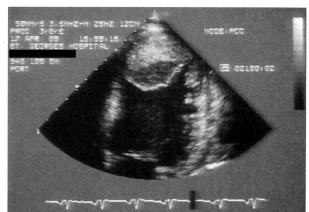

a)

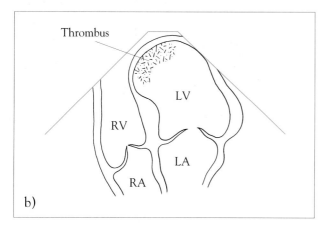
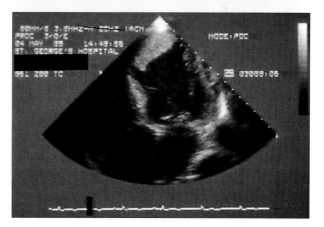

b)

(a) Apical four-chamber view from a patient with a recent apical myocardial infarction showing a jelly-like mass of thrombus accumulating over the site of injury. (b) The same case four weeks later showing shrinkage and consolidation of the thrombus.

46 Spin echo transaxial image showing a thinned apex of the left ventricle (arrows) following myocardial infarction.

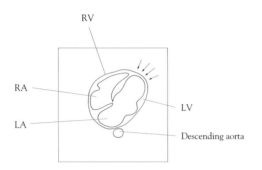

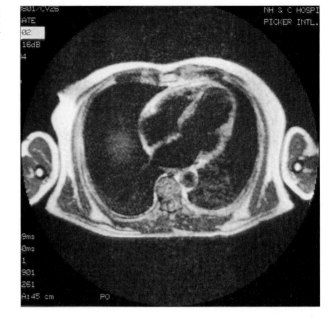

47

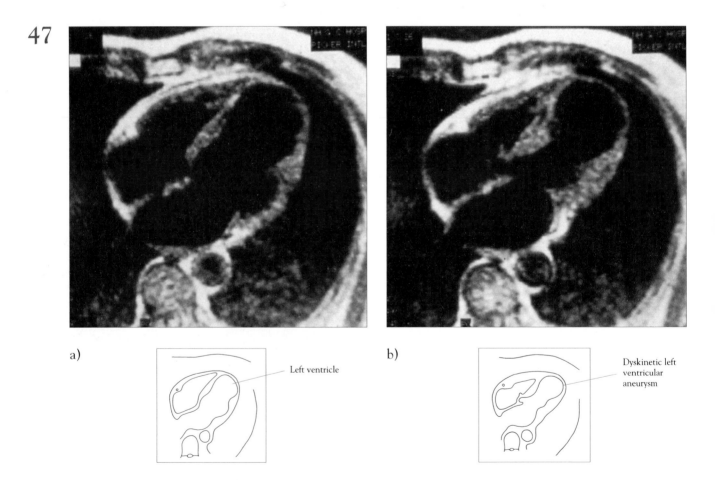

a)

Left ventricle

b)

Dyskinetic left ventricular aneurysm

Transverse section at end-diastole (a) and end-systole (b) in a patient with previous myocardial infarction and an apical left ventricular aneurysm. The basal myocardium contracts, but the whole of the apex is thin and dyskinetic.

48

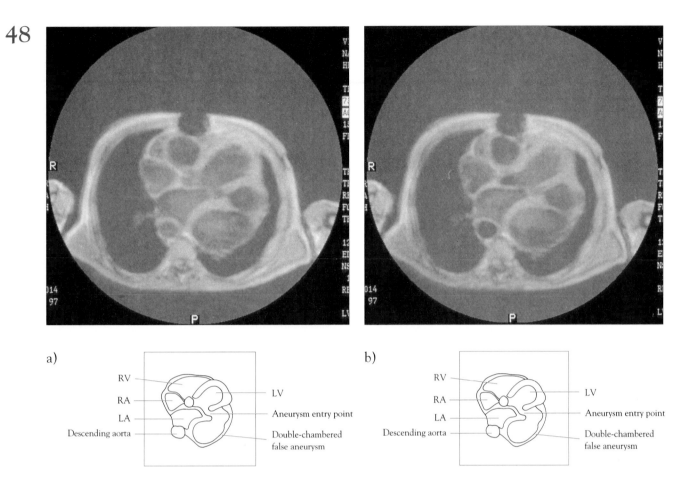

a)

RV
RA
LA
Descending aorta

LV
Aneurysm entry point
Double-chambered
false aneurysm

b)

RV
RA
LA
Descending aorta

LV
Aneurysm entry point
Double-chambered
false aneurysm

False aneurysm of the left ventricle following lateral wall myocardial infarction. Gradient-echo images in the transaxial plane: (a) diastole, (b) systole. The entry site to the aneurysm is clearly shown just below the mitral valve. The aneurysm has two chambers, and on the cine loop blood can be seen circulating within the aneurysm. The systolic image (b) demonstrates left atrial tamponade.

49 Left ventricular thrombus. Transaxial spin echo image showing a filling defect in the apex of the left ventricle.

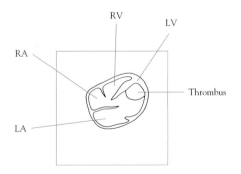

RV
LV
RA
Thrombus
LA

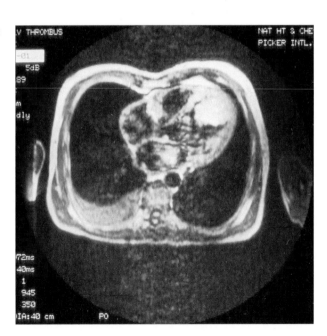

50 Ultrafast CT of the left ventricle showing antero-apical myocardial infarction and apical thrombus.

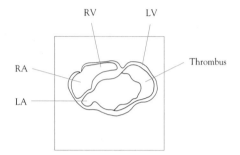

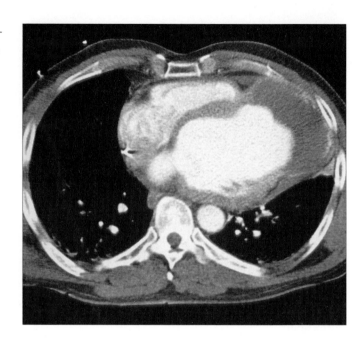

51 Hemodynamic findings in complications of acute myocardial infarction.

Subset	Pulmonary capillary wedge pressure	Right atrial pressure	Cardiac output
Uncomplicated	Normal	Normal	Normal
Heart failure	Elevated	Normal	Normal
Cardiogenic shock	Elevated	Normal or elevated	Low
Right ventricular infarction	Normal	Elevated	Low or normal
Hypovolemic shock	Low	Low	Low

52

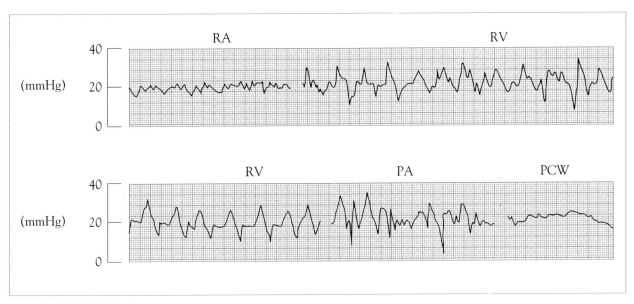

Hemodynamic abnormalities in severe right ventricular myocardial infarction. Mean right atrial (RA) and pulmonary capillary wedge pressures are similar, indicating disproportionate elevation of RA pressure and equalization of right heart and left heart pressures. Right ventricular (RV) pressure pulse shows dip and plateau diastolic wave form due to pericardial constraining effect. Pulmonary artery (PA) pressure wave form is frequently distorted.

53

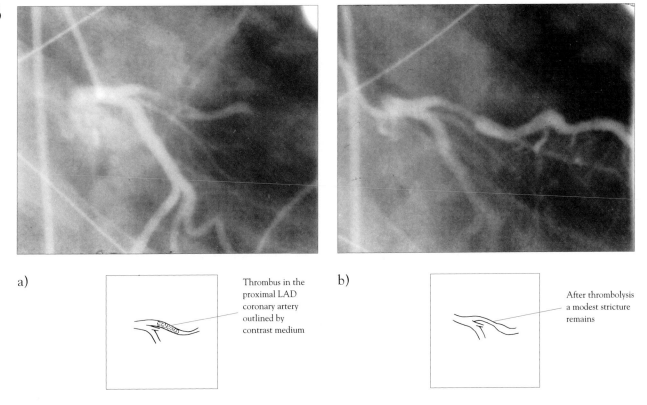

a)   Thrombus in the proximal LAD coronary artery outlined by contrast medium

b)   After thrombolysis a modest stricture remains

Successful thrombolysis in a patient with acute myocardial infarction. Before thrombolysis (a), there is a large thrombus, outlined by the contrast medium, in the proximal descending coronary artery. There is no forward flow. After thrombolysis (b), coronary arteriography showed modest coronary artery stenosis following recanalization of the infarct-related artery, illustrating that acute thrombosis and occlusion of the coronary artery can occur in the presence of a hemodynamically insignificant stenotic lesion due to atheromatous plaque.

54

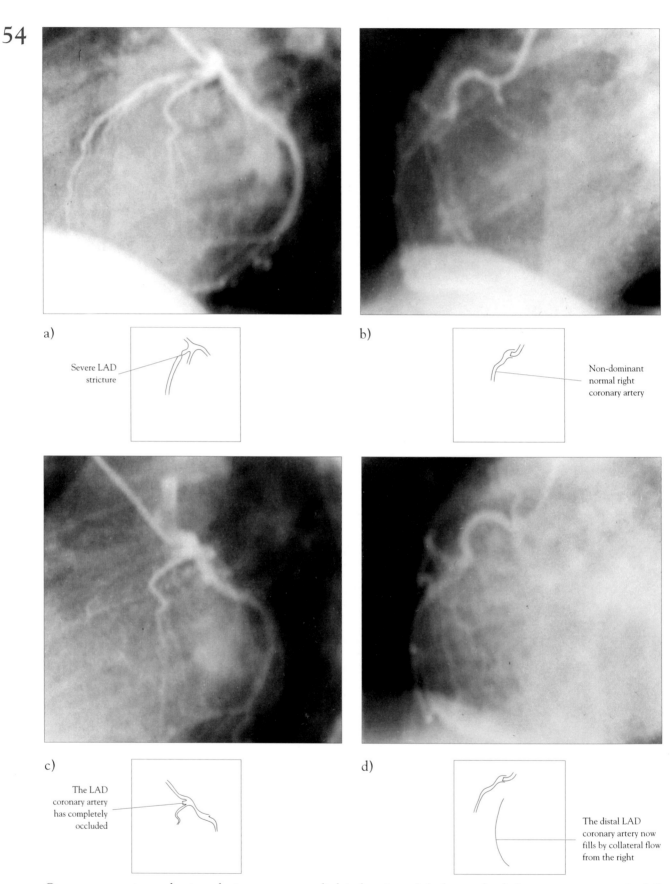

a)

Severe LAD
stricture

b)

Non-dominant
normal right
coronary artery

c)

The LAD
coronary artery
has completely
occluded

d)

The distal LAD
coronary artery now
fills by collateral flow
from the right

Coronary arteriography in relation to myocardial infarction: (a) shows the left coronary artery in left lateral view with a severe stricture in the anterior descending branch; (b) shows a non-dominant right coronary artery and a normal appearance. After myocardial infarction (c) the left coronary artery injection shows that the anterior descending branch is now completely obstructed at the point of the previous stricture. The right coronary artery after injection (d) revealed collateral opacification of the distal anterior descending coronary artery.

55

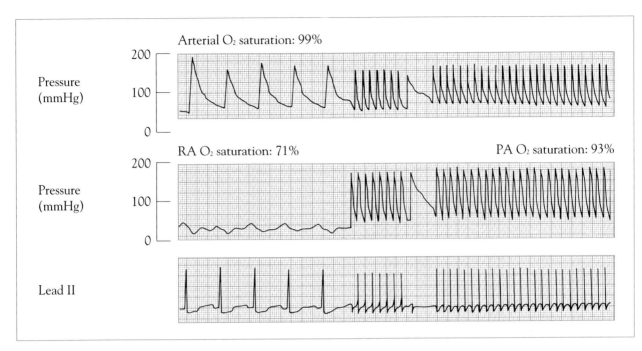

Arterial O₂ saturation: 99%

Pressure (mmHg)

RA O₂ saturation: 71%   PA O₂ saturation: 93%

Pressure (mmHg)

Lead II

Higher O₂ saturation in the pulmonary arterial (PA) blood compared with O₂ saturation in the right atrial (RA) blood indicates left-to-right shunt as in this patient with post-infarction ventricular septal rupture.

Adapted from: Parmley WW, Chatterjee K (Editors). *Cardiology*. Philadelphia: JB Lippincott Publishing Company, 1988.

56 Left ventricular angiogram in the left anterior oblique projection showing a shunt from the left ventricle into the right ventricle due to rupture of the muscular septum.

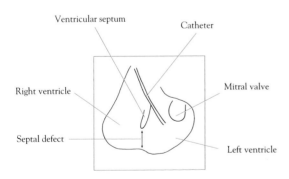

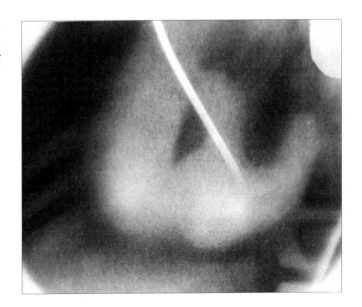

57 Pulmonary capillary wedge and pulmonary artery pressure tracings obtained during right heart catheterization by balloon flotation catheter in a patient with a papillary muscle infarct. A giant peaked 'v' wave in the pulmonary capillary wedge pressure tracing after balloon inflation and a reflected 'v' wave in the pulmonary artery pressure tracing before balloon inflation confirms the diagnosis of severe mitral regurgitation.

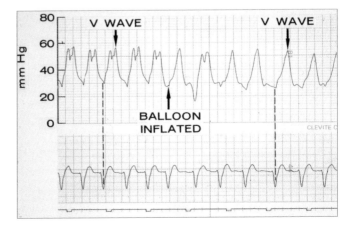

58

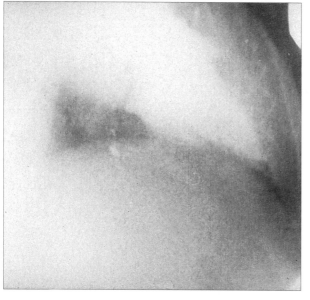
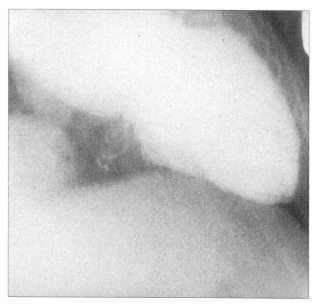

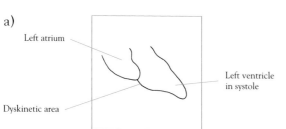

Left ventricular angiogram in the right anterior oblique projection with systolic (a) and diastolic (b) frames. It shows reduced contraction of the inferior wall of the left ventricle and dense opacification of the left atrium due to mitral regurgitation.

59 Potential decrease in the risk of mortality with beta-adrenergic blocking agents, angiotensin converting enzyme (ACE) inhibitors, and lipid-lowering agents in patients with acute myocardial infarction.

PHARMACOLOGIC RISK MODIFICATION IN ISCHEMIC HEART DISEASE	
Intervention	**Approximate % risk reduction of death and/or non-fatal myocardial infarction**
Beta-blockers	13 – 23%
ACE inhibitors	19 – 37%
Lipid-lowering agents	30 – 42%

60

Study	Number of patients randomized	Time of initiation	Drug used	Duration of follow-up	% of patients* receiving thrombolytic therapy	% risk reduction in mortality
CONSENSUS II	6090	<24 hours	Enalapril	6 months	56	NS
SAVE	2231	3–16 days	Captopril	42 months	33	19
ISIS-4	54,824	<24 hours	Captopril	35 days	70	6
GISSI-3	18,985	<24 hours	Lisinopril	6 weeks	71	11
AIRE	2006	3–10 days	Ramipril	15 months	58	27
CHINESE	13,634	<36 hours	Captopril	28 days	27	NS
TRACE	1749	3–7 days	Trandolapril	26 months	45	22
SMILE	1556	<24 hours	Zofenopril	12 months	0	29

CONSENSUS II: Cooperative New Scandinavian Enalapril Survival Study II
SAVE: Survival and Ventricular Enlargement
ISIS-4: International Study of Infarct Survival-4
GISSI-3: Gruppo Italiano Per Lo Studio Della Sopravvivenza Nell'Infarto Mio Cardico-3
AIRE: Acute Infarction Ramipril Efficacy
TRACE: Trandolapril Cardiac Evaluation
SMILE: Survival of Myocardial Infarction Long-term Evaluation

NS = Not significant
* Survival benefits were observed irrespective of thrombolytic therapy

Reported survival benefits with angiotensin converting enzyme inhibitors in patients with acute myocardial infarction in large prospective randomized trials.

61 Principles of management of acute myocardial infarction.

1. Bed rest, analgesia, supplemental oxygen

2. Intravenous thrombolytic agents and aspirin unless specifically contraindicated

3. ACE inhibitors, particularly in patients with reduced left ventricular ejection fraction and heart failure

4. Beta-blockers in the absence of overt heart failure

5. Consider nitrates and beta-blockers for post-infarction ischemia, and magnesium for ventricular arrhythmias

6. Intravenous heparin in patients with antero-apical infarction, particularly with mural thrombi

7. Modify risk factors of coronary heart disease, and particularly lipid-lowering agents in those with hypercholesterolemia

62 Principles of management of dysrhythmias in acute myocardial infarction.

a) Bradyarrhythmias

1. Atropine for symptomatic sinus bradycardia

2. No treatment for first degree- and Mobitz type I heart block

3. Temporary pacing for Mobitz type II- and complete atrioventricular block

4. Bifascicular and trifascicular block require prophylactic temporary pacing

b) Tachyarrhythmias

1. Atrial fibrillation, flutter, or tachycardia require digitalization or DC version if hemodynamic compromise

2. Sustained ventricular tachycardia or ventricular fibrillation require DC version followed by antiarrhythmic agents

63

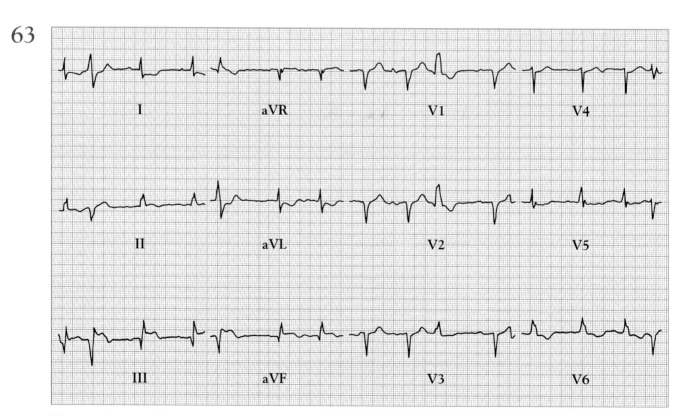

Electrocardiogram illustrating ectopic QRS complexes in a patient with acute myocardial infarction.

64

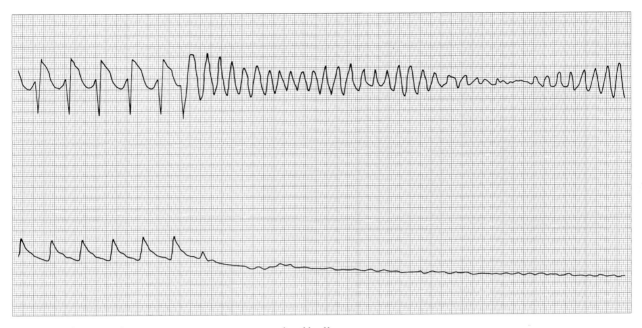

Electrocardiogram showing spontaneous ventricular fibrillation.

65

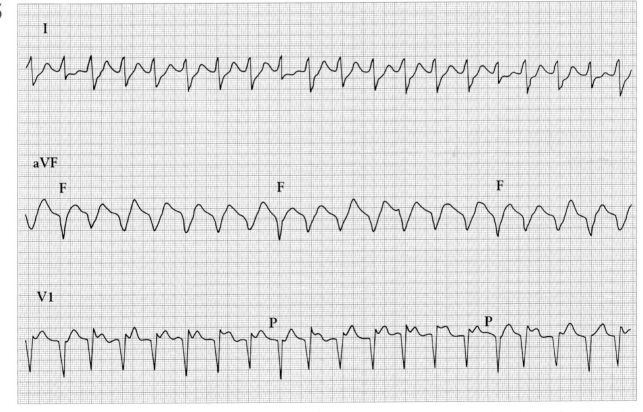

Simultaneous recordings of leads I, aVF and V1, showing monomorphic ventricular tachycardia. The QRS complexes are wide, and atrioventricular dissociation and fusion complexes are present. P=P-waves. Intermittent different QRS morphologies represent fusion complexes (F).

66

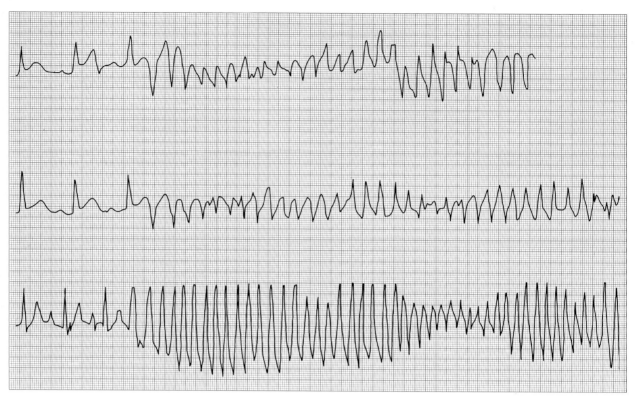

Polymorphous ventricular tachycardia (VT) in acute myocardial infarction. Note that it is not pause dependent and QT is not prolonged. Note also the variable QRS morphology and axis. It can be seen that ST-segment elevation, indicating acute infarction, precedes the onset of polymorphous VT.

67

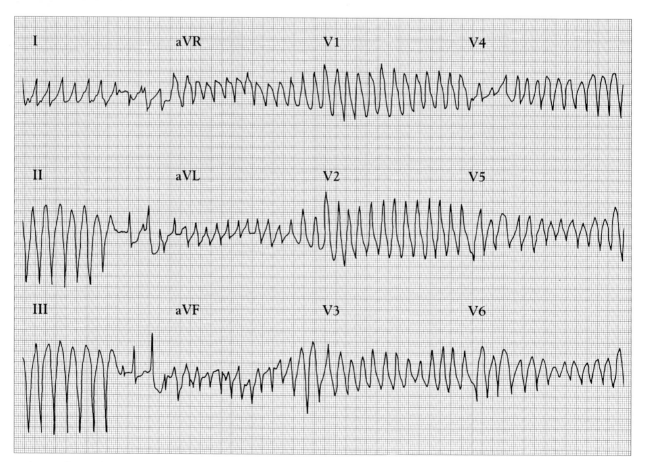

Polymorphous ventricular tachycardia, with a fast ventricular rate and changing QRS morphology and axis.

68

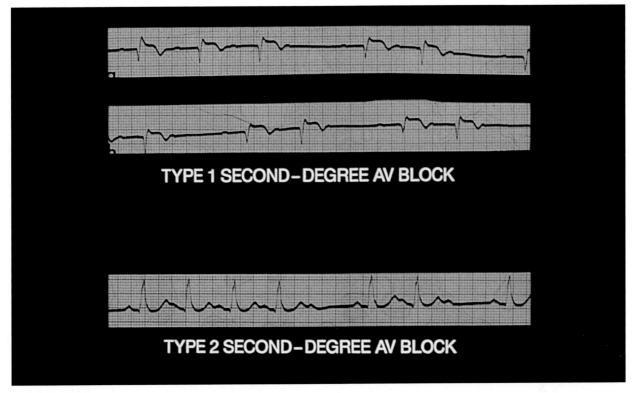

Rhythm strips showing Mobitz type I and Mobitz type II second-degree atrioventricular (AV) block in a patient with inferior myocardial infarction. Mobitz type I (Wenckebach phenomenon) is characterized by the gradual prolongation of PR interval followed by a dropped beat. Mobitz type II AV block is characterized by fixed PR interval and presence of dropped beats, with the P-wave falling beyond the refractory period of the preceding QRS complex.

69

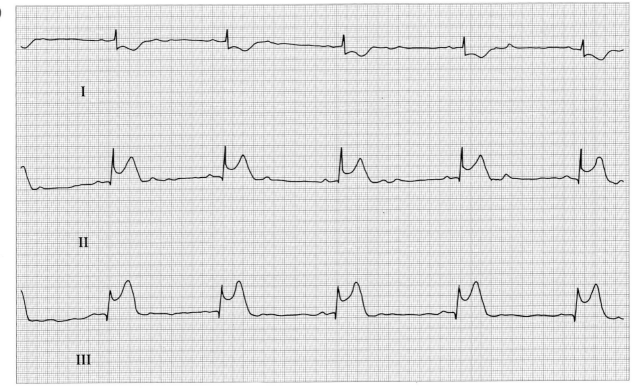

A rhythm strip showing atrioventricular block in a patient with inferior myocardial infarction. QRS rates are slower than sinus rates. ST elevations suggest acute infarction.

70

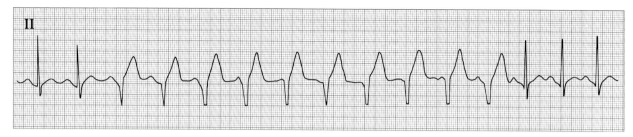

Accelerated idioventricular rhythm with atrioventricular dissociation. The QRS complex is wide indicating a ventricular origin of the escape pacemaker. The ventricular escape rate is less than 100 beats/min.

71

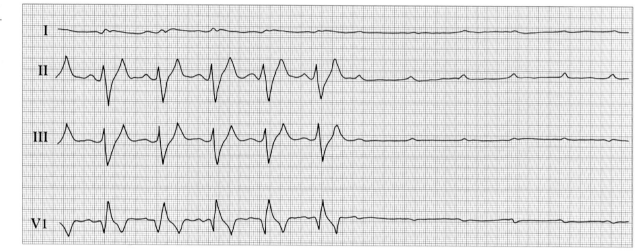

An example of bifascicular block with right bundle branch block and the frontal plane QRS axis exceeding −30° in a patient with acute myocardial infarction. Sudden ventricular asystole (P-waves) without QRS complexes occurred in this patient.

72

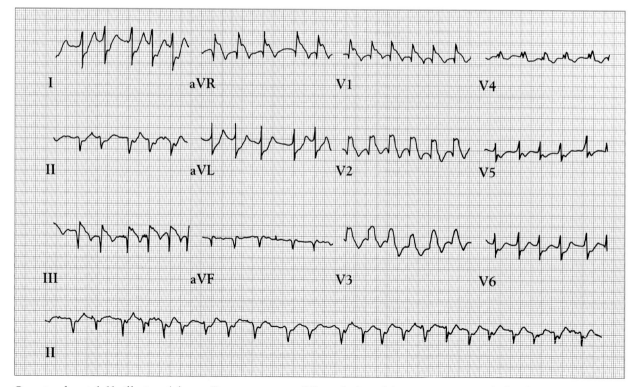

Sustained atrial fibrillation (absent P-wave, varying RR cycle length) in acute myocardial infarction. The wide QRS complex is due to aberrant conduction.

73 Principles of management of acute pulmonary edema.

1. Supplemental oxygen (60 – 100%) by face mask; intubation in patients remaining hypoxic

2. Intravenous morphine, diamorphine

3. Intravenous frusemide

4. Sublingual nitroglycerin followed by intravenous nitroglycerin

5. Echo-Doppler to exclude the presence of mechanical defects

6. Hemodynamic monitoring for maintenance vasodilator and/or inotropic therapy

7. Consider coronary arteriography and primary angioplasty if no response to treatment as above

74 Principles of management of acute cardiogenic shock.

1. Coronary angiography with a view to primary angioplasty of the infarct-related artery

2. Vasopressors to maintain arterial pressure

3. Intra-aortic balloon counterpulsation therapy as soon as feasible

4. Supportive pharmacotherapy according to hemodynamics

5. Treat pulmonary edema

6. Echo-Doppler to exclude mechanical defects

7. Left ventricular assist devices as a bridge to cardiac transplant in refractory patients

75 Principles of management of mechanical complications of acute myocardial infarction.

a) Papillary muscle rupture

   1. Supportive therapy with vasodilators in normotensive patients

   2. Intra-aortic balloon counterpulsation in hypotensive patients. Subsequently, vasodilators and/or inotropic agents may be required

   3. Corrective surgery following stabilization

b) Ventricular septal rupture

   1. Intra-aortic balloon counterpulsation

   2. Arterial vasodilators

   3. Inotropic agents may be required

   4. Corrective surgery following stabilization

76 Principles of management of acute ventricular infarction.

1. Intravenous thrombolytic agents in uncomplicated patients;
   in patients with cardiogenic shock, primary angioplasty rather than thrombolysis should be considered

2. Asymptomatic patients: avoid nitroglycerin and diuretics

3. Hypotension with normal right atrial pressure: intravenous fluids

4. Hypotension with elevated right atrial pressure: inotropic agents

5. AV block: consider atrioventricular sequential pacing

CHAPTER 2
Heart Failure

Abbreviations

Ao	Aorta	MPA	Main pulmonary artery
AoV	Aortic valve	MV	Mitral valve
Eff	Effusion	MVL	Mitral valve leaflet
IAS	Interatrial septum	PVW	Posterior ventricular wall
IVC	Inferior vena cava	RA	Right atrium
IVS	Interventricular septum	RV	Right ventricle
LA	Left atrium	TV	Tricuspid valve
LV	Left ventricle		

Definition

The generally accepted definition of heart failure is 'a clinical syndrome caused by an abnormality of the heart and recognized by a characteristic pattern of hemodynamic, neural, and hormonal responses'.

Pathophysiology

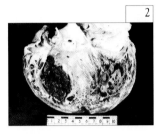

The clinical syndrome of heart failure consists of breathlessness, evidence of poor tissue perfusion (fatigue, oliguria, drowsiness), and the consequences of stimulation of the sympathetic and renin-angiotensin-aldosterone systems (tachycardia, peripheral vaso-constriction, salt and water retention). The clinical syndrome may result from myocardial, pericardial, valvular, or congenital heart disease. Both predominant systolic and pre-dominant diastolic myocardial dysfunction can cause clinical heart failure. Impaired left ventricular systolic function is the more common cause of heart failure, and ischemic heart disease is the most frequent pathophysiologic condition causing left ventricular systolic dysfunction.

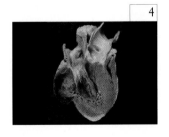

In ischemic heart disease (acute myocardial infarction [1] and chronic ischemic myocardial damage [2] including left ventricular aneurysm [3,4]) and dilated cardio-myopathy [5] both systolic and diastolic dysfunction may coexist. In so-called 'ischemic cardiomyopathy', replacement fibrosis of the left ventricular myocardium and extensive narrowing in the coronary arteries are usually present. In non-ischemic cardiomyopathy, myocardial fibrosis is diffuse and coronary artery disease is absent. Specific causes of cardiomyopathy include alcohol, myocarditis, peripartum cardiomyopathy, and thyroid disease, all of which induce clinical syndromes indistinguishable from dilated cardiomyopathy for which no cause has been established.

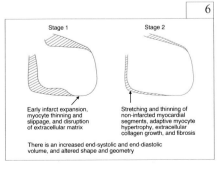

In ventricular remodeling [6] following ischemic injury or acute myocarditis, there may be progressive ventricular dilatation with increased end-systolic and end-diastolic volumes. Soon after myocardial infarction, thinning and stretching of the infarcted segment (infarct expansion) occurs. Infarct expansion is also caused by myocyte slippage along with disruption of the extracellular matrix. Subsequently, replacement fibrosis occurs in areas of myocyte necrosis. The non-infarcted myocardial segments stretch and thin concurrently. Adaptive hypertrophy of the myocytes and changes in the extracellular matrix, with increased collagen, occur in the non-infarcted segments. Increased regional and global left ventricular wall stress serve as the stimulus for ventricular remodeling, with ventricular enlargement and altered geometry and shape.

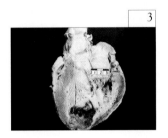

Neurohormonal changes consist of activation of both vasodilatory, natriuretic, and antimitogenic agents (such as atrial natriuretic and brain natriuretic peptides) and vaso-constrictive, antinatriuretic, and mitogenic agents (such as catecholamines, angiotensins, aldosterone, and cytokines). A balance between these two systems has the potential to attenuate development of clinical heart failure; an imbalance on the other hand may cause progressive clinical heart failure [7].

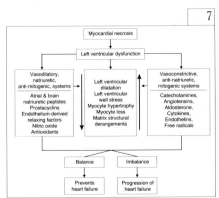

Impaired left ventricular systolic function can establish a vicious cycle of heart failure [8]. Decreased stroke volume and cardiac output activate several neurohormonal systems. Enhanced sympathetic activity increases systemic vascular resistance and impairs renal perfusion. Increased angiotensin II also increases systemic vascular resistance which is

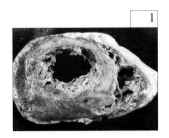

Stage 1

Stage 2

Early infarct expansion, myocyte thinning and slippage, and disruption of extracellular matrix

Stretching and thinning of non-infarcted myocardial segments, adaptive myocyte hypertrophy, extracellular collagen growth, and fibrosis

There is an increased end-systolic and end-diastolic volume, and altered shape and geometry

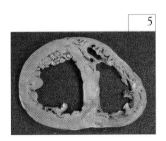

Myocardial necrosis → Left ventricular dysfunction

Vasodilatory, natriuretic, anti-mitogenic, systems → Atrial & brain natriuretic peptides, Prostacyclins, Endothelium-derived relaxing factors, Nitric oxide, Antioxidants

Left ventricular dilatation, Left ventricular wall stress, Myocyte hypertrophy, Myocyte loss, Matrix structural derangements

Vasoconstrictive, anti-natriuretic, mitogenic systems ← Catecholamines, Angiotensins, Aldosterone, Cytokines, Endothelins, Free radicals

Balance → Prevents heart failure

Imbalance → Progression of heart failure

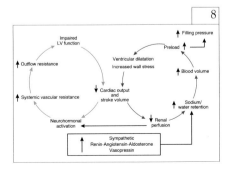

Impaired LV function, ↑ Filling pressure, Preload ↑, ↑ Outflow resistance, Ventricular dilatation, Increased wall stress, ↑ Blood volume, ↑ Systemic vascular resistance, Cardiac output and stroke volume, Sodium/water retention, Neurohormonal activation, Renal perfusion, Sympathetic Renin-Angiotensin-Aldosterone Vasopressin

associated with increased left ventricular outflow resistance, causing further impairment of left ventricular systolic function. Activated renin-angiotensin-aldosterone systems, resulting from decreased cardiac output and impaired renal perfusion, promote sodium and fluid retention and increased left ventricular volume (preload) and diastolic pressure. Increased left ventricular volume causes an increase in its wall stress (afterload) which causes a further reduction in cardiac output.

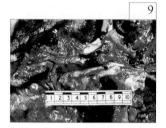

High output states such as Paget's disease, arteriovenous fistula, anemia, beriberi, and hyperthyroidism can result in clinical syndromes similar to heart failure. Right ventricular dysfunction may be secondary to left ventricular dysfunction, usually due to post-capillary pulmonary hypertension. Any cause of pulmonary hypertension, either acute (massive pulmonary embolism [9]) or chronic (chronic obstructive airways disease, primary pulmonary hypertension, chronic thromboembolic disease), may result in right ventricular myocardial dysfunction and clinical heart failure.

Presentation

Symptoms

Acute heart failure presents with acute breathlessness and impaired perfusion to vital organs. Breathlessness is mainly caused by pulmonary congestion due to increased left ventricular filling pressure. Lying flat increases pulmonary venous pressure further and causes orthopnea; this may progress to the development of frank pulmonary edema causing attacks of breathlessness at night which wake the patient (paroxysmal nocturnal dyspnea). Pulmonary edema is often incorrectly diagnosed as bronchitis.

Acute heart failure may be precipitated by an alteration of cardiac rhythm in patients with pre-existing myocardial dysfunction, fresh damage to the myocardium (e.g. myocardial infarction or myocarditis), myocardial ischemia ('hibernating' myocardium), inappropriate alterations of therapy, and, rarely, infection or pulmonary infarction. Occasionally, no precipitating cause can be found.

Exertional dyspnea and fatigue are the two most common symptoms of chronic heart failure. Unlike acute heart failure, the cause of breathlessness in chronic heart failure is not well understood, but may be related to reduced perfusion of the tissues, abnormal function of the cardiopulmonary receptors, and respiratory muscle fatigue rather than to pulmonary congestion due to increased pulmonary capillary wedge pressure. Occasionally, a non-productive cough may be the only symptom in heart failure. Fatigue in chronic heart failure may be due to the reduced cardiac reserve on exercise, inadequate blood flow to exercising muscles, and abnormal skeletal muscle metabolism. Palpitation and syncope are rare presenting symptoms except in patients with right ventricular cardiomyopathy. Angina-like chest pain as a sole presenting symptom is uncommon, but occurs, in association with other symptoms, in 20–40% of patients with ischemic or non-ischemic cardiomyopathy.

Patients with chronic heart failure may notice the development of fluid retention with swollen ankles and abdominal distention due to ascites or hepatic congestion. The patient with chronic heart failure may complain of nausea, vomiting, and abdominal discomfort due to gastrointestinal and hepatic congestion; such patients are frequently thought to have other abdominal pathology.

Acute right ventricular failure due to massive pulmonary embolism presents with circulatory collapse or acute breathlessness.

Signs

The physical signs may indicate whether heart failure is due to myocardial dysfunction or to some other abnormality. Myocardial diastolic dysfunction renders the ventricles stiff and gives rise to a double apical impulse, a gallop rhythm (fourth and/or third heart sounds), and secondary mitral or tricuspid regurgitation (pansystolic murmur); primary valvular abnormalities, congenital cardiac abnormalities, or pericardial disease have distinctive clinical features.

Low cardiac output with stimulation of the sympathetic and renin-angiotensin-aldosterone systems is associated with sinus tachycardia, peripheral vasoconstriction, and fluid retention, causing a raised jugular venous pressure, pulmonary edema, hepatic congestion, ascites, and peripheral edema. Renal, hepatic, and cerebral impairment may also occur. In patients with compensated chronic heart failure from a myocardial abnormality, the signs of systemic and pulmonary venous congestion may be absent. A sustained double apical impulse and a gallop rhythm may be the only abnormal findings. Pulsus alternans, which almost always indicates impaired left ventricular systolic function, may also be present.

Investigations

Investigation of patients with clinical heart failure is essential in order to diagnose the cause. Evidence of valvular, congenital, and pericardial diseases may be detected and should be further investigated. The text which follows deals with the investigatory aspects of patients whose heart failure is due to myocardial disease.

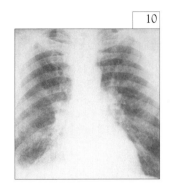

Radiology
In patients presenting with 'acute' heart failure and breathlessness, heart size may be normal [10,11] or enlarged. An enlarged heart implies pre-existing heart disease. The chest X-ray will show evidence of raised pulmonary venous pressure, such as dilatation of the upper zone pulmonary vessels, perihilar shadowing, left atrial enlargement [12], Kerley B-lines (short horizontal lines in the peripheral lung fields [13]), and, occasionally, unilateral or bilateral pleural effusions [14]; these findings correlate well with the elevation of left ventricular filling pressure and left atrial pressure and the consequent high pulmonary capillary wedge pressure in acute heart failure. Pulmonary edema is usually bilateral [15] but, occasionally, may be unilateral [16]. In 'chronic' heart failure the heart is usually enlarged and there may [17] or may not [18] be radiologic features associated with raised pulmonary venous pressure. Characteristic radiologic abnormalities are seen in acute pulmonary embolism, cor pulmonale, primary pulmonary hypertension, and chronic thromboembolic disease. Features suggestive of a left ventricular aneurysm may also be seen [19].

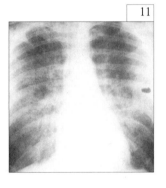

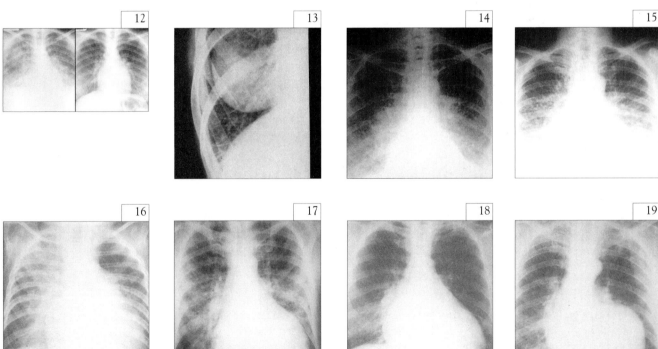

Electrocardiography

The ECG may show acute [20] or old [21] myocardial infarction, evidence of left ventricular aneurysm [22], or left ventricular hypertrophy [23]. Common abnormalities associated with chronic left ventricular dysfunction include left atrial configuration of the 'P'-waves, left bundle branch block [24], or only ST-T abnormalities [25]. Patients with heart failure due to myocardial disease often have rhythm abnormalities which may be seen on the routine ECG [26,27] or may be detected only during 24-hour ambulatory monitoring [28]. Right ventricular dysfunction may be associated with right axis deviation and right bundle branch block or evidence of right ventricular hypertrophy. In right ventricular cardiomyopathy (arrhythmogenic right ventricular dysplasia) the resting electrocardiogram usually shows T-wave inversion in leads V1-V4 [29], and incomplete or complete right bundle branch block with variable frontal plane QRS axis. In right ventricular cardiomyopathy, ventricular premature beats usually have left bundle branch block pattern with right axis deviation.

Echocardiography

The echocardiographic features will reflect the underlying cardiac abnormality. In patients with ischemic heart disease, there is likely to be an increase in left ventricular dimensions and a reduction in wall motion which may be regional [30] or generalized [31,32]. Global reduction in the amplitude of wall motion is more frequent in idiopathic dilated cardiomyopathy [33]. The appearances of the left ventricle either in extensive ischemic heart disease or in idiopathic dilated cardiomyopathy are frequently difficult to assess because of the presence of left bundle branch block, which in itself causes dyskinetic contraction. Systolic wall thinning and/or dyskinesia are readily apparent from inspection of the systolic and diastolic images. Enlargement of the left atrium due to chronic elevation of the left ventricular filling pressure is common [34].

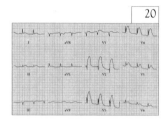

20

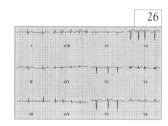

21

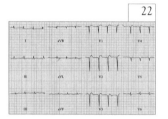

22

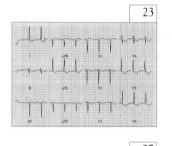

23

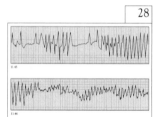

24

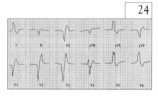

25

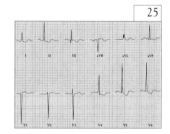

26

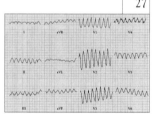

27

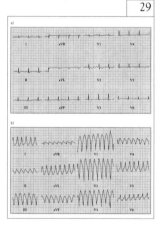

28

29

30

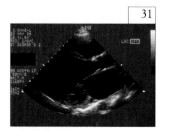

31

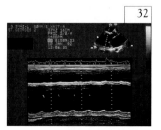

32

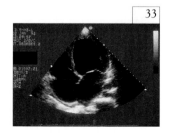

33

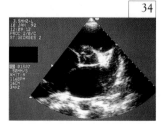

34

A localized left ventricular aneurysm (in patients who have had a previous myocardial infarct) may be detected by echocardiography [35]. Thrombus within the abnormal left ventricle can sometimes be visualized [36].

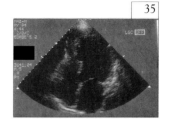

Doppler echocardiography is useful in excluding primary valvular heart disease as the cause of heart failure. The Doppler technique may reveal secondary mitral regurgitation (due to dominantly left ventricular myocardial disease) of varying severity [37].

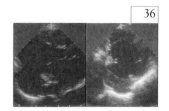

Doppler transmitral flow patterns in patients with heart failure and sinus rhythm are variable. In the early stages, impaired relaxation leads to decreased amplitude and prolonged duration of the early filling ('e') wave with a compensatory increase in the atrial filling ('a') wave; hence, a decreased e/a ratio may be seen [38]. In the late stages, accentuated 'e' wave amplitude and reduced 'a' wave amplitude implying a restrictive physiology may be seen [39]. In dilated cardiomyopathy, an abbreviated 'e' wave with decreased deceleration time and reduced 'a' wave amplitude is associated with a poor prognosis. In patients whose heart failure is due to dominant diastolic dysfunction (as in systemic hypertension), the 'e' wave is decreased and the 'a' wave accentuated while the left ventricle is seen to be hypertrophied, but contracts normally [40].

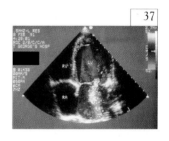

The presence of tricuspid regurgitation in patients with heart failure allows non-invasive measurement of the pulmonary artery systolic pressure [41,42]. If the cause of the heart failure is left ventricular disease, the level of the pulmonary artery systolic pressure will reflect the left ventricular filling pressure.

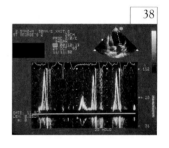

If tricuspid regurgitation is due to a right ventricular cardiomyopathy or acute massive pulmonary embolism, the right ventricle is dilated and contracts poorly, and the pulmonary artery systolic pressure is only slightly elevated in contrast to cases of long-standing pulmonary hypertension from any cause. In patients with heart failure due to pulmonary hypertension but without left heart disease, there may be paradoxical septal motion on M-mode echocardiography, and right ventricular hypertrophy and dilatation seen on two-dimensional echocardiography [43].

Nuclear Techniques

An important nuclear cardiologic procedure in patients with heart failure is radionuclide ventriculography using technetium-99m to label the intracardiac blood pool. Imaging is performed either during the first passage of the bolus through the central circulation or when it has reached equilibrium [44,45]. Left ventricular volumes, ejection fraction, and

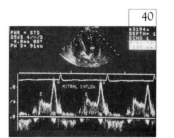

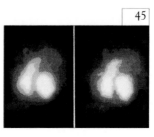

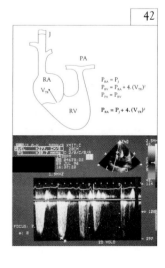

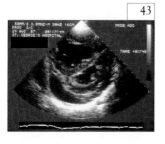

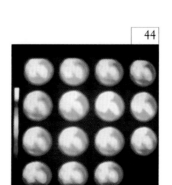

parameters of diastolic function, such as filling rates, can be measured [46]. Unfortunately, the ejection fraction is only an approximate indicator of ventricular performance and is poorly related to the severity of symptoms in heart failure. However, the degree of reduction in left ventricular ejection fraction correlates well with prognosis. Right ventricular systolic function can also be assessed; this correlates with the severity of exercise intolerance.

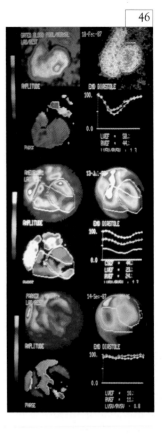

Thallium-201 imaging may show extensive ischemia. Significant thallium uptake in areas of wall motion abnormality suggests hibernation [47]. To demonstrate this, thallium reinjection may be required [48]. If significant reversible myocardial perfusion defects are detected, coronary arteriography is indicated because revascularization may improve the state of heart failure. Entirely normal myocardial perfusion images virtually exclude an ischemic etiology. Myocardial perfusion and metabolism can be assessed by positron emission tomography to enable a diagnosis of hibernating myocardium to be made [49].

Cardiac Catheterization and Angiography
Bedside monitoring of right heart hemodynamic variables can be useful in the management of patients with acute heart failure.

A balloon-tipped thermodilution catheter [50] positioned with its tip in the pulmonary artery [51] allows accurate measurement of pulmonary artery and wedge pressures and cardiac output, facilitating assessment of the severity of the hemodynamic abnormalities and the results of therapeutic interventions. In heart failure due to left ventricular disease, the left ventricular end-diastolic pressure is usually elevated, often with a prominent 'a' wave [52].

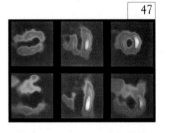

Left ventricular angiography is often unnecessary in patients with heart failure as non-invasive techniques will have defined the nature and degree of dysfunction. Localized hypokinesis [53] or left ventricular aneurysm may be seen following myocardial infarction. Alternatively, the left ventricle may be globally hypokinetic in generalized ischemic heart disease or dilated cardiomyopathy [54]. The presence and the severity of mitral regurgitation can be assessed by contrast ventriculography.

Coronary arteriography is performed to demonstrate whether heart failure is due to coronary artery disease and, if so, to assess the possibilities of treatment. Localized stenoses or, more often, widespread coronary disease may be found [55] even in the absence of a history of myocardial infarction or angina.

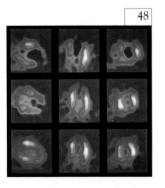

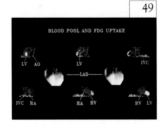

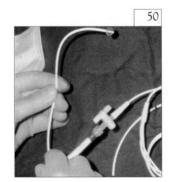

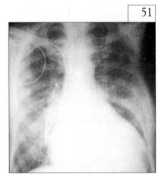

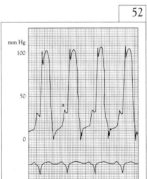

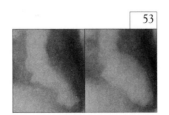

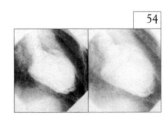

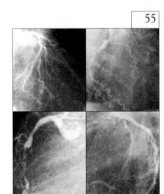

Exercise Testing

All of the investigations referred to above assess the type and degree of left ventricular dysfunction rather than the clinical state of the patient. Exercise testing provides an objective measure of functional impairment in heart failure. Maximal or submaximal tests on a treadmill or bicycle ergometer, with measurement of exercise time or oxygen consumption [56], can be useful in the assessment and follow-up of patients. Maximal oxygen consumption ($\dot{V}O_2$ max) can be used to assess the severity of heart failure. In patients with mild or no heart failure, $\dot{V}O_2$ exceeds 20 ml/kg/min, and in severe heart failure, $\dot{V}O_2$ is 6 ml/kg/min or less. When $\dot{V}O_2$ max is less than 14 ml/kg/min the prognosis is grave and is used as an indication for cardiac transplantation.

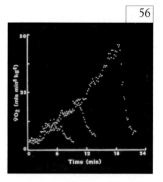

Magnetic Resonance Imaging (MRI) and Computed Tomography (CT)

MRI and CT reveal cardiac anatomy non-invasively and without the injection of contrast media. Accurate measurements of ventricular volumes [57], wall thickness, and wall motion [58] can be made, and filling defects such as thrombus are readily detectable. Both MRI and CT are useful in excluding pericardial disease.

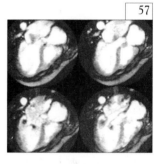

Principles of Management

Patients who have left ventricular systolic dysfunction, but do not have symptoms, may be considered for treatment with angiotensin converting enzyme (ACE) inhibitors [59]. ACE inhibitors have been shown to delay the development of heart failure and subsequent ischemic events in those whose left ventricular dysfunction is due to ischemic heart disease. Patients with mild to moderate heart failure have been shown to improve symptomatically with diuretics and ACE inhibitors. Chronic diuretic therapy alone is associated with a decreased cardiac output and neurohormonal activation. The addition of either the vasodilator combination, hydralazine and nitrates, or an ACE inhibitor has been shown to reduce mortality, but the greater effect is achieved with the ACE inhibitor. In severe heart failure, diuretics and ACE inhibitors should be used. ACE inhibitors have been shown to reduce mortality in this group. The use of digoxin in addition to diuretics and ACE inhibitors in patients with sinus rhythm may result in symptomatic improvement and increased left ventricular ejection fraction. Overall mortality, however, may not change, as mortality due to heart failure may decline with a concurrent increase in mortality due to arrhythmias. Nevertheless, hospitalization frequency for treatment of heart failure significantly decreases with digoxin therapy. Survival benefit of low-dose amiodarone in patients with refractory heart failure has not been firmly established. It may, however, improve symptoms, left ventricular ejection fraction, and the prognosis of selected patients with severe heart failure, particularly due to non-ischemic dilated cardiomyopathy. Vasoselective long-acting dihydropyridine calcium channel blockers may also improve symptoms in patients with heart failure already treated with diuretics, digitalis, and ACE inhibitors. Some of these agents may also improve prognosis if heart failure results from non-ischemic dilated cardiomyopathy.

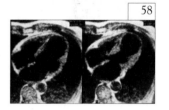

1. Asymptomatic left ventricular systolic dysfunction
   (ejection fraction of 45% or less):
   ACE inhibitors
2. Mild to moderate symptomatic heart failure:
   Diuretics
   ACE inhibitors
   Angiotensin II receptor antagonists, particularly when ACE inhibitors are not tolerated because of cough
   Hydralazine-isosorbide dinitrate in those who cannot tolerate ACE inhibitors or angiotensin receptor antagonist
3. Severe heart failure - medical treatment:
   Diuretics
   ACE inhibitors
   Digoxin
   Low-dose amiodarone in selected patients
   Beta-blocking agents in selected patients with idiopathic dilated cardiomyopathy
4. Severe heart failure - surgical treatment:
   Aneurysmectomy for localized left ventricular aneurysm
   Revascularization in selected patients with hibernating myocardium
5. Refractory heart failure:
   Combination vasodilators
   Non-glycosidic inotropic agents
   DDD pacemaker
   Cardiomyoplasty
   Cardiac transplantation

Cardioselective and non-selective beta-blockers, and beta-blockers with additional pharmacologic effects (vasodilatory, antioxidant properties), can improve symptoms, left ventricular function, and prognosis of patients with heart failure due to systolic dysfunction.

Beta-adrenergic agonists and other non-glycosidic inotropic agents, such as phospho-diesterase inhibitors, are used only for short-term treatment of refractory heart failure, as long-term treatments with these agents are associated with increased mortality. Ultrafiltration, hemodialysis, and DDD pacing with short P-R interval may improve symptoms in selected patients although they do not improve prognosis.

Cardiac surgery may be worthwhile in certain patients who have ischemic heart disease. Aneurysmectomy can be performed in those with a localized left ventricular aneurysm, and revascularization can be attempted in those with hibernating myocardium in order to improve heart failure. Other surgical procedures, such as cardiomyoplasty, may be considered in selected patients. The surgical treatment of choice, however, is cardiac transplantation.

1   Transverse slice (fresh) of the ventricles. A recent (four-day-old) full-thickness myocardial infarction is present in the anterior wall of the left ventricle which extends into the interventricular septum.

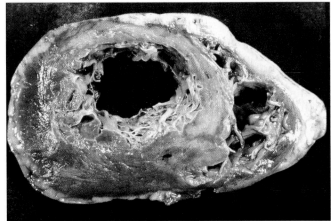

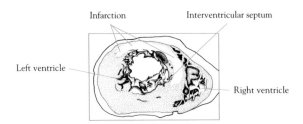

2   Widespread ischemic scarring of the myocardium producing a dilated thin-walled ventricle. A thrombus has formed in one area in relation to the aneurysmal bulge of the ventricular wall.

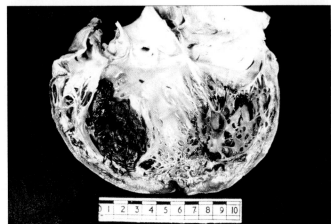

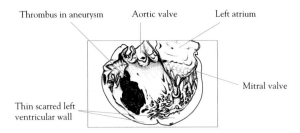

3   Localized left ventricular aneurysm due to previous myocardial infarction. The aneurysm does not contain more than a fine deposit of thrombus and has a larger central cavity opening into the ventricle.

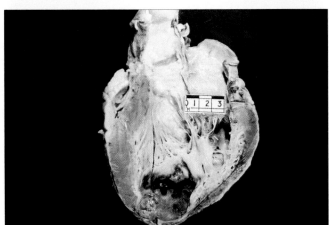

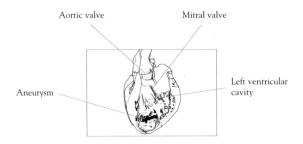

4   Longitudinal slice through the heart showing a lateral aneurysm containing thrombus.

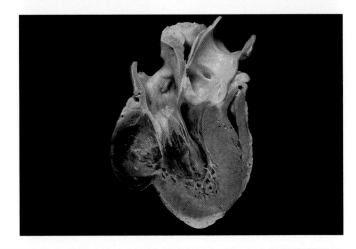

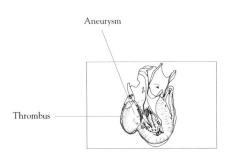

5 Transverse section in dilated cardiomyopathy showing bilateral cavity dilatation and thinning of the ventricular walls.

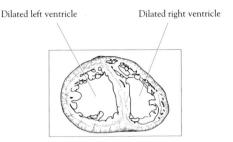

Dilated left ventricle   Dilated right ventricle

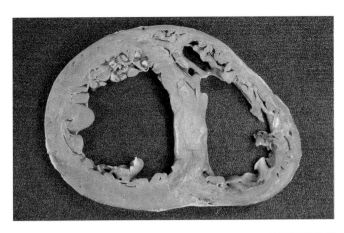

6 Schematic illustration of left ventricular re-modeling following myocardial injury, showing infarct expansion and changes in the non-infarcted segments.

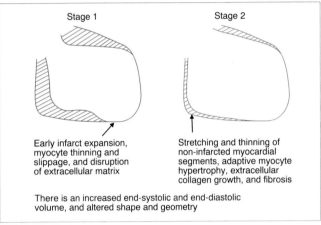

7 Left ventricular systolic dysfunction, resulting from myocardial necrosis, activates vasodilatory, natriuretic, anti-mitogenic systems which tend to decrease ventricular dilatation, left ventricular wall stress, myocyte hypertrophy, myocyte loss, and matrix structural derangements. Activation of vasoconstrictive, antinatriuretic, mitogenic systems tends to produce the opposite effects, i.e. ventricular dilatation, increased myocyte hypertrophy and loss, and matrix structural derangements.

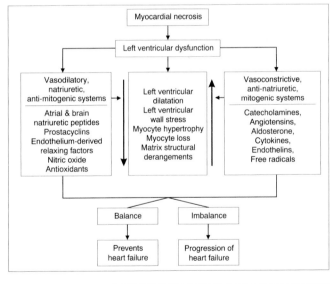

8 Vicious cycle of heart failure.

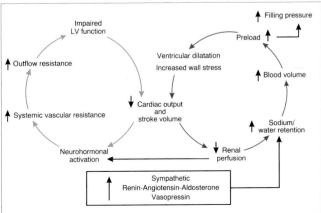

9   Large saddle embolus is seen astride both right and left pulmonary arteries.

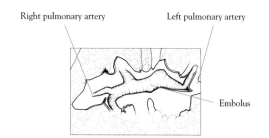

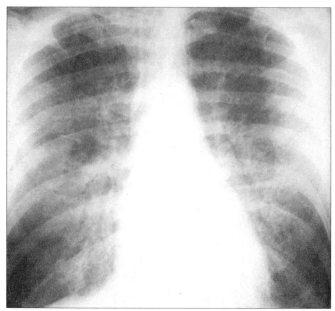

10   Chest X-ray showing a normal sized heart with upper lobe venous distention and a small right pleural effusion.

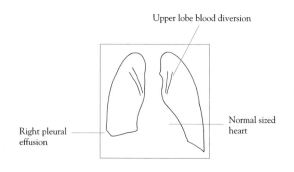

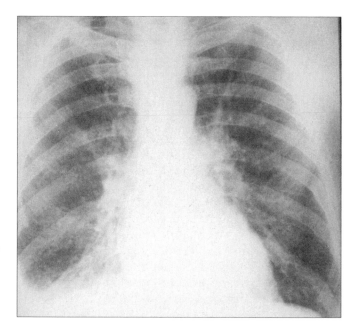

11   Chest X-ray showing a normal sized heart with pulmonary edema.

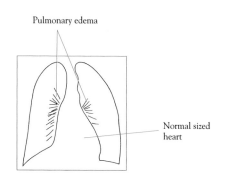

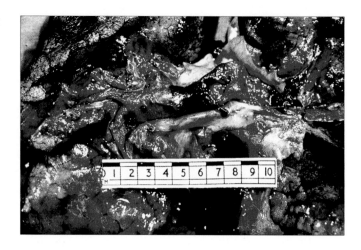

12 (a) Acute pulmonary edema with a normal sized heart. Note the classic perihilar shadowing. After treatment (b) the heart is virtually normal in size but with left atrial enlargement typical of mitral disease. Distended upper lobe veins are now clearly seen.

a)

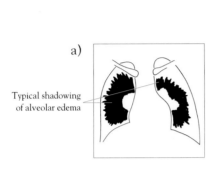

Typical shadowing of alveolar edema

b)

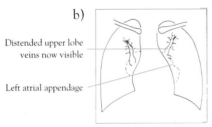

Distended upper lobe veins now visible

Left atrial appendage

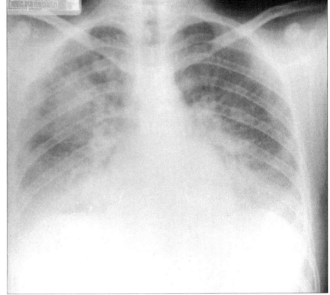

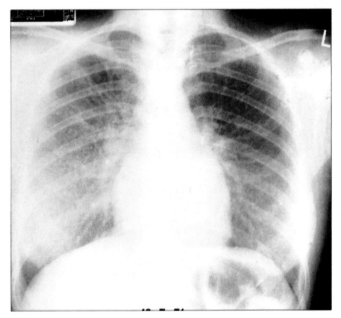

13 Detail from chest X-ray showing septal lines (Kerley B-lines) and pleural effusion.

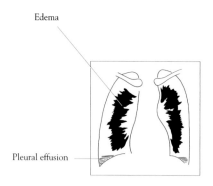

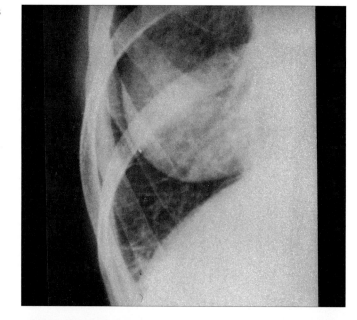

14 Chest X-ray showing pulmonary edema and bilateral pleural effusions following acute myocardial infarction.

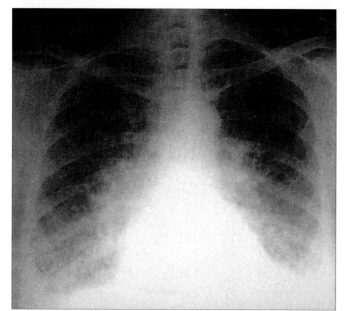

15 Chest X-ray in acute heart failure due to acute myocardial infarction. There is gross pulmonary edema.

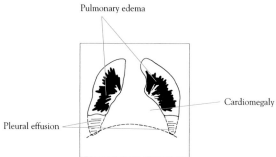

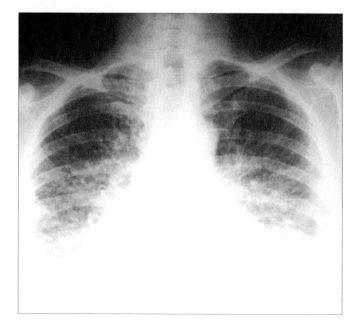

16   Chest X-ray showing cardiomegaly and
pulmonary edema of the right lung only.

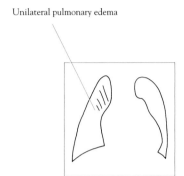

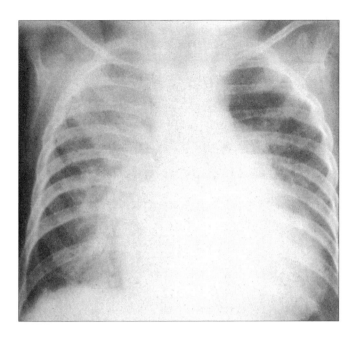

17   Chest X-ray showing cardiomegaly with features
of raised pulmonary venous pressure (enlarged
veins and upper zone blood diversion).

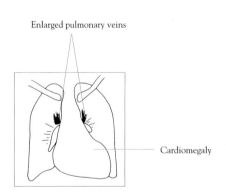

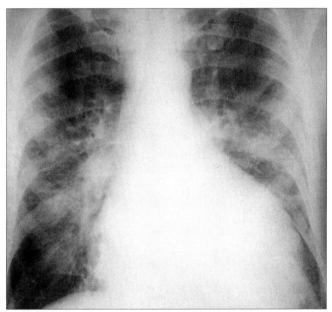

18   Chest X-ray showing an enlarged heart without
upper zone blood diversion.

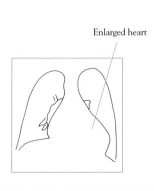

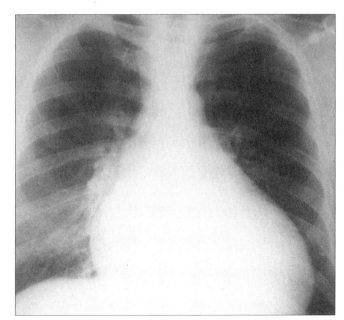

19 Chest X-ray showing a bulge on the left heart border suggestive of a left ventricular aneurysm.

Left ventricular bulge

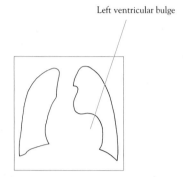

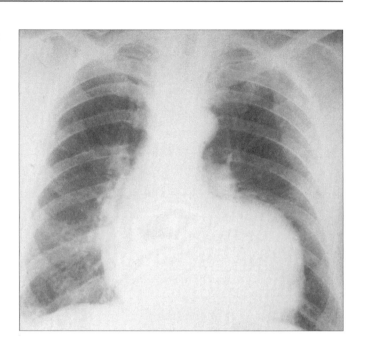

20

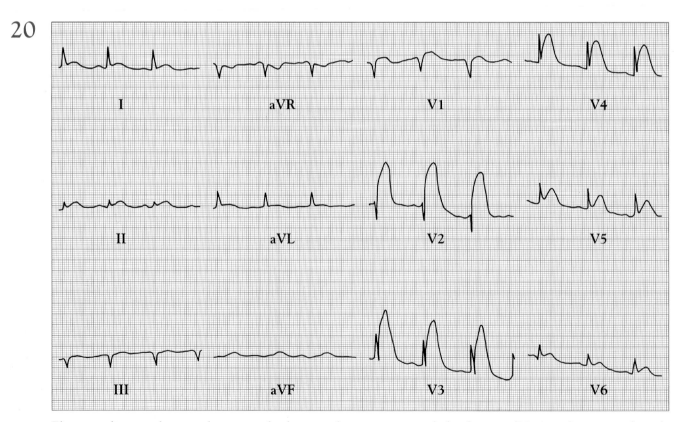

Electrocardiogram showing the very early changes of anterior myocardial infarction (30 min after onset of pain). There is ST-segment elevation in leads I, II, and across all the V leads, but no Q-wave development yet.

21

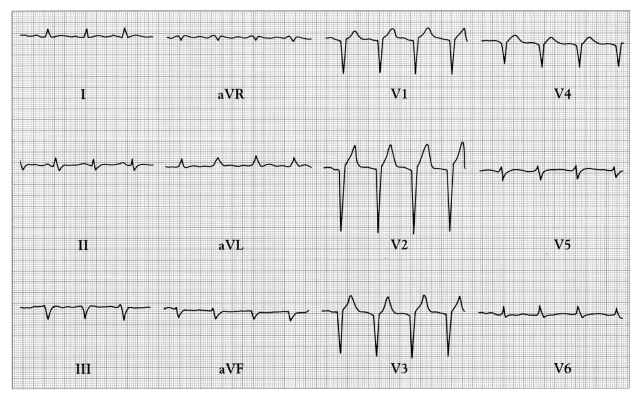

Electrocardiogram of a patient with chronic ischemic heart disease, showing old anterior infarction, with Q-waves in V1-V4 and poor R-wave progression in V5-V6.

22

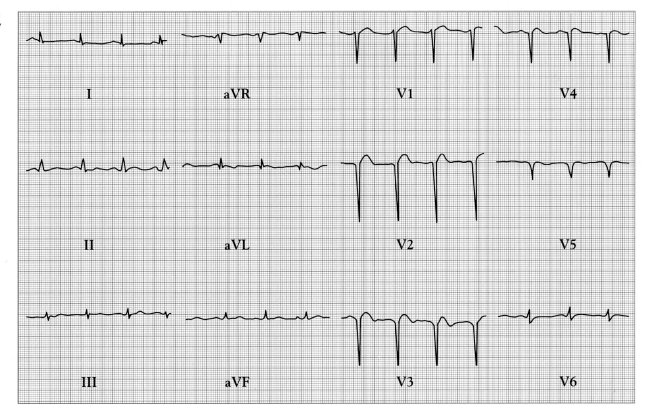

Electrocardiogram in a patient with left ventricular aneurysm, showing Q-waves and persistent ST-segment elevation in the anterior chest leads, six months after myocardial infarction.

23

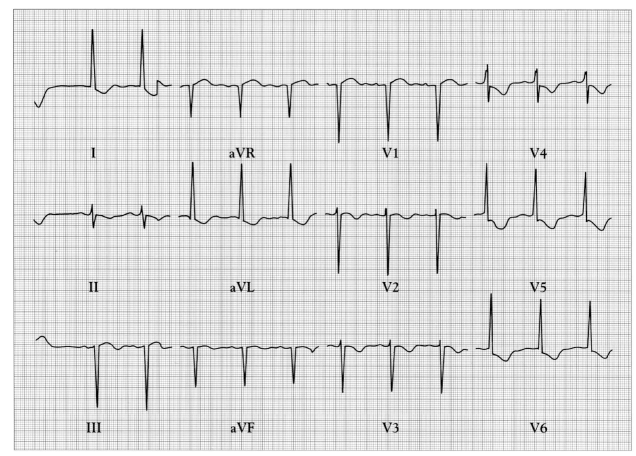

Electrocardiogram showing both increased voltage and ST-T abnormalities consistent with left ventricular hypertrophy.

24

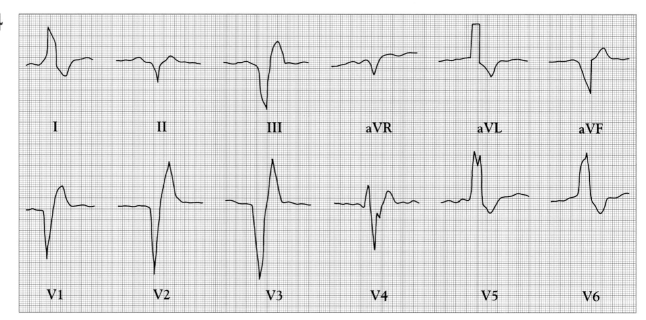

Electrocardiogram in a patient with dilated cardiomyopathy showing left bundle branch block.

25

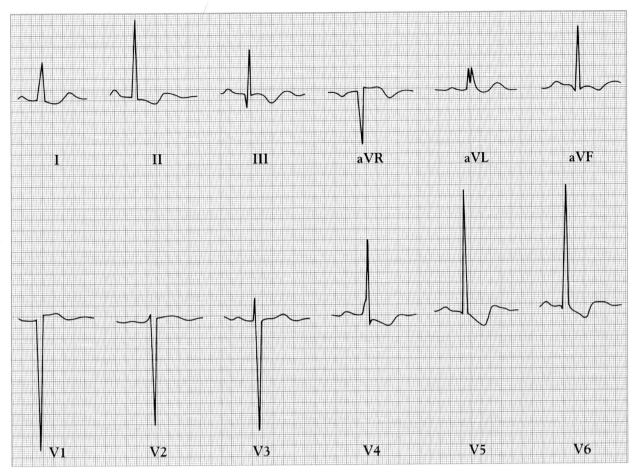

Electrocardiogram in a patient with dilated cardiomyopathy showing non-specific ST-T abnormalities.

26

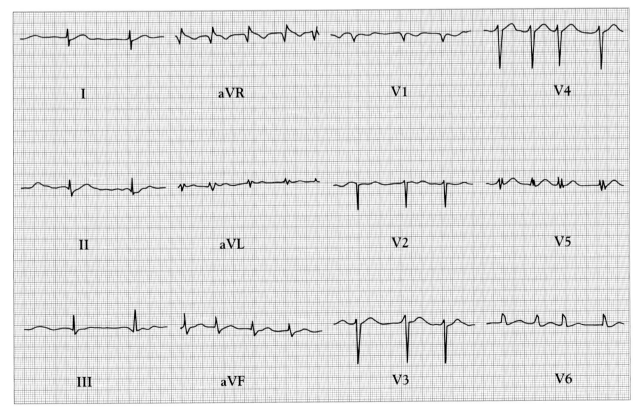

Electrocardiogram of a patient with dilated cardiomyopathy, showing atrial fibrillation, poor R-wave progression in the chest leads, partial left bundle branch block, but no Q-waves.

27
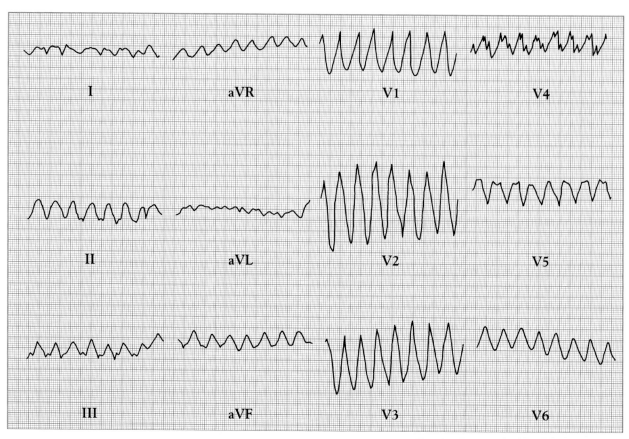

Electrocardiogram recorded from a patient with dilated cardiomyopathy, taken when he complained of dizziness. The 12-lead ECG shows ventricular tachycardia.

28

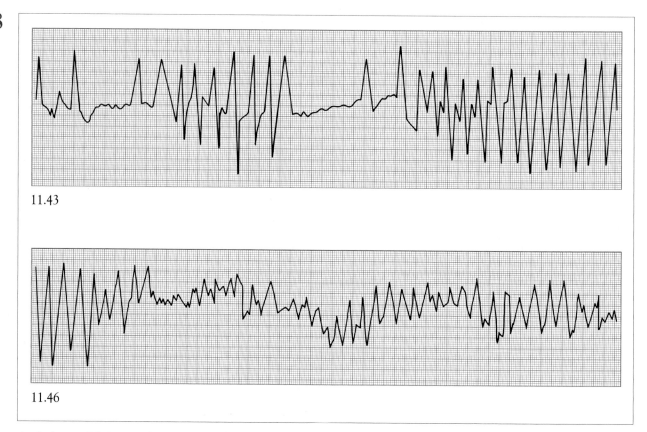

11.43

11.46

Ambulatory ECG recording from a patient with heart failure. On returning home with the recorder at 11.35, the patient sat down to drink a cup of coffee. At 11.43 he developed ventricular tachycardia and collapsed. At 11.46 ventricular fibrillation developed and the patient died.

29

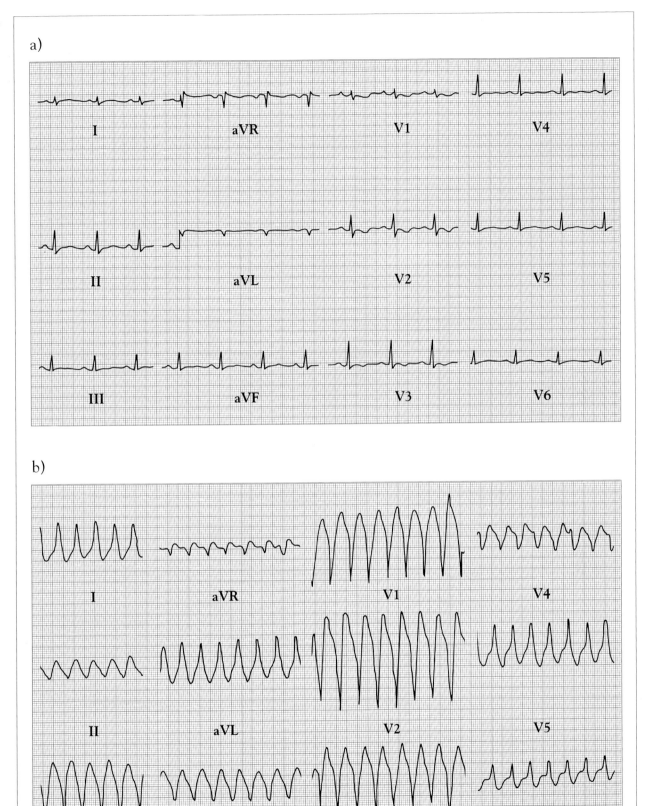

(a) Electrocardiogram of a patient with right ventricular cardiomyopathy showing T-wave inversions in right precordial leads. (b) Monomorphic ventricular tachycardia in the same patient.

30

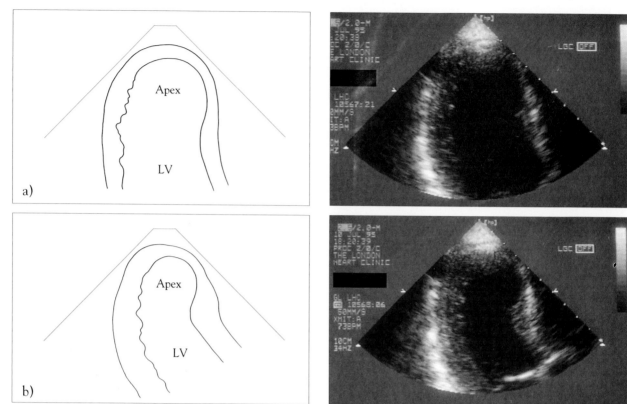

Apical long-axis views at end-diastole (above) and end-systole (below) in a patient with heart failure secondary to myocardial infarction. The antero-apical segment is thin and scarred and plays no part in the contractile process.

31

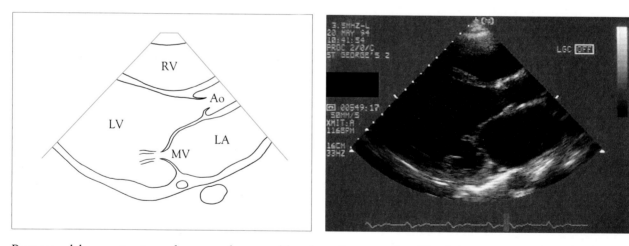

Parasternal long-axis view of a case of severe dilated cardiomyopathy. The left atrium is enlarged. The left ventricle is large, thin-walled, and globally hypocontractile.

32   M-mode recording showing the enlarged, thin-walled left ventricle with almost no difference between the systolic and diastolic cavity dimensions.

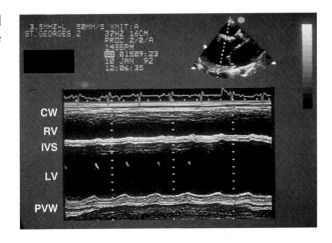

33

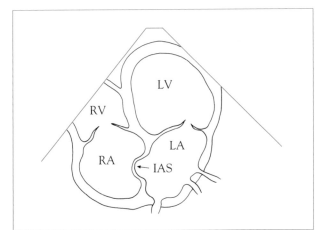

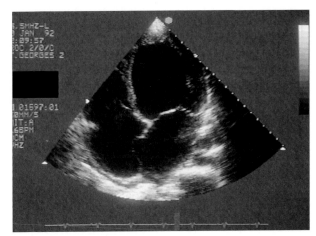

Apical four-chamber view from the same patient as in [32]. The left ventricle is globular in shape. The left atrium is enlarged and the region of the fossa ovale (arrow) stretched by the elevated filling pressure.

34

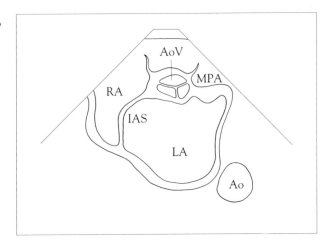

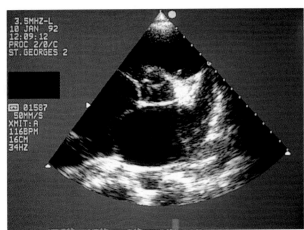

Parasternal short-axis view of the same patient as in [32] and [33], showing the enlarged left atrium and tense interatrial septum.

35

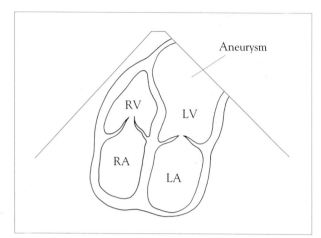 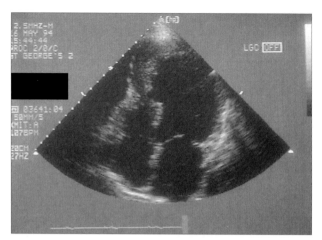

Apical four-chamber view showing the enlarged apical region with abnormal cavity contour in a patient with a left ventricular aneurysm.

36

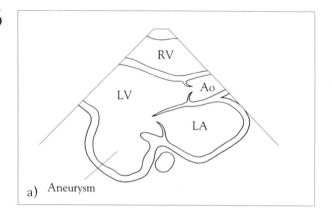 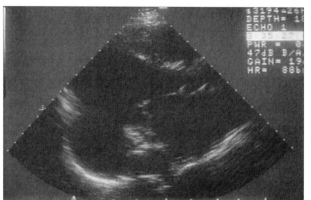

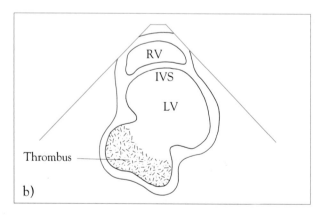 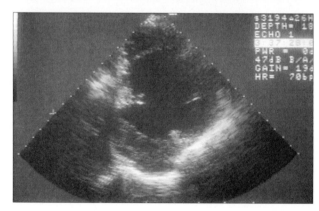

Parasternal long-axis (a) and parasternal short-axis (b) views of a large postero-basal left ventricular aneurysm. Echo densities shown in the short-axis view are strongly suggestive of layered thrombus in the aneurysm.

37

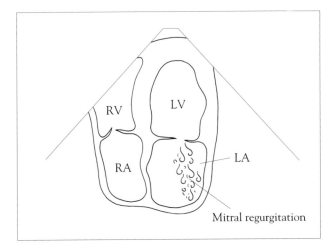

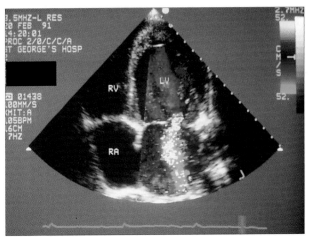

Apical four-chamber view with color-flow Doppler showing severe functional mitral regurgitation caused by dilatation of the valve annulus in a patient with left ventricular disease.

38 Pulsed Doppler recording taken from the apex, showing the transmitral flow in a patient with severely deranged diastolic function. The middle complex is a post-ectopic beat with adequate filling time but there is poor early relaxation and the majority of filling occurs with atrial contraction. The left and right complexes are sinus beats but with a single 'summation' filling pattern.

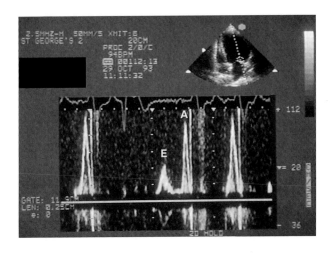

39 Pulsed Doppler recording of transmitral flow showing a restrictive filling pattern. There is a brief early-filling phase with rapid flow deceleration and little or no late filling despite sinus rhythm and a relatively long P-R interval.

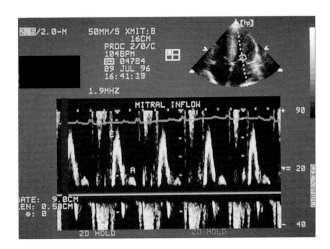

40 Pulsed Doppler recording of transmitral flow in a patient with chronic hypertension. As a result of impaired relaxation, the 'e' wave velocity is reduced and early filling time prolonged in a pattern similar to that of mild mitral stenosis. The majority of filling occurs only as a result of atrial contraction.

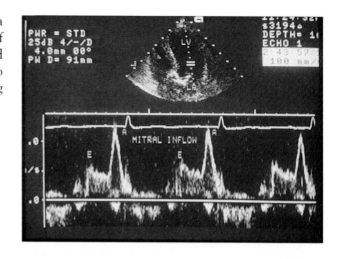

41

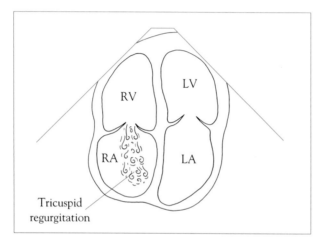

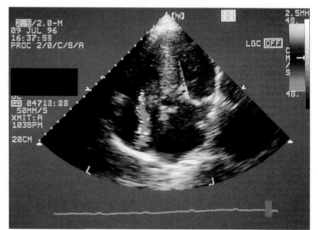

Apical four-chamber view with color-flow Doppler showing a systolic jet of tricuspid regurgitation entering the right atrium.

42

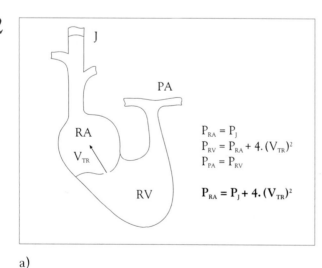

$$P_{RA} = P_J$$
$$P_{RV} = P_{RA} + 4.(V_{TR})^2$$
$$P_{PA} = P_{RV}$$

$$P_{RA} = P_J + 4.(V_{TR})^2$$

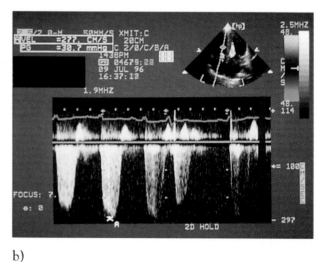

a)   b)

(a) Diagram showing the basis for assessment of pulmonary hypertension using continuous-wave spectral Doppler. Pressure in the right atrium (P_{RA}) can be determined from inspection of the jugular venous pulse. If any tricuspid regurgitation is present, the Bernoulli equation ($\Delta P = 4 \times V^2$) allows the (RV-RA) pressure gradient to be calculated from the velocity of the jet (V_{TR}). Systolic pressure in the right ventricle (P_{RV}) equals that in the pulmonary arteries (P_{PA}) as long as there is no right ventricular outflow obstruction. (b) Continuous-wave spectral Doppler of tricuspid regurgitation. The peak jet velocity is 2.8 m/s, corresponding to a (RV-RA) gradient of 31 mmHg. Pulmonary artery pressure is thus equal to (RA pressure + 31) mmHg.

43

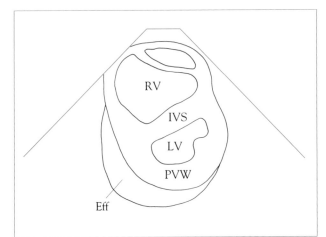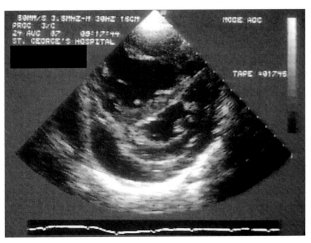

Parasternal short-axis view in a case of severe pulmonary hypertension, showing the characteristic distortion of the interventricular septum leading to a 'D-shaped' appearance of the short-axis section of the left ventricle. There is also some fluid in the pericardial sac.

44 Gated blood pool scan in a normal subject: 15 frames have been acquired (end-systole at frame 4, end-diastole at frame 1).

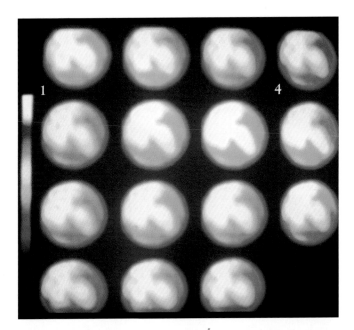

45 Gated blood pool scan in dilated cardiomyopathy showing little difference in the size of the ventricular cavities between end-diastole (left) and end-systole (right).

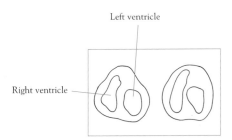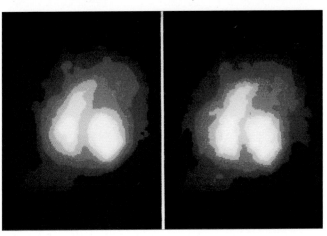

46 End-diastolic frames of equilibrium gated blood pool scans (top right) with regions of interest outlining the right and left ventricular cavities. By measuring the counts in these regions throughout the cardiac cycle, an accurate measure of the change in cavity volume can be made, to yield volume curves and calculated ejection fractions (EF) (bottom right); (a) normal (LVEF 58%, RVEF 44%), (b) LV aneurysm (LVEF 23%, RVEF 24%), (c) dilated cardiomyopathy (LVEF 10%, RVEF 11%).

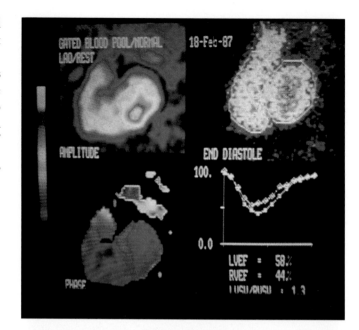

a)

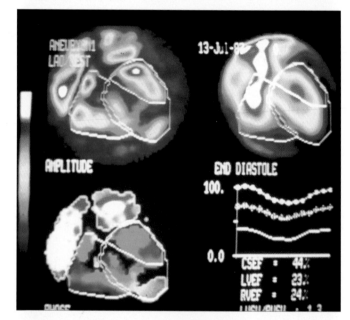

b)

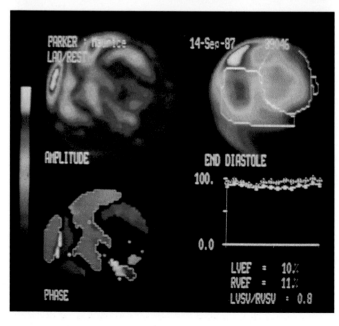

c)

47 Thallium tomography of severe coronary artery disease with infarction and poor left ventricular function. The upper row shows the stress images where perfusion is only present in the lateral wall. In addition, the left ventricle is dilated. There is some improvement in most territories following three hours' redistribution, suggesting that viable ischemic myocardium is present.

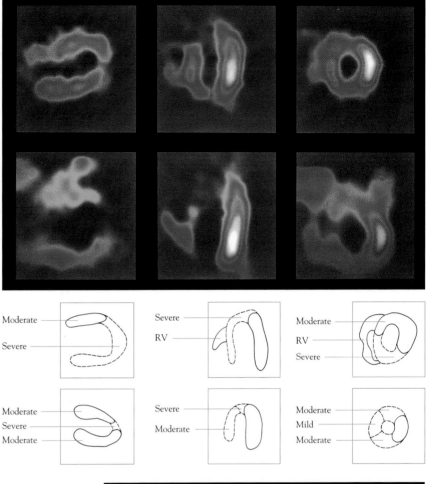

48

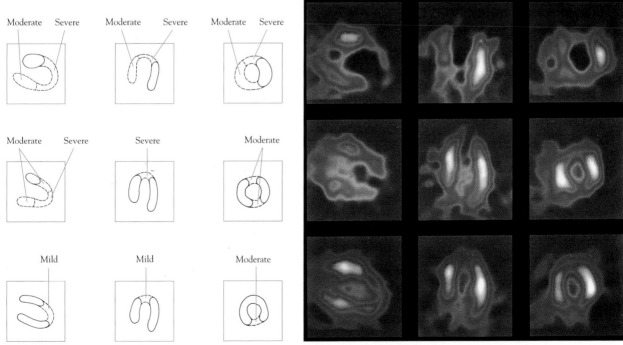

Thallium tomography following reinjection for the detection of hibernating myocardium. The upper three images show myocardial perfusion after stress. There is greatly reduced uptake in the anterior wall, septum and apex, and the inferior wall. The middle row shows images after three hours' redistribution. There is considerable improvement in the septum, confirming reversible ischemia, but only minor changes in the apex, inferior wall, and distal anterior wall. The bottom row shows images acquired after reinjection of thallium. There is considerable improvement in the tracer uptake in all parts of the myocardium, confirming that the anterior wall, inferior wall, and apex also contain viable myocardium.

49 Positron emission tomography assessment of hibernating myocardium. The figure illustrates the case of a patient with chronic dysfunction of the antero-apical wall of the left ventricle (LV) which is subtended by an occluded left anterior descending (LAD) coronary artery (two central panels). The top and bottom panels are positron emission tomographic images (obtained after three-dimensional reconstruction) showing, in different projections, the heart and big vessels. The blood pool, obtained after inhalation of a tracer amount of $C^{15}O$, is shown in red and the myocardial uptake of ^{18}F-fluorodeoxyglucose (FDG), during fasting conditions, is superimposed in white. The distal part of the anterior wall and the apex of the LV show a considerable uptake of FDG which indicates the presence of viable tissue.

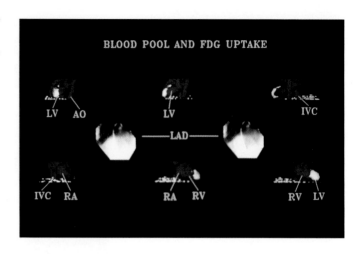

50 A balloon-tipped thermodilution catheter for right heart hemodynamic monitoring.

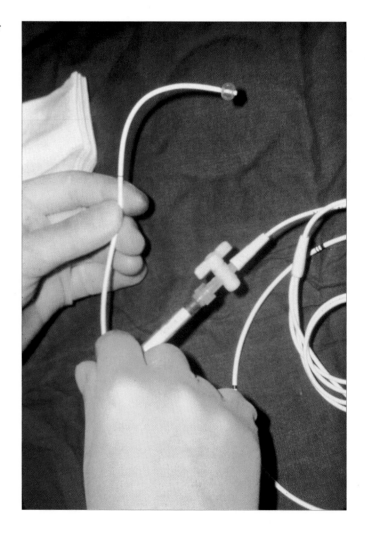

51 Chest X-ray showing a catheter inserted via the right subclavian vein, positioned with its tip in the right pulmonary artery for measurement of wedge pressure.

Balloon-tipped catheter

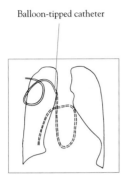

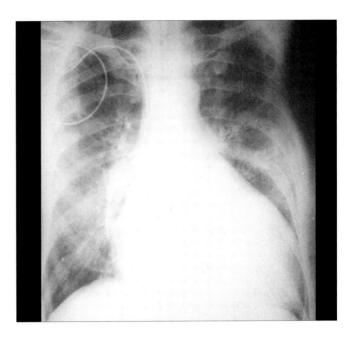

52 Pressure recording from the left ventricle in a patient with heart failure. The end-diastolic pressure is raised and there is a prominent 'a' wave.

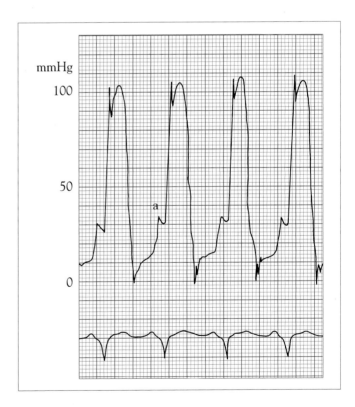

53

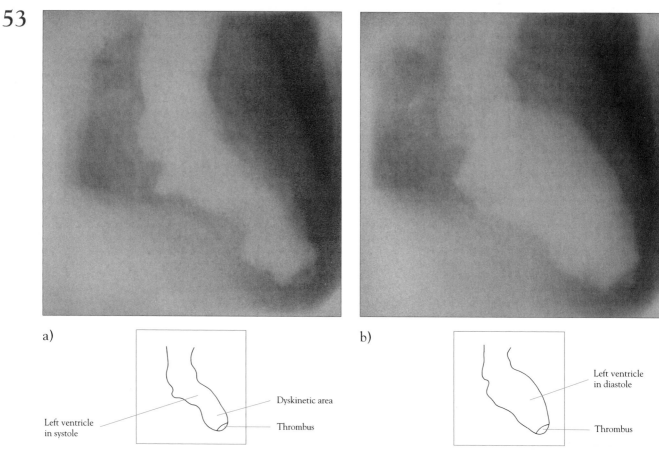

Left ventricular angiogram in the right anterior oblique projection. (a) Systolic and (b) diastolic frames reveal the presence of apical dyskinesis and thrombus.

54

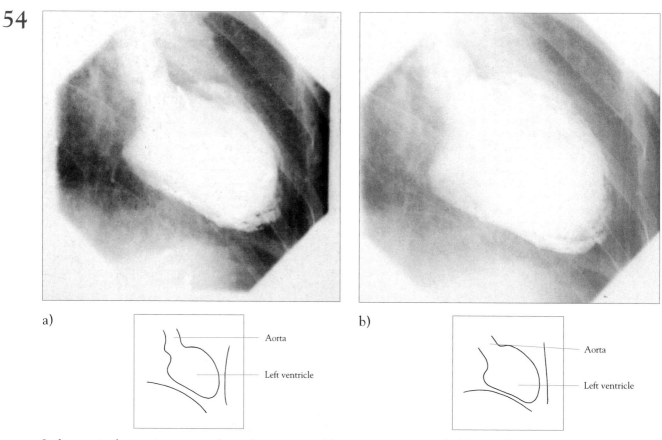

Left ventricular angiogram in the right anterior oblique projection with (a) systolic and (b) diastolic frames showing global hypokinesis and ventricular dilatation.

55

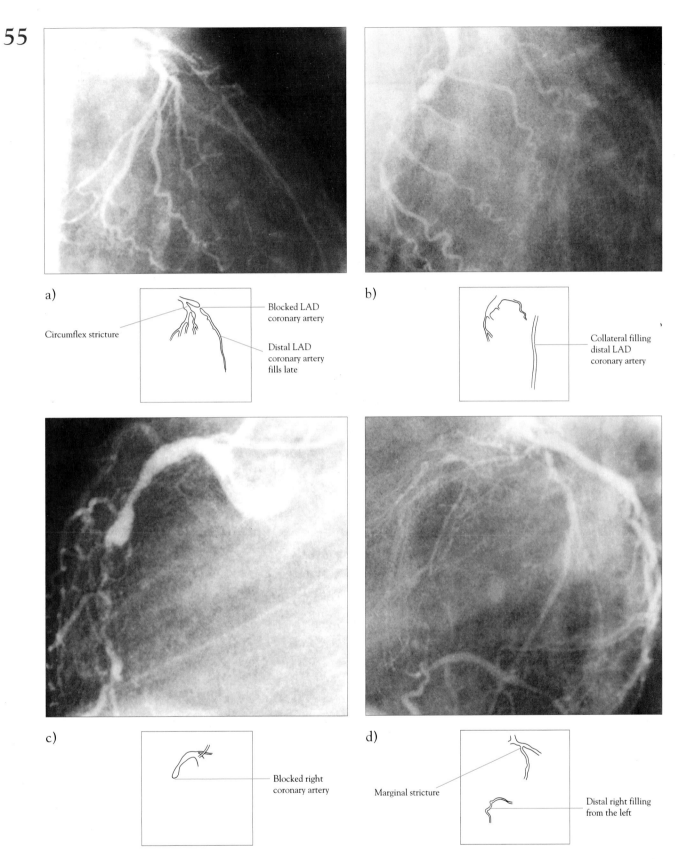

a)

Circumflex stricture

Blocked LAD
coronary artery

Distal LAD
coronary artery
fills late

b)

Collateral filling
distal LAD
coronary artery

c)

Blocked right
coronary artery

d)

Marginal stricture

Distal right filling
from the left

Coronary arteriograms in ischemic cardiomyopathy showing coronary artery stenoses in all three major vessels. (a) Left coronary injection in RAO projection shows a blocked anterior descending and a strictured circumflex vessel. (b) Right coronary injection in RAO projection shows the blocked right coronary artery. (c) The right coronary injection in LAO projection confirms the irregularly dilated coronary artery with a complete block of the mid-right heart border. (d) The left coronary artery injection in LAO projection shows the blocked anterior descending, with some collateral flow through the septum to the distal anterior descending artery beyond the block. It also shows the terminal branch of the right filling from the left.

56 Oxygen consumption ($\dot{V}O_2$) during symptom limited treadmill exercise and on recovery, in a normal subject (right), a patient with moderate heart failure (middle) and a patient with severe heart failure (left). At rest and during the first five minutes of exercise all three subjects have similar oxygen consumption, but peak $\dot{V}O_2$ is progressively reduced with increasing heart failure.

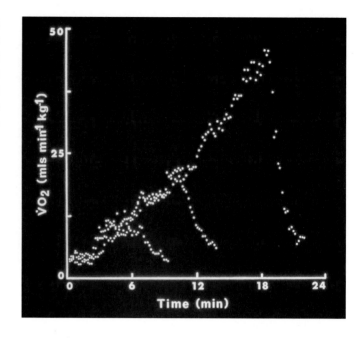

57 Magnetic resonance imaging in dilated cardiomyopathy. Four frames from a cine acquisition in the horizontal long-axis plane using a field echo sequence where blood appears with high signal (white) except where there is turbulence. There is global left ventricular hypokinesia.

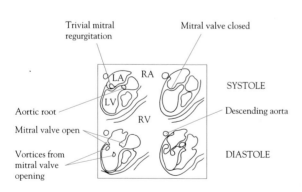

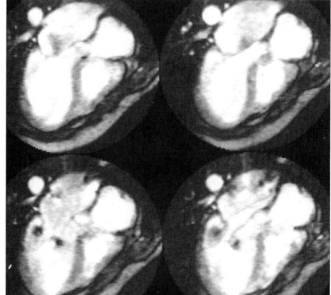

58

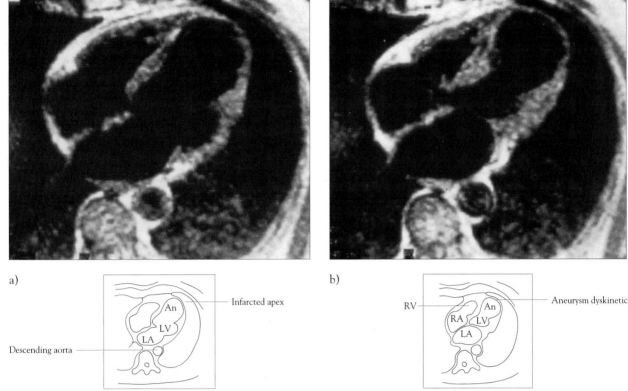

a)

Infarcted apex

An
LV
LA

Descending aorta

b)

RV

An
RA   LV
LA

Aneurysm dyskinetic

Magnetic resonance imaging in left ventricular aneurysm (An). (a) Diastolic and (b) systolic transverse sections in a patient with previous infarction and an apical left ventricular aneurysm. The basal myocardium contracts well while the apical myocardium is thin and dyskinetic.

HEART FAILURE   **Principles of Management**

59   Principles of management of systolic ventricular failure.

1. Asymptomatic left ventricular systolic dysfunction (ejection fraction of 45% or less):

   ACE inhibitors

2. Mild to moderate symptomatic heart failure:

   Diuretics
   ACE inhibitors
   Angiotensin II receptor antagonist, particularly when ACE inhibitors are not tolerated because of cough
   Hydralazine-isosorbide dinitrate in those who cannot tolerate ACE inhibitors or angiotensin receptor antagonist

3. Severe heart failure - medical treatment:

   Diuretics
   ACE inhibitors
   Digoxin
   Low-dose amiodarone in selected patients
   Beta-blocking agents in selected patients with idiopathic dilated cardiomyopathy

4. Severe heart failure - surgical treatment:

   Aneurysmectomy for localized left ventricular aneurysm
   Revascularization in selected patients with hibernating myocardium

5. Refractory heart failure:

   Combination vasodilators
   Non-glycosidic inotropic agents
   DDD pacemaker
   Cardiomyoplasty
   Cardiac transplantation

CHAPTER 3
Hypertension

Abbreviations

Ao	Aorta		LV	Left ventricle
BP	Blood pressure		PVW	Posterior ventricular wall
IVS	Interventricular septum		RA	Right atrium
LA	Left atrium		RV	Right ventricle

Introduction

High blood pressure is a major cardiovascular risk factor. Indeed, it is the major risk factor for strokes and an important risk factor for ischemic heart disease, peripheral vascular disease, and congestive cardiac failure. Risk for these conditions is continuously related to blood pressure, i.e. there is no threshold blood pressure above which patients are at risk [1]. Thus, patients whose blood pressure lies at the bottom of the blood pressure distribution curve have a lower risk of cardiovascular morbidity and mortality than those whose blood pressure is close to the population mean. There is now strong evidence that much of this risk is reversible. Large multicenter trials have demonstrated that the increased probability of having a stroke in patients with high blood pressure is completely reversed by anti-hypertensive drug treatment, and the benefits of treatment are probably seen in the sharp decline in the incidence of stroke in many countries, although this is not seen in, for instance, eastern Europe.

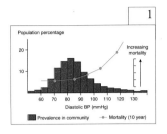

The situation with regard to ischemic heart disease is less clear. Pooling all the trials the overall fall of 6 mmHg observed would be expected to reduce fatal and non-fatal myocardial infarction by 20–25%. The observed figure is, however, 14–16%. Whether this is due to the fact that coronary artery disease is already established before treatment or whether the shortfall is due to the particular agents used in these trials is unknown. However, this residual uncertainty should not detract from the major success story presented by the management of hypertension over the last few decades. The importance of hypertension and its high prevalence impose a heavy responsibility, not only on doctors but on health services across the world. Blood pressure can be lowered in most cases where patients will accept therapy [2]. Despite this, there are many individuals with high blood pressure who are either unrecognized or are not receiving adequate treatment.

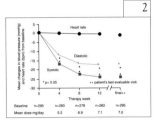

Prevalence

Systolic blood pressure rises with age; diastolic blood pressure rises up to the age of 50–60 years, then stabilizes and subsequently falls slightly. Blood pressure in pre-menopausal women is lower than that in men of the same age; after the menopause it is slightly higher [3]. There is no natural dividing line between hypertensive and normotensive individuals [4]. The fact that risk is spread right across the blood pressure distribution means that there are advantages in lowering blood pressure, particularly by population measures, even in patients who fall below any arbitrary cut-off point used to define hypertension. Nevertheless, for clinical purposes cut-off points are often adopted. The most widely used was formerly that chosen by the Expert Sub-Committee of the World Health Organization, i.e. 160/95 mmHg or above. The recent Joint National Committee report from the USA uses a more refined classification which takes account of the increased risks associated even with marginal elevation of blood pressure [5]. Using the WHO criterion the prevalence of hypertension ranges from about 3% in subjects below the age of 20 to over 40% of the male population in the older age groups. The overall prevalence on single readings lies between 15% and 20%. This figure falls by about one-third to one-half when the average of repeated measurements is taken, since blood pressure usually falls with repeated measurement.

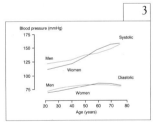

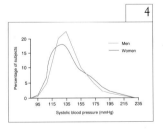

Genetic factors contribute about 30% to blood pressure variance under normal circumstances. The important environmental factors are stress and diet. Thus, hypertension is more common in obese subjects and in those consuming large amounts of alcohol. Stress is more difficult to measure, but some investigations have shown that blood pressure is elevated in individuals in whom pressure at work exceeds the individual's ability to meet those pressures. Blood pressure is higher at all ages in American Blacks and the risk of cardiac and cerebrovascular disease is greater, although when adjusted for blood pressure level and adequacy of treatment, there is no additional risk.

Hypertension is commonly classified according to its cause. Individuals in whom the only apparent cause is a genetic predisposition (usually shown by a strong family history) and those with no predisposing factors, apart from family history, are regarded as

Category	Systolic (mmHg)	Diastolic (mmHg)
Normal	<130	<85
High normal	130–139	85–89
Hypertension		
Stage 1 (mild)	140–159	90–99
Stage 2 (moderate)	160–179	100–109
Stage 3 (severe)	180–209	110–119
Stage 4 (very severe)	≥ 210	≥ 120

having primary or essential hypertension. Individuals in whom a specific cause can be identified are regarded as having secondary hypertension. The true prevalence of the two classes of hypertension is difficult to establish because most reported figures come from highly selected populations in special clinics. However, it is unlikely that more than 5–10% of the hypertensive population suffers from secondary hypertension. The most common causes of secondary hypertension are probably the contraceptive pill, obesity, and alcohol. The association between salt intake and blood pressure is controversial and the evidence from epidemiologic studies is rather weak. It has been suggested that long-standing exposure to high salt intake is necessary, although this is by no means proven. The true prevalence of secondary hypertension excluding obesity, the contraceptive pill, and alcohol excess is probably less than 1%.

Hypertension used to be classified into so-called benign or 'accelerated' (malignant) hypertension. The term 'benign' has now been abandoned since any chronic elevation of blood pressure carries increased cardiovascular risk. The terms 'accelerated' and 'malignant' hypertension are now used synonymously.

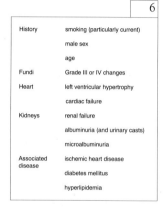

		6
History	smoking (particularly current)	
	male sex	
	age	
Fundi	Grade III or IV changes	
Heart	left ventricular hypertrophy	
	cardiac failure	
Kidneys	renal failure	
	albuminuria (and urinary casts)	
	microalbuminuria	
Associated disease	ischemic heart disease	
	diabetes mellitus	
	hyperlipidemia	

Symptoms and Signs

Hypertension causes no symptoms in the majority of patients until target organ damage occurs [6]. There is, however, an increased incidence of nocturia, epistaxis, and headaches in hypertensive patients. Characteristically, hypertensive headaches are situated in the occiput, throbbing in character, and occur in the early morning. Many hypertensive patients complain of less specific headaches, however, and in a proportion of cases these are unrelated to high blood pressure. Nevertheless, studies in hypertensive clinics have shown a significant reduction in headaches as a result of blood pressure control. While symptoms such as tiredness and vertigo are common, these probably reflect anxiety and not high blood pressure.

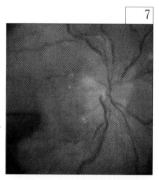

Examination of the cardiovascular system may be normal, but left ventricular hypertrophy may cause a forceful displaced apex beat. The presence of this sign in a hypertensive patient pinpoints high cardiovascular risk. There may be an accentuation of the aortic component of the second sound, a fourth heart sound, and an ejection systolic murmur in the aortic area. Left ventricular failure or aortic regurgitation are an indication of advanced hypertensive heart disease.

Other signs reflect target organ damage, i.e. evidence of cerebrovascular disease in the form of focal neurologic signs or loss of cerebral function. Peripheral vascular disease may be shown by diminished peripheral pulses or ischemic changes in the toes and feet.

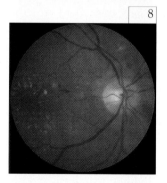

Fundal appearances provide the best assessment of the vascular tree during clinical examination. The earliest change is narrowing of the arterial lumen, decreasing the ratio of arterial to venous diameter. Thickening of the arterial wall gives rise to an increased reflection of light (light reflex) and the appearance of silver wiring. The veins may be nipped at the point where they cross an artery (arteriovenous nipping) [7]. Silver wiring and arteriovenous nipping may also be seen in normotensive elderly patients, and the presence of either sign is therefore of little significance in patients from their late 50s onwards. Nevertheless, they are conventionally graded according to the Keith-Wagener classification as Grade I and Grade II changes, respectively. Grade III retinopathy is associated with hemorrhages and exudates. The latter comprise two types. Hard exudates are small discrete white lesions caused by small amounts of denatured protein [8]. Cotton-wool spots are larger white lesions with a less distinct outline. They are due to retinal infarction secondary to arterial blockage. Grade IV changes are characterized by papilledema [9]. Both Grade III and Grade IV changes are associated with a poor prognosis in untreated patients. There is little difference in prognosis between patients with Grade III and Grade IV changes and consequently the difference between accelerated (Grade III) fundal changes and malignant (Grade IV) changes has now been abandoned. The most important prognostic feature in patients with accelerated or malignant hypertension is the presence of significant renal impairment.

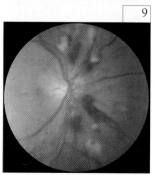

Pathologic Consequences

Hypertension causes changes throughout the arterial tree and in the organs supplied by the vasculature ('target organ').

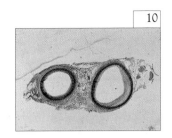

Large Arteries and Arterioles

The aorta and larger vessels arising from it are slightly dilated and lose some of their elasticity. Histologically, the smooth muscle component of the vascular media is increased, the internal elastic lamina becomes duplicated, and there is fibrous thickening of the sub-intimal part of the artery [10,11]. The peripheral large arteries become elongated and tortuous so that the visible pulsations may be noticeable, particularly in older patients. Atheroma is more commonly seen in hypertensive patients [12,13]. This is largely a hemodynamic effect as it is not seen in the arteries not exposed to increased pressure, e.g. in the pulmonary circulation.

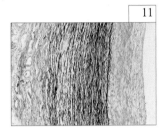

Small Arteries and Arterioles

The key change at this level is an increase in the wall-to-lumen ratio, which increases the resistance to flow. This is a characteristic feature of hypertension. Medial hypertrophy occurs in association with increased collagen content in the media and there is some sub-intimal thickening [14]. Some vessels show a decrease in luminal diameter with no increase in overall wall mass ('remodeling'). The relative contributions of remodeling and genuine hypertrophy are subject to vigorous debate at present. Arterioles also characteristically show hyaline thickening, which develops gradually from patchy deposition until, in long-standing hypertension, it may replace the structure of the arteriolar wall, leaving only the endothelium intact [15]. It is most frequently seen in the afferent arterioles of the kidney.

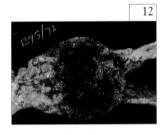

Patients with accelerated (malignant) hypertension typically have fibrinoid necrosis of the small arteries [16]. This is believed to be due to damage caused by a rapid increase in blood pressure resulting in increased permeability of the vascular endothelium to plasma proteins. The vessel wall is replaced by a structureless, fibrin-like material containing plasma protein component. The access of growth factors to the vessel wall causes proliferation of collagen resulting in extreme intimal thickening (onion skinning).

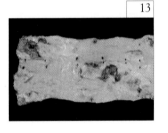

The Heart

Sustained hypertension is associated with left ventricular hypertrophy [17]. This, in part at least, reflects the increased load against which the left ventricle has to contract, since there is a close correlation between 24-hour blood pressure measurement and the degree of left ventricular hypertrophy. However, in this process other neural and humoral growth factors probably play an important role. With the development of sensitive, non-invasive imaging methods, such as echocardiography, it has become apparent that a mild degree of left ventricular hypertrophy occurs quite early in the development of hypertension. This is associated with a reduction in the volume of the left ventricular cavity and in overall compliance. Left ventricular failure is associated with dilatation of the left ventricle. Pulmonary edema and pleural effusions occur as a late complication [18]. The presence of left ventricular hypertrophy on echocardiography, electrocardiography, or chest X-ray is associated with a much worse cardiac prognosis.

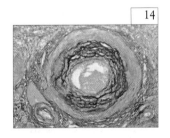

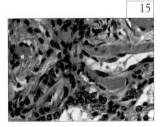

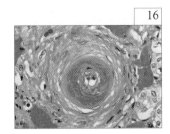

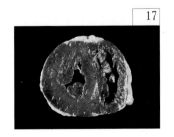

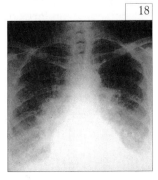

Coronary atheroma is a frequent finding in hypertensive patients [19] and myocardial infarction is the most frequent cause of death. Myocardial infarction is three times as common as stroke in hypertensive patients, although the contribution of other risk factors (e.g. hyperlipidemia and smoking) to coronary heart disease is greater.

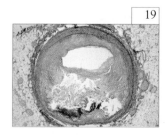

The Brain

Hypertension has several effects on the cerebral blood vessels. An increased prevalence of atheroma in both extra-cranial and intra-cranial vessels increases the risk of cerebral infarction, either as a result of in-situ thrombosis (particularly in the territory of the middle cerebral artery), or embolization from a distal site causing multiple infarction. Intra-cerebral hemorrhage occurs as a result of rupture of a Charcot–Bouchard aneurysm [20]. These are degenerative lesions of the wall of small perforating arteries supplying the basal ganglia, thalamus, and internal capsule. Thrombosis of these aneurysms may also occur, giving rise to small lacunar infarctions in the brain, causing minor strokes and progressive dementia (lacunar state).

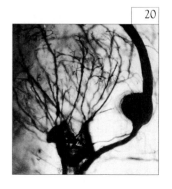

Aneurysms of the circle of Willis are congenital lesions giving rise to sub-arachnoid hemorrhage [21,22]. Although they are more frequent in hypertensive patients, they also often cause sub-arachnoid hemorrhage in normotensive subjects.

Sudden acute rises in cerebral perfusion pressure give rise to focal areas of vaso-dilatation in the smaller arteries and arterioles of the brain. The dilated areas are abnormally permeable and cause local cerebral edema, giving rise to focal neurologic signs and fits. This is the pathologic basis of hypertensive encephalopathy. Encephalopathy is more common in patients who have not developed protective structural changes in the vessels as a result of long-standing blood pressure elevation [23]. It is also responsible for the fits in eclampsia of pregnancy.

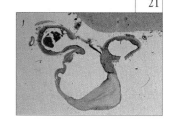

The Kidneys

Renal failure is rare in patients with essential hypertension unless they have entered the accelerated phase. Nevertheless, histologic changes are commonly seen. Atheroma of the renal vessels, or renal embolization from the aorta or renal arteries, may cause infarction and scarring. Bilateral severe renal atheroma may cause renal failure, particularly in elderly patients. The renal vessels show the structural changes seen in vessels from other tissues. Hyaline degeneration is particularly evident, most commonly in the afferent glomerular arterioles. The normal loss of nephrons with aging is accelerated in essential hypertension so that, histologically, nephrosclerosis becomes evident. There is frequently a moderate reduction in renal size with diffuse cortical thinning [24]. Scarring of the surface of the kidney leads to an adherent capsule with an irregular sub-capsular surface. Although vascular disease often produces a slight reduction in renal blood flow, the glomerular filtration rate is usually maintained. Both renal blood flow and glomerular filtration rate are reduced in accelerated hypertension as a result of fibrinoid necrosis. Renal failure may progress rapidly under these circumstances. The afferent arterioles are particularly susceptible. The wall is disrupted, the lumen is often completely obliterated, and the glomerulus supplied by that arteriole is destroyed. Since this is a relatively acute process, the kidneys are usually normal in size and the sub-capsular space is spotted with tiny hemorrhages [25].

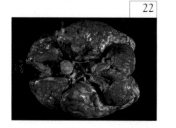

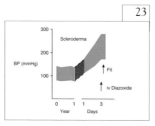

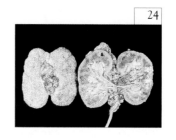

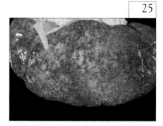

Secondary Hypertension

A number of diseases cause secondary hypertension (see Table 1).

Table 1. Causes of Secondary Hypertension.

Renal	Dietetic (alcohol and obesity)
– Vascular	Endocrine
– Parenchymal	– Primary aldosteronism
Pregnancy	– Pheochromocytoma
	– Acromegaly
Medications and the contraceptive pill [26]	– Myxedema
Coarctation	– Hyperparathyroidism
Neurologic	

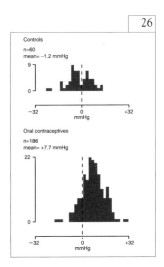

Renal Hypertension

Diseases of the renal blood vessels may cause hypertension (renovascular hypertension), as may diseases of the kidney itself (renal parenchymal hypertension).

Renovascular hypertension is produced by unilateral or bilateral renal ischemia [27,28]. The two most common causes of this are atheroma of the renal arteries and fibromuscular dysplasia. The former causes discrete areas of narrowing associated with atheromatous plaques, usually situated at the mouth of the renal artery. The most common form of fibromuscular dysplasia gives rise to regular fibromuscular ridges separated by thin segments of the vessel wall (corkscrew appearance). The cause is unknown but it usually occurs in a younger age group than atheroma and is more common in female patients and smokers. In addition to these intrinsic diseases of the renal artery, ischemia may be produced by fibrous bands compressing the vessel, by tumors [29], or by neurofibromatosis.

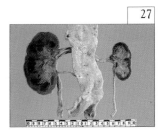

The three most common forms of renal parenchymal disease giving rise to hypertension are chronic pyelonephritis [30], chronic glomerulonephritis, and polycystic kidney. Hypertension may also be seen in less common diseases that affect the kidney, such as scleroderma [31], polyarteritis nodosa, disseminated lupus erythematosus, and analgesic nephropathy.

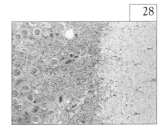

Hypertension is a common feature of acute glomerulonephritis and is seen in most patients with proliferative glomerulonephritis [32] at some stage in the course of their disease. It is less common in membranous glomerulonephritis [33] and is not observed in minimal change nephropathy [34]. Macroscopically, in the acute stage of glomerulo-

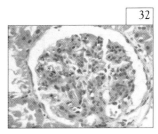

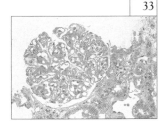

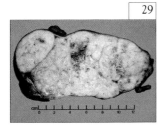

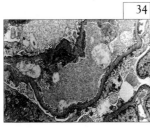

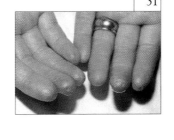

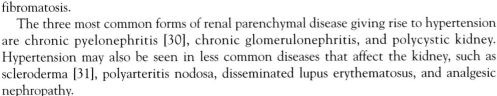

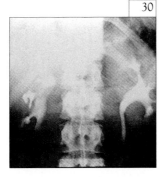

nephritis the kidneys may be swollen but, as chronic glomerulonephritis proceeds, they become shrunken. The more florid proliferative glomerular changes are associated with more severe degrees of hypertension.

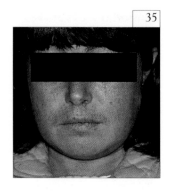

Endocrine Causes of Hypertension

Both the glucocorticoid and mineralocorticoid adrenal secretions produce hypertension. Glucocorticoids produce the characteristic appearance of Cushing's syndrome [35], which may be due either to adrenal tumors or to bilateral adrenal hyperplasia [36]. The latter may be secondary to stimulation of the adrenal gland as a result of a basophil pituitary tumor. Primary aldosteronism [37] results from hypersecretion of aldosterone which, in addition to producing hypertension, gives rise to a characteristic hypokalemic alkalosis. The majority of cases of primary aldosteronism are due to tumor, but a substantial minority are caused by bilateral multinodular hyperplasia. The biochemical changes are usually less marked in this condition. In both cases, however, the diagnosis is made by the finding of a high plasma aldosterone and suppressed plasma renin. This distinguishes primary from secondary hyperaldosteronism, where both renin and aldosterone levels are elevated.

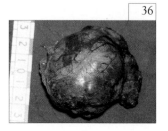

Adrenal medullary tumors produce hypertension through secretion of excessive amounts of the catecholamines, noradrenaline, and adrenaline (pheochromocytoma) [38]. Occasionally, these tumors may lie outside the adrenal glands, developing in the sympathetic tissue in, for instance, the urinary bladder, thorax, organs of Zuckerkandl, or other sites within the abdomen. These tumors are loaded with stored catecholamines [39], and manipulation, for example by palpation of the abdomen or during surgery, may cause the release of catecholamines and disastrous paroxysmal hypertension.

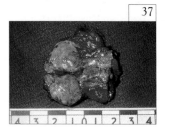

There is a complex association between hypertension and diabetes [40] that is independent of the obesity frequently seen in Type II (non-insulin-dependent) diabetes mellitus. Patients with essential hypertension have slightly increased insulin resistance associated with dyslipidemia (elevated triglycerides and low HDL-cholesterol). This has been described as 'syndrome X' (Reavan's syndrome). These patients are at particular risk of cardiovascular disease. Although hypertension is often present in patients with diabetic nephropathy, the renal disease is probably not responsible for the high blood pressure. It has been suggested that patients genetically predisposed to essential hypertension (i.e. with a strong family history) are particularly liable to develop nephropathy if they have associated diabetes. However, this has been challenged in recent studies.

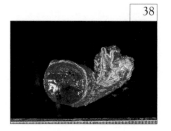

Hypertension is frequently seen in endocrine conditions such as acromegaly, myxedema, or hyperparathyroidism. It frequently regresses when these conditions are treated medically or surgically.

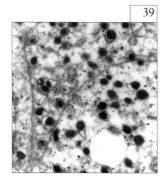

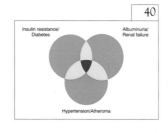

Coarctation
This is a congenital narrowing of the aorta just below the origin of the left subclavian artery, causing hypertension proximal to the lesion [41,42]. Clinically, suspicion is raised by radio-femoral delay in the pulse and the presence of pulsatile collateral vessels over the inner margin of the scapula posteriorly.

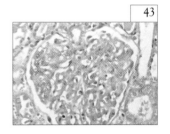

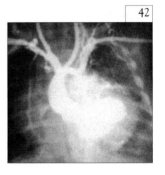

Hypertension of Pregnancy
Hypertension may occur in pregnancy as a result of pre-existing renal disease or essential hypertension. In addition, hypertension may occur (particularly in first pregnancies) after the 30th week of gestation, in association with proteinuria and edema (pre-eclamptic toxemia). Renal biopsy in such patients has shown enlarged edematous glomeruli with narrowing of the capillary lumina and swelling of endothelial cells [43]. The major importance to the mother in hypertension of pregnancy is the possibility of developing eclampsia, which carries a high mortality rate. Uncontrolled blood pressure is associated with increased risk of fetal loss, placental infarction, and small birthweight.

Medication
Hypertension may be iatrogenic, e.g. due to steroid treatment or as a result of the contraceptive pill. Elevated blood pressure is associated with the estrogen content of the pill and there is little evidence that progestogen-only pills cause hypertension. A slight elevation of blood pressure is produced by medication which causes fluid retention, e.g. carbenoxolone or non-steroidal anti-inflammatory drugs. It can also be produced by drugs that mimic the action of the sympathetic nervous system, such as ephedrine, amphetamine, and monoamine oxidase inhibitors taken with tyramine-containing foods. Withdrawal of clonidine may cause hypertension through increased sympathetic activity. The immunosuppressant, cyclosporin A, frequently causes hypertension although the mechanism is unknown. Erythropoietin administered to patients with renal failure to raise their hemoglobin levels increases whole blood viscosity and blood pressure.

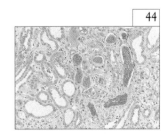

Investigation of Hypertension

In the majority of hypertensive patients, there is no advantage in carrying out detailed investigations to find the cause. Investigations should be confined to clinical situations where there is increased likelihood of a cause, i.e. unusual age of onset (below 30 years or above 55 years), clinical evidence of a cause (e.g. renal artery bruit), or where the patient stands to gain substantially (e.g. when blood pressure is difficult to control, or in the presence of advanced retinopathy).

Routine Tests
The vast majority of patients with essential hypertension have normal serum bio-chemistry. Renal impairment is usually evidence of either a renal cause of hypertension or hypertension which has entered the accelerated phase. Urine testing may also be normal. Abnormal proteinuria suggests either primary renal disease or accelerated hypertension. Microalbuminuria (i.e. protein excretion up to 200 mg a day) is frequently seen in hyper-tensive patients, is a marker of target organ damage, and therefore helps to identify high-risk patients. The presence of casts and red cells [44] suggests acute renal damage and is frequently seen in patients with primary renal disease or accelerated hypertension. Increased numbers of white cells suggest renal parenchymal disease, e.g. pyelonephritis.

   The decision to treat a patient with anti-hypertensive drugs may be aided by the demonstration of the presence of other risk factors on routine screening, e.g. elevated blood glucose, hyperlipidemia, or left ventricular hypertrophy.

Electrocardiogram
The electrocardiogram may be normal or show left-axis deviation in patients with mild hypertension in whom more sensitive investigations show significant left ventricular hypertrophy. More marked long-standing hypertension is associated with electro-cardiographic evidence of left ventricular hypertrophy, i.e. an increase in the R-wave

voltage in the left chest leads and the S-waves in the right chest leads so that the sum of the two exceeds 35 mm. Later, T-wave flattening, ST-segment depression, and T-wave inversion occur in the antero-lateral chest leads (left ventricular strain) [45].

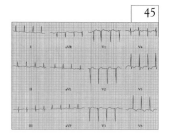

Chest X-ray

Mild to moderate hypertension is frequently associated with a normal chest X-ray. Left ventricular enlargement may be manifested by an increased cardiothoracic ratio [46], although this is a comparatively insensitive measure. In addition, the aortic shadow becomes 'unfolded'. Left ventricular failure is manifested by a 'bat's wing' appearance of the pulmonary vessels, cardiomegaly, small pleural effusions, and Kerley B-lines [47]. Rib notching may be visible in patients with coarctation of the aorta [48]. This is produced by collateral vessels bypassing the coarctation.

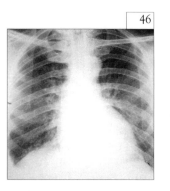

Ambulatory Blood Pressure Monitoring

A number of devices enable blood pressure to be measured over 24 hours. Those involving direct arterial cannulation are exclusively used for research purposes, but non-invasive, automatically inflating instruments are now entering clinical practice [49]. These show variations in blood pressure over the course of the day, and in healthy individuals will show the normal blood pressure fall with sleep [50]. The role of these devices in routine patient management is still under assessment. However, they are useful in demonstrating spurious ('white coat') hypertension in which blood pressure only becomes elevated when being measured, usually by a doctor [51]. Absence of the normal nocturnal fall in blood pressure (non-dipping) identifies a group at high risk of cardio-vascular disease.

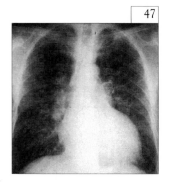

Renal Radiology

Intravenous urography is usually normal in patients with essential hypertension. In patients with renal artery stenosis [52a & b] the affected kidney may be smaller and there is delay in the appearance of the urogram, which may persist longer on the affected side and be more dense. Rapid sequence films are therefore necessary to time the first appearance of the urogram on the two sides. Routine intravenous urography is not generally used in screening for renovascular hypertension, because of both cost and a relatively high false-negative rate (20–30%); however, it is useful in the diagnosis of chronic renal disease. Chronic pyelonephritis [53] may be associated with scarring of the renal cortex and clubbing of calyces. Chronic glomerulonephritis causes bilateral smooth contraction of both kidneys [54], while polycystic kidneys give rise to distortion and

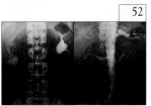
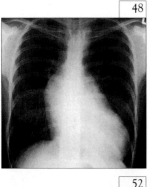
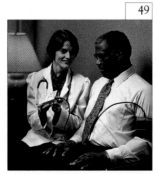
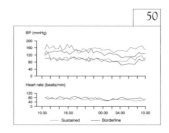
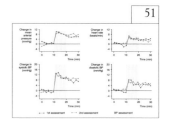
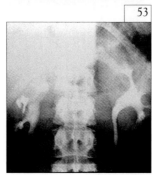
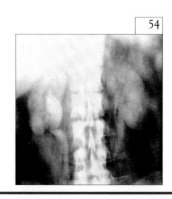

stretching of the calyces around the large cysts [55]. Analgesic nephropathy may be apparent as distorted calyces: necrotic papillae cause characteristic 'ring' shadows [56].

Renal angiography is still the gold standard for demonstrating the lesion in renal artery stenosis. Digital subtraction angiography yields excellent pictures with a higher degree of resolution [57]. Atheromatous plaques may be visible on the angiogram as small discrete lesions causing luminal narrowing and post-stenotic dilatation. Fibromuscular dysplasia causes a characteristic corkscrew appearance with alternate areas of narrowing and dilatation [58]. Pheochromocytoma can be demonstrated by arteriography, although computerized axial tomography (CAT) scanning is a safer and preferable option. In cases where the diagnosis is uncertain, angiography can be combined with vena caval sampling for plasma catecholamines, to identify the source.

Adrenal adenomata can be demonstrated by either arteriography or adrenal phlebography [59]. These lesions can also be seen on CAT scanning, although they are more difficult to demonstrate.

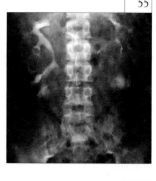

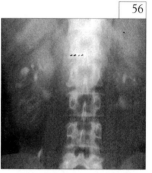

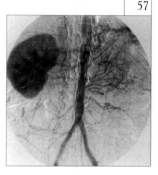

Ultrasound Scanning

This may help to demonstrate transsonic renal cysts in polycystic renal disease [60] and may help in the assessment of renal size in patients with parenchymal disease. Ultrasound scanning is also extensively used to demonstrate contraction in glomerulonephritis.

Isotope Scanning

Radiolabeled cholesterol is taken up preferentially by the adrenal gland and used in the synthesis of adrenal steroids. This provides an excellent method for demonstrating tumors, e.g. in Conn's syndrome, and lateralizing them for surgery [61]. ^{131}I metaiodobenzylguanethidine localizes both intra- and extra-adrenal pheochromocytomata.

Isotope renography is useful in the demonstration and lateralization of renovascular disease. Technetium-labeled diethylenetriamine penta-acetic acid (DTPA) or glucoheptinate act as a marker of glomerular filtration rate on the two sides while dimercaptosuccinic acid (DMSA) or radiolabeled sodium iodohippurate serve as markers of renal plasma flow [62]. In the presence of renovascular hypertension, angiotensin converting enzyme inhibitors, by dilating the efferent arteriole, cause a reduction in glomerular filtration rate without having a major influence on renal plasma flow. This is the basis of the captopril renogram, in which captopril is administered to a patient shortly before a second

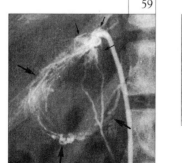

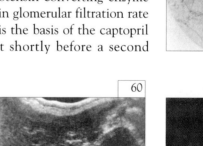

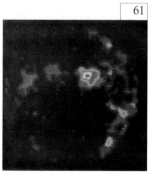

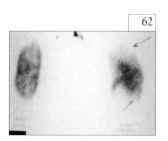

renogram is carried out. The captopril renogram [63] is widely used as the investigation of choice in the initial diagnosis of renovascular disease.

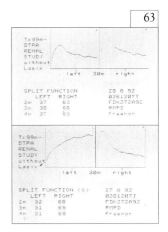

Echocardiography
Although magnetic resonance imaging represents the 'gold standard' for measuring cardiac chamber dimensions and wall thicknesses, from which left ventricular mass can be calculated, the lower cost and wide availability make echocardiography the preferred method in routine clinical practice [64a & b, 65]. It also provides assessment of associated pathology such as valve lesions.

Systolic function is usually well preserved, even with significant hypertrophy. However, the thickened interventricular septum can bulge into the left ventricular outflow tract and generate some turbulence, resulting in an audible murmur mimicking that of aortic stenosis or hypertrophic cardiomyopathy [66a & b]. Chronic hypertension can lead to systolic failure with chamber enlargement and reduction in systolic shortening fraction [67a & b, 68]. This is usually accompanied by functional aortic and/or mitral regurgitation.

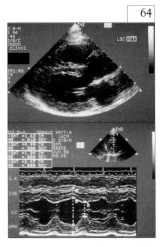

Diastolic function is frequently affected by even quite mild hypertension. Doppler studies can document transmitral flow and its time relationship to aortic outflow. From these recordings, a number of functional parameters can be derived, including the isovolumic relaxation time (IVRT) [69]; the ratio of the early filling wave ('e' wave) and the atrial systolic filling wave ('a' wave) amplitudes; and the decleration time of the 'e' wave [70,71]. The validity of these measurements has been demonstrated in numerous controlled studies, but it is frequently hard to apply the findings in routine practice as there are so many other factors, notably the patient's age, which affect them.

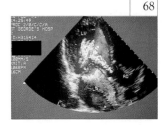

Magnetic Resonance Imaging (MRI)
Magnetic resonance images can be used to calculate atrial and ventricular volumes, and these measurements can be used to derive very accurate values for stroke volume and ejection fractions. The ventricular myocardium is well shown on magnetic resonance

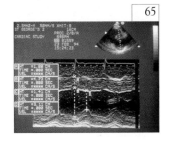

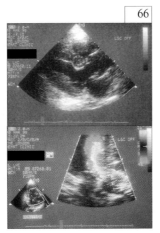

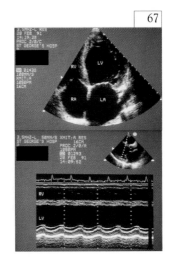

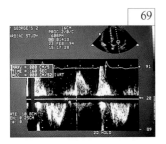

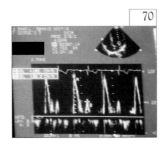

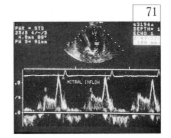

images and its thickness can be accurately measured [72]. Some of the causes of hypertension, such as renal disease [73], renal artery stenosis [74], and coarctation [75] are clearly demonstrated. In addition, some of the sequelae are also seen [76]. The value of assessing the hypertensive patient is still a matter for research, and techniques have not entered routine clinical practice yet. The use of MRI scanning to demonstrate cerebral blood vessels also carries great promise for the future management of the hypertensive patient.

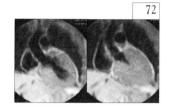

Management of the Hypertensive Patient

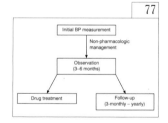

All patients should have a full clinical history taken and undergo examination before treatment is initiated. Clinical assessment will occasionally show a cause for hypertension (e.g. the contraceptive pill or a previous renal history) and it may also help treatment selection (e.g. dietary management for an obese patient).

Severe hypertension associated with fundal hemorrhages, exudates, or papilledema is a medical emergency and demands early treatment. Milder degrees of hypertension should be assessed by several blood pressure measurements. The duration of the period of observation depends upon the severity of hypertension, but in patients with borderline or mild blood pressures (e.g. diastolic blood pressures from 90 to 105 mmHg), blood pressure should be followed for three to six months before treatment is initiated [77].

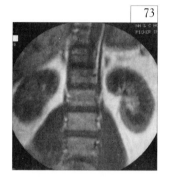

Except where urgent investigation or treatment is required, the first therapeutic interventions should be non-pharmacologic management [78], i.e. dietary weight reduction, avoidance of heavy alcohol intake (more than 21 units per week in a man or 14 units per week in a woman), regular physical exercise, and dietary salt restriction. Drug treatment should be reserved for patients whose blood pressure remains elevated despite these interventions. National therapeutic guidelines for the threshold blood pressure level at which drug treatment should be initiated differ slightly, but lie in the range diastolic blood pressure >90–100 mmHg and systolic blood pressure >140–160 mmHg. These levels should be lowered in the presence of other risk factors (e.g. hyperlipidemia, left ventricular hypertrophy, glucose intolerance, or continued smoking). The aim of treatment should be to secure target blood pressures of less than 140/90 mmHg in a patient free of adverse effects.

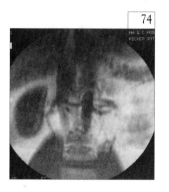

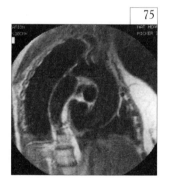

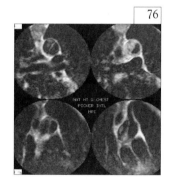

1 Blood pressure distribution in the population and the risk of cardiovascular mortality.

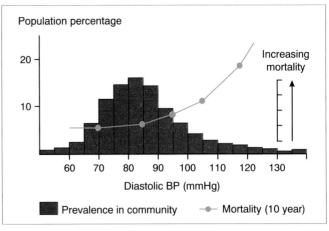

2 In an open multicenter general practice study, 320 patients with sitting diastolic blood pressure (DBP) in the range of 95–115 mmHg were treated with amlodipine (5–10 mg) once daily. Amlodipine treatment significantly reduced the mean BP throughout the study without significantly affecting heart rate. Of the patients receiving amlodipine monotherapy, 90.2% were therapy successes (sitting DBP reduced ≥10 mmHg or to ≤90 mmHg). Investigators' global evaluation of toleration was excellent or good in 92% of patients.

From Varrone J *et al.* The efficacy and safety of amlodipine in the treatment of mild and moderate essential hypertension in general practice. *J Cardiovasc Pharmacol* 1991; **17** (suppl 1): S30–S33.

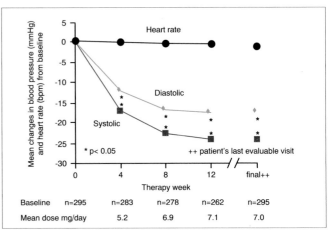

3 Mean systolic and diastolic blood pressures in relation to age.

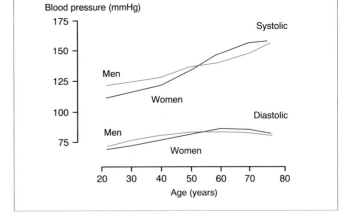

4 Systolic blood pressure distribution in men and women.

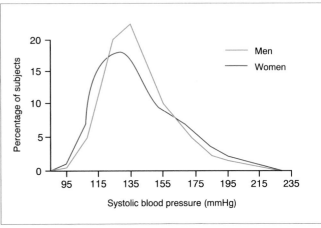

5   Joint National Committee classification of hypertension.

Category	Systolic (mmHg)	Diastolic (mmHg)
Normal	<130	<85
High normal	130–139	85–89
Hypertension		
Stage 1 (mild)	140–159	90–99
Stage 2 (moderate)	160–179	100–109
Stage 3 (severe)	180–209	110–119
Stage 4 (very severe)	≥ 210	≥ 120

6   Prognostic features in the hypertensive patient.

History	smoking (particularly current)
	male sex
	age
Fundi	Grade III or IV changes
Heart	left ventricular hypertrophy
	cardiac failure
Kidneys	renal failure
	albuminuria (and urinary casts)
	microalbuminuria
Associated disease	ischemic heart disease
	diabetes mellitus
	hyperlipidemia

7   Fundus from a hypertensive patient presenting with a sub-arachnoid hemorrhage. A large sub-hyaloid hemorrhage with an upper fluid level is seen on the left. There is also silver wiring with arteriovenous nipping and hard and soft exudates.

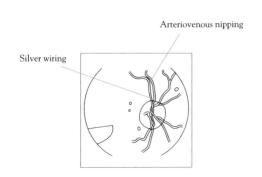

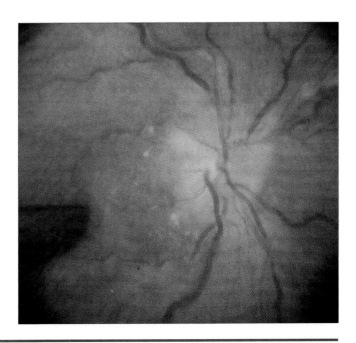

8   Fundus from a patient with accelerated hypertension. Note 'macular starring' of hard exudates and some small hemorrhages.

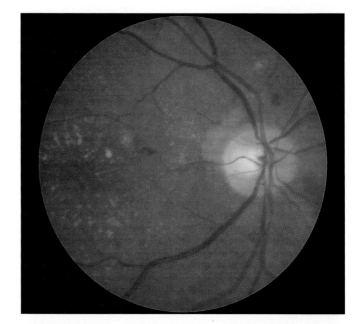

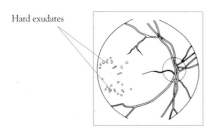

9   Fundus from a patient with malignant hypertension. Note presence of extensive hemorrhages, soft exudates, and papilledema. Blood pressure was treated medically and the patient remains well.

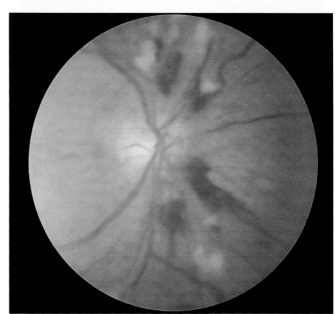

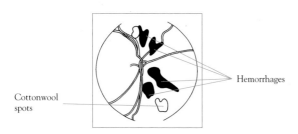

10 Carotid bifurcation showing marked intimal thickening in the sinus associated with hypertension.

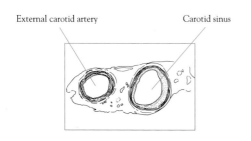

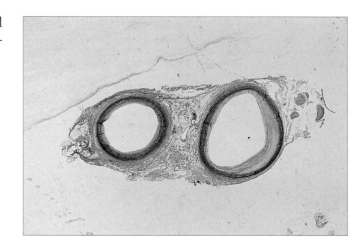

11   Higher magnification of carotid sinus wall from same patient as in [10], confirming intimal thickening, irregular elastic laminae, and some medial collagen increase.

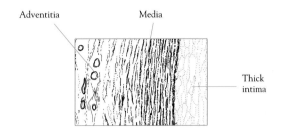

Adventitia   Media

Thick intima

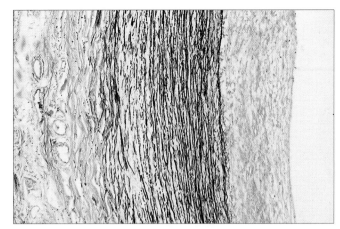

12   An atheromatous abdominal aortic aneurysm at the typical site below the renal arteries and proximal to the bifurcation. The aneurysm contains thrombus.

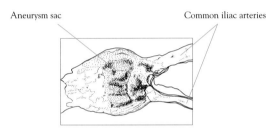

Aneurysm sac   Common iliac arteries

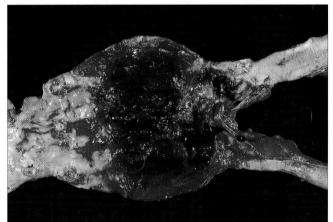

13   Aorta with severe atheroma. The plaques are ulcerated and calcified.

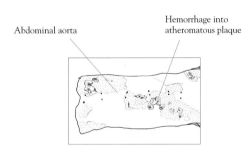

Abdominal aorta   Hemorrhage into atheromatous plaque

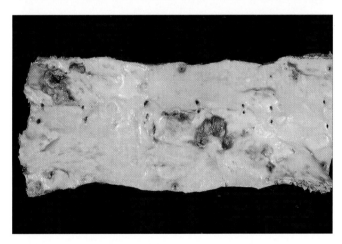

14   Section through a renal interlobular artery in essential hypertension showing reduplication of the internal elastic lamina. The lumen is reduced but patent.

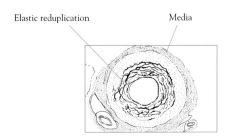

Elastic reduplication   Media

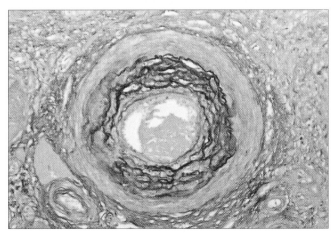

15 Microscopic appearance of hyaline arteriolar change in afferent glomerular arteriole due to essential hypertension. The hyaline deposit is sharply defined and the vessel lumen is patent.

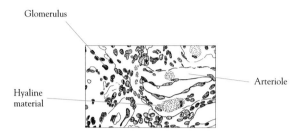

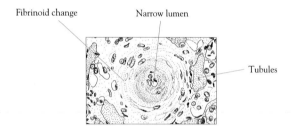

16 High-power photomicrograph of renal arteriole showing fibrinoid necrosis in malignant hypertension. The fibrin deposits are blurred and poorly localized compared with the hyaline deposits in essential hypertension.

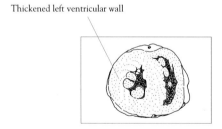

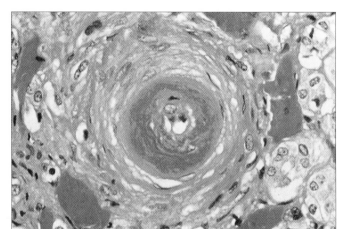

17 Transverse section of heart with concentric left ventricular hypertrophy due to hypertension. Small left ventricular cavity indicates absence of cardiac failure.

Thickened left ventricular wall

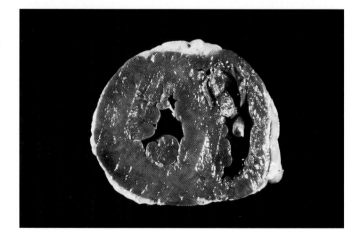

18 Chest X-ray showing pulmonary edema and bilateral pleural effusions following acute myocardial infarction.

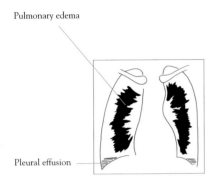

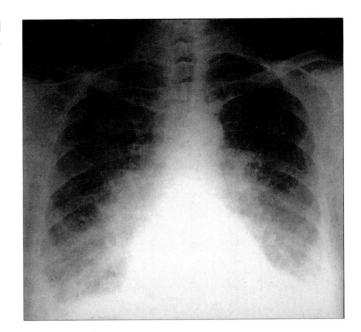

19 Transverse section of atheromatous coronary artery. The intima shows fibrous thickening with a large lipid deposit on one side leaving a reduced slit-like lumen.

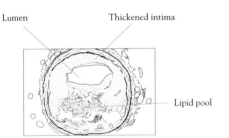

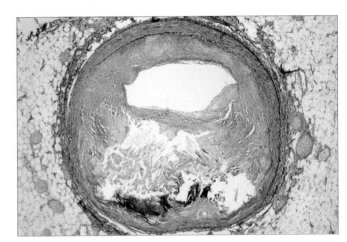

20 Charcot–Bouchard aneurysm lying along the course of a small intracerebral artery.

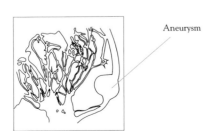

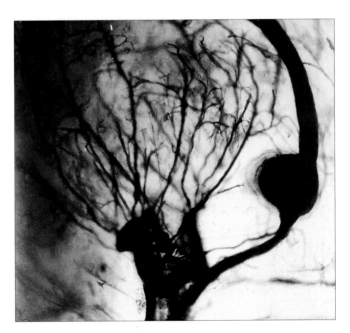

21   Microscopic section through an intact berry aneurysm on the circle of Willis. The aneurysm has a fibrous wall with no elastic tissue present.

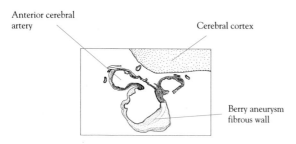

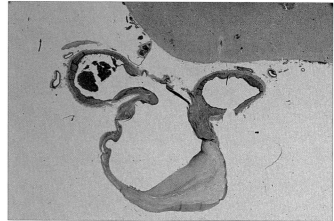

22   Inferior surface of the brain from a patient dying after extensive sub-arachnoid hemorrhage due to rupture of a large berry aneurysm.

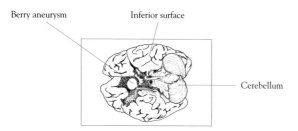

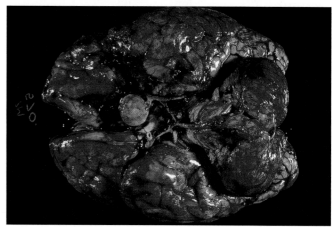

23   Hypertensive encephalopathy in a patient with severe hypertension of recent origin due to scleroderma.

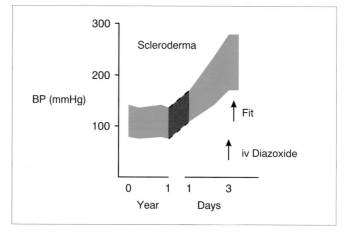

24   Nephrosclerosis due to essential hypertension causing cortical thinning with a granular capsular surface. The kidneys are atrophic due to ischemia.

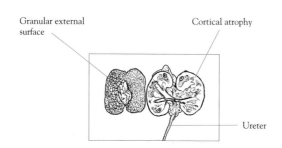

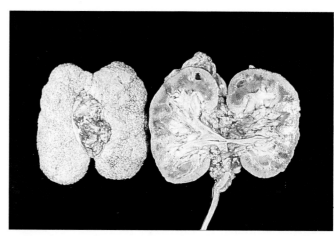

25 External surface of a kidney in malignant hypertension (BP 210/130 mmHg) showing 'flea-bitten' appearance due to tiny sub-capsular hemorrhages.

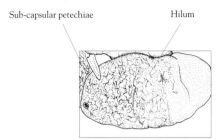

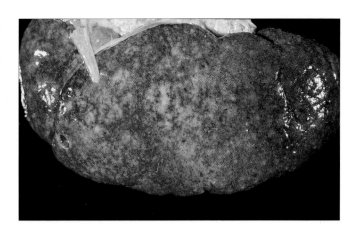

26 Changes in systolic blood pressure after two years in women aged 21–30 years taking estrogen–progestogen oral contraceptives and in controls.

Reproduced from the *Handbook of Hypertension*, Vol 2, 1983, with the permission of Dr RJ Weir and Elsevier Science Publishers.

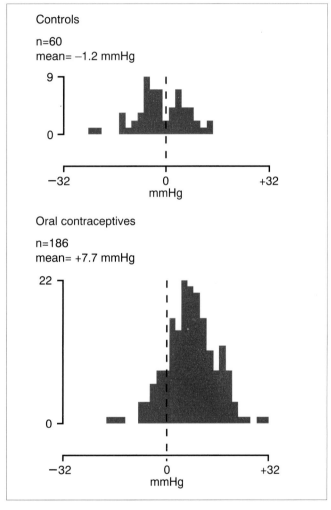

27 Left renal artery stenosis due to atheroma causing left renal atrophy and compensatory hypertrophy of the right kidney, which has three patent arteries. There is mild aortic atheroma.

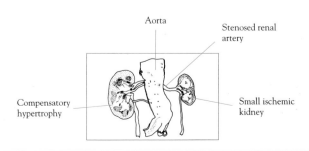

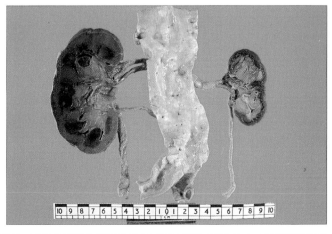

28 Long-standing renal artery stenosis has caused almost total tubular atrophy in the kidney with relative sparing of the glomeruli, which are protected from the effects of systemic hypertension by the renal artery stenosis.

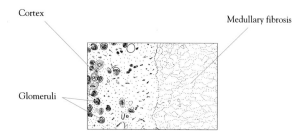

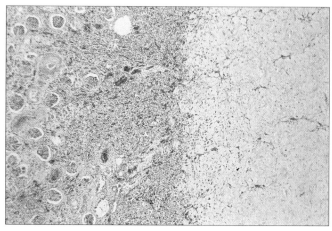

29 Large Wilms' tumor compressing the kidney from a 5-year-old child. The child presented with hypertension.

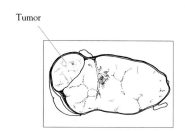

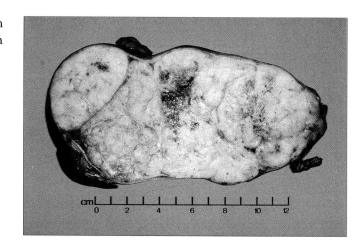

30 Intravenous urogram from hypertensive patient with contracted right kidney due to chronic pyelonephritis.

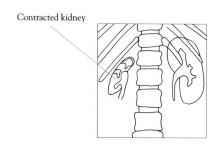

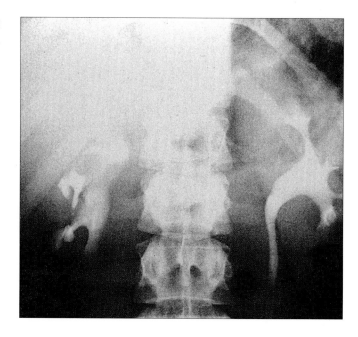

31 Fingers of a patient with scleroderma. The patient had been treated for Raynaud's disease for several years when she presented with a fit secondary to malignant hypertension. The patient died of renal failure two weeks later.

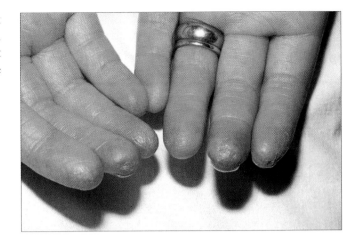

32 Proliferative glomerulonephritis. The glomerular tuft is hypercellular and swollen. Only a few glomerular capillary loops appear patent. The hypercellularity is due to increased numbers of mesangial and endothelial cells and to an infiltrate of neutrophil polymorphonuclear leukocytes. The latter are recognized by their lobed nuclei. There is no epithelial proliferation and Bowman's space remains clear.

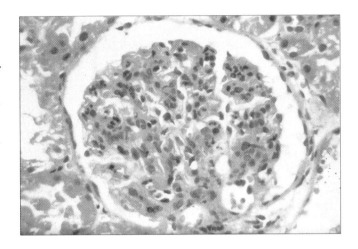

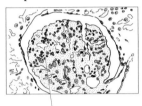

Neutrophil polymorphonuclear leukocytes

33 Advanced membranous glomerulonephritis. Resin section stained with hematoxylin and eosin shows uniform thickening of the glomerular capillaries on the edge of this biopsy. The glomerulus is of normal cellularity.

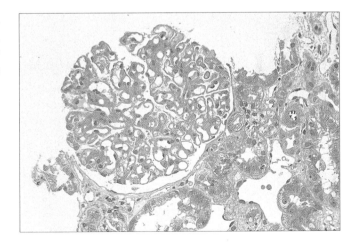

Thickened glomerular capillaries

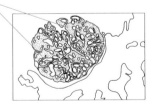

34 Minimal change glomerulonephritis. Electron micrograph from a male with nephrotic syndrome due to minimal change glomerulonephritis. There is total foot process fusion (arrows) of the epithelial cells on the outer surface of the glomerular capillary loops. There is no immune complex deposition or any other abnormality of the basement membrane.

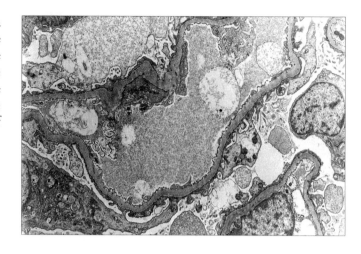

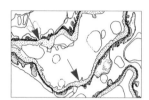

35 Facial appearance of patient who presented with moderate hypertension (BP 180/110 mmHg). She commented that her face had recently become rounded, which had been noted by her friends. A diagnosis of Cushing's syndrome with bilateral adrenal hyperplasia was subsequently made.

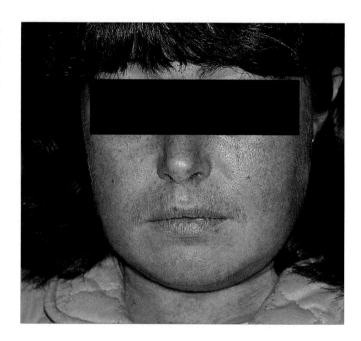

36 Adrenal adenoma in Cushing's syndrome. Removal resulted in resolution of Cushing's syndrome and restoration of blood pressure to normal.

Adrenal adenoma

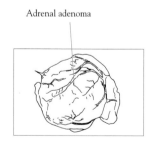

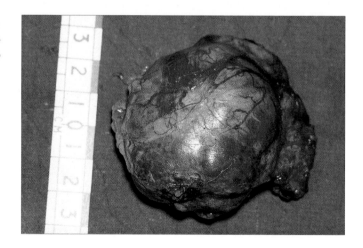

37 Adrenal gland removed at operation from a patient with primary aldosteronism. The orange tumor has been cut open.

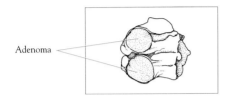

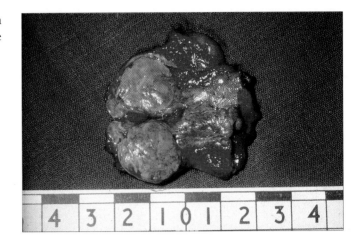

38 A typical adrenal pheochromocytoma forming a round brown nodule within the medulla and quite distinct from the yellow cortical layer.

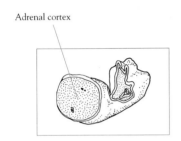

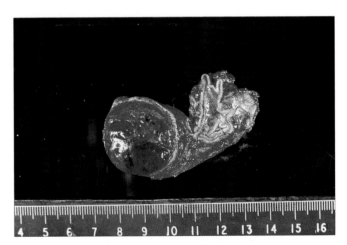

39 Electron micrograph (×33,000) of pheochromocytoma showing stored secretory granules.

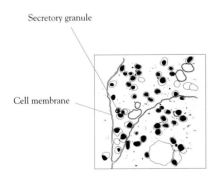

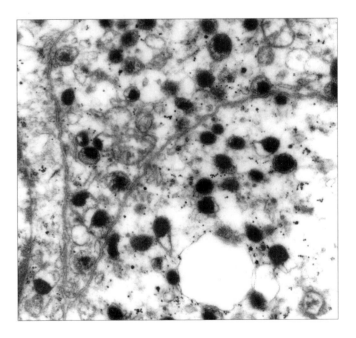

40 The overlap between diabetes, renal failure, and hypertension. There is an association between glucose intolerance, diabetes, obesity, and hypertension. These constitute a group at high cardiovascular risk. When diabetic nephropathy develops, the risk is increased further.

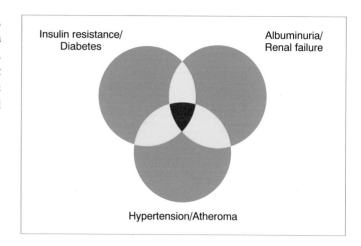

41 Coarctation of the aorta just distal to the left subclavian artery. A red probe is present through the coarctation and also through a coincidental ventricular septal defect.

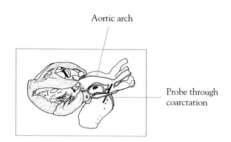

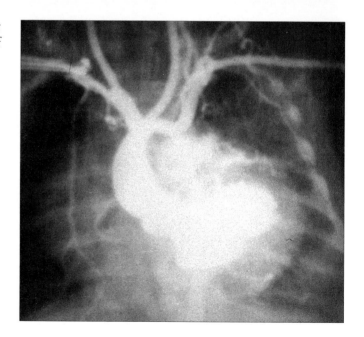

42 Left ventricular angiogram (antero-posterior projection) showing severe tubular hypoplasia of the aortic arch.

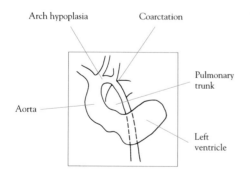

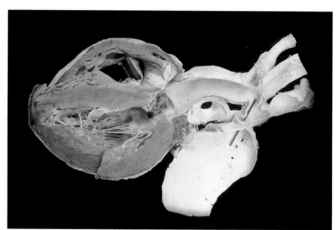

43 A swollen glomerulus from a patient dying of eclampsia shows thickening of the capillary walls due to cell swelling. The capillary loops are patent.

Swollen endothelial cells and narrowing capillary lumen

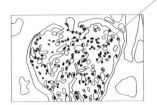

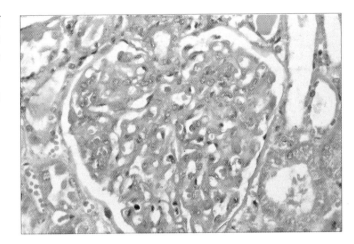

44 Red cell casts fill renal tubules and may be seen by microscopy of urine passed by patients with necrotizing glomerulonephritis and in some cases of malignant hypertension that cause glomerular bleeding.

Red cell casts

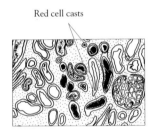

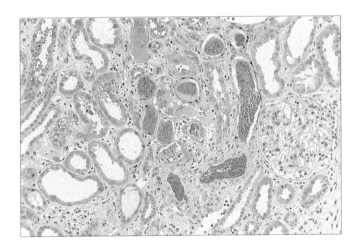

45

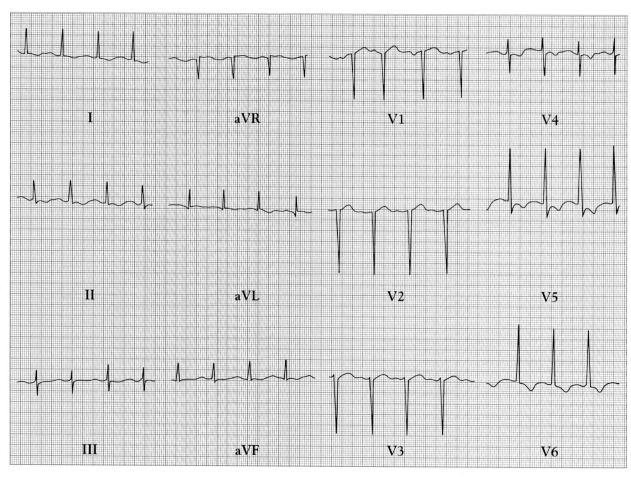

Electrocardiogram from patient with malignant hypertension. Voltage charges of left ventricular hypertrophy (deep S-waves in the right ventricular leads and tall R-waves in the left ventricular leads) are seen together with a 'strain' pattern (inverted T-waves in the left ventricular leads).

46 Chest X-ray showing left ventricular enlargement in a hypertensive patient. Note the increased cardiothoracic ratio.

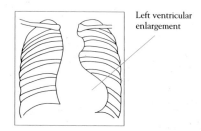

Left ventricular enlargement

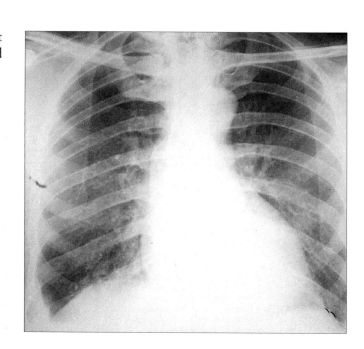

47 Chest X-ray from patient with left ventricular failure due to hypertension. Vascular engorgement gives rise to a 'bat's wing' appearance and distended lymphatics give rise to Kerley B-lines.

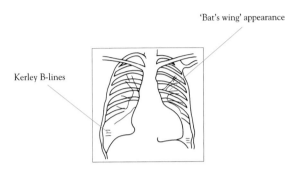

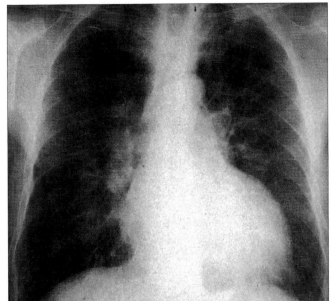

48 Chest X-ray from 20-year-old hypertensive patient. Coarctation is suggested by rib notching, bulging ascending aorta, and absence of aortic knuckle.

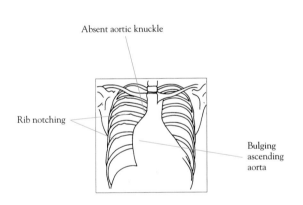

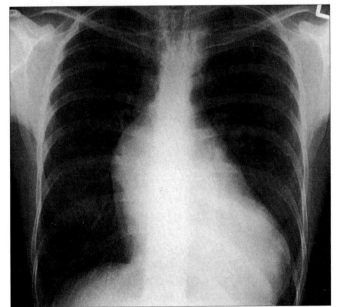

49 Ambulatory blood pressure monitor records patient's blood pressure reading during the course of the day.

Photograph courtesy of SpaceLabs Medical, Inc. 1994.

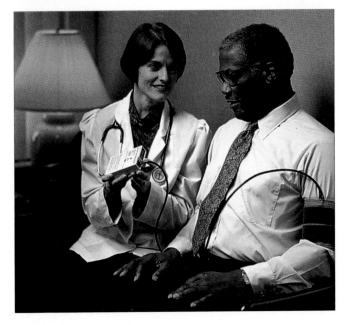

50 Twenty-four-hour ambulatory blood pressure recording using a non-invasive monitor in borderline and sustained hypertension.

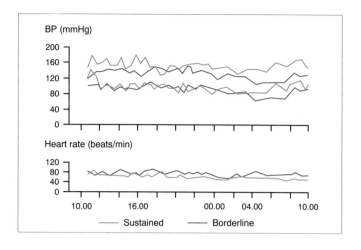

51

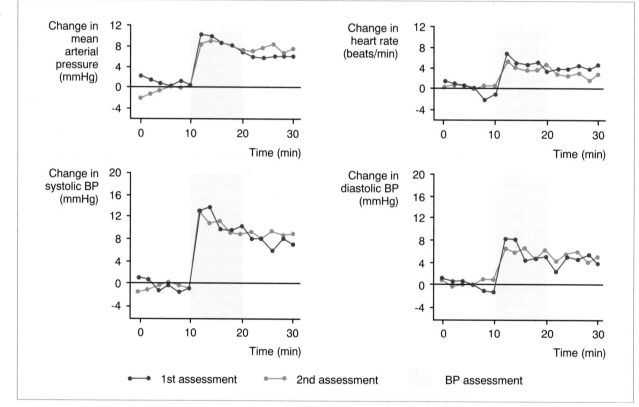

'White coat' hypertension. In this experiment, patients were visited twice by the same doctor. Each visit had the same, unmistakable effect, raising systolic and diastolic blood pressure.

Reproduced with the permission of Dr G Mancia.

52

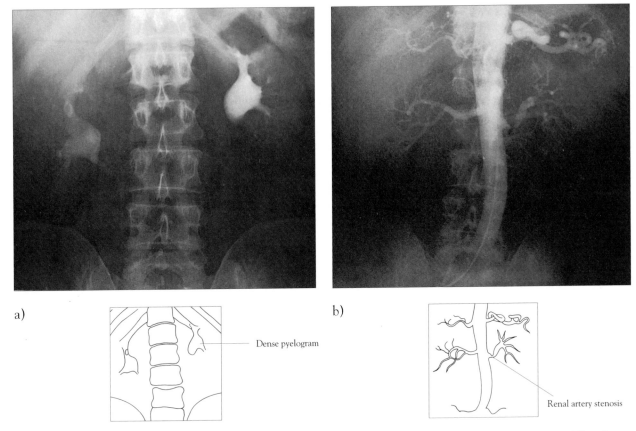

a)

Dense pyelogram

b)

Renal artery stenosis

(a) Intravenous urogram from patient with left renal artery stenosis at 20 minutes after injection. The dye is more concentrated in the pelvis of the left kidney. (b) Renal angiogram from the same patient. A tight stenosis is seen at the mouth of the left renal artery.

53 Intravenous urogram from hypertensive patient. Clubbing of the calyces is clearly visible on the contracted kidney.

Clubbed calyces

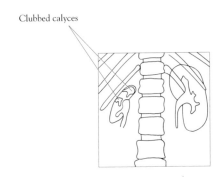

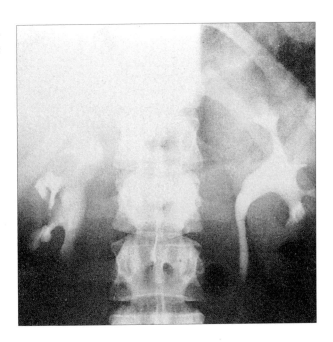

54 Intravenous urogram with tomography from hypertensive patient with contracted kidneys due to chronic glomerulonephritis.

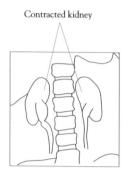

Contracted kidney

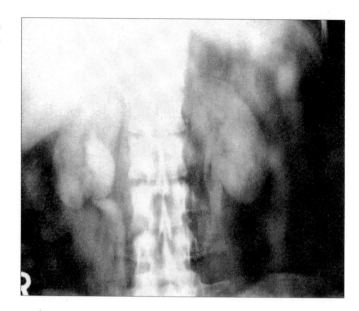

55 Intravenous urogram from patient with polycystic kidney showing calyces stretched over cysts.

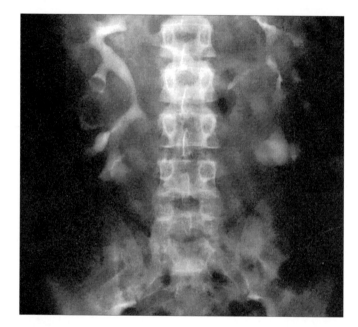

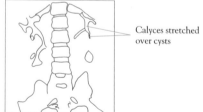

Calyces stretched over cysts

56 Intravenous urogram from patient with papillary necrosis due to analgesic nephropathy. Characteristic 'ring' shadows are caused by necrotic papillae.

'Ring' shadow

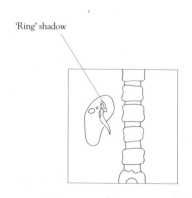

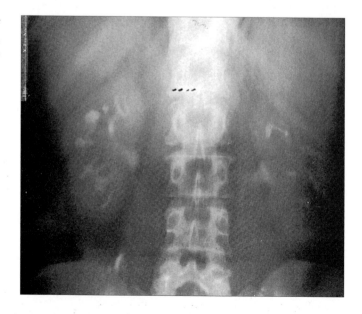

57 Digital subtraction angiogram from patient with left renal artery stenosis. A tight stenosis is present at the mouth of the left renal artery.

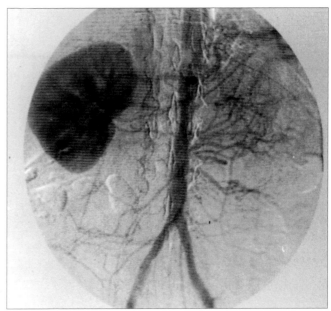

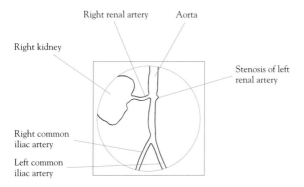

58 Arteriogram showing characteristic 'corkscrew' appearance from patient with fibromuscular dysplasia.

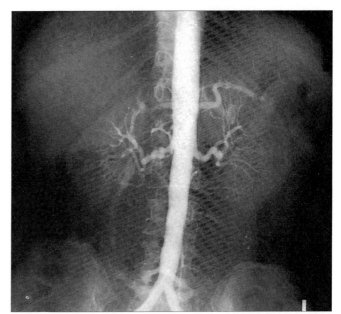

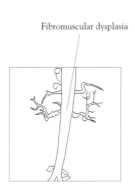

59 Right adrenal venogram from a patient with a pheochromocytoma. The vessels are displaced by the tumor.

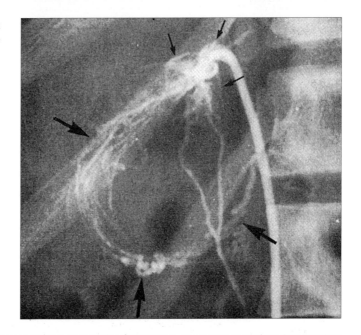

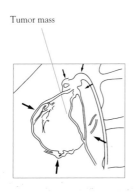

60 Ultrasound scan of kidney from patient with polycystic renal disease. Note the multiple large cysts.

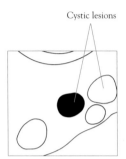

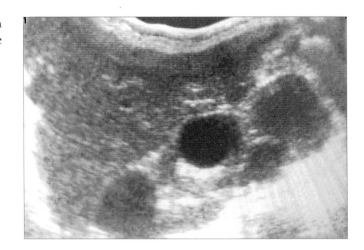

61 Isotope scan from patient with a right adrenal adenoma. Note the high concentration of isotope (shown by a brown 'hot spot' over the right adrenal).

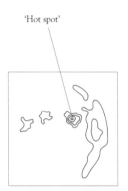

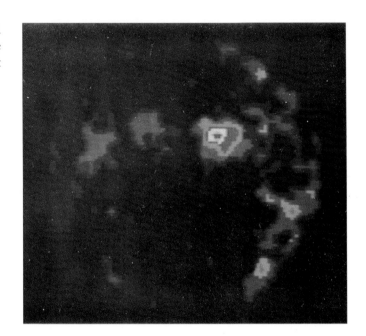

62 Patchy impairment of right renal blood flow (arrows) in a patient who suffered multiple embolization (technetium-labeled glucoheptinate scan).

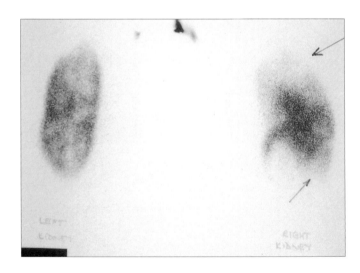

63

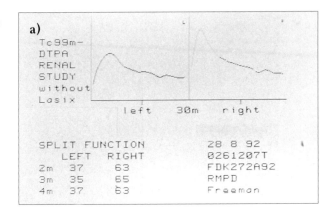
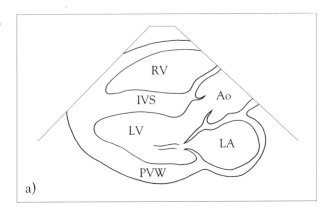

(a) Captopril renogram showing left renal artery stenosis in a man of 70 with hypertension which proved difficult to control. The peak activity is slightly delayed on the left. (b) After captopril the curve is further flattened so that no peak is obtained.

64

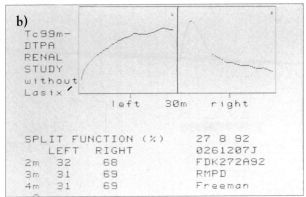

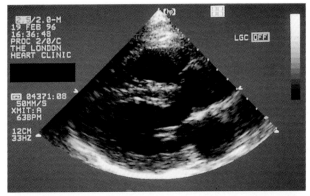

(a) Parasternal long-axis view showing moderately severe concentric left ventricular hypertrophy caused by hypertension. (b) M-mode recording from the same patient showing measurements of wall thicknesses and end-diastolic and end-systolic cavity dimensions.

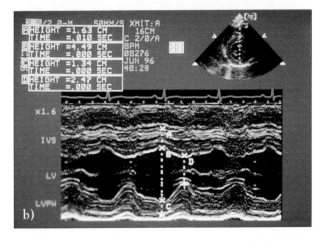

65 M-mode recording showing severe left ventricular hypertrophy. Both the interventricular septum and the posterior ventricular wall are more than 1.6 cm thick. The left ventricular cavity is relatively small, particularly the end-systolic dimension. Systolic shortening fraction remains within normal limits.

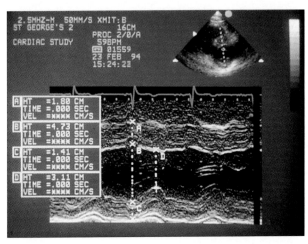

66

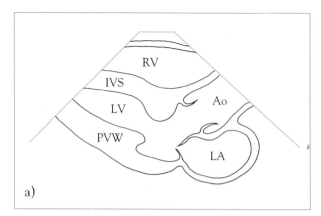

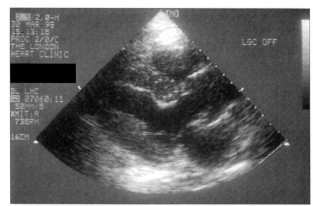

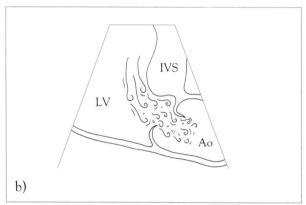

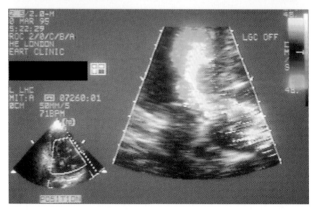

(a) Parasternal long-axis view showing a prominent 'upper septal bulge', or 'sigmoid septum' in a patient who also has moderately severe concentric hypertrophy due to hypertension. This is a relatively common finding, particularly in elderly subjects, and is considered benign. (b) Magnified apical long-axis view with color-flow Doppler showing flow acceleration in the left ventricular outflow tract which is causing an ejection systolic murmur.

67

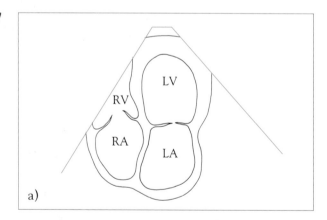

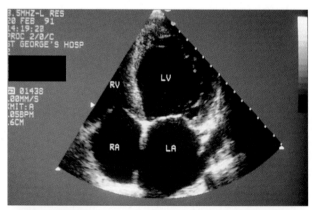

Hypertensive heart failure. (a) Apical four-chamber view showing enlargement of all four cardiac chambers, particularly on the left side. (b) M-mode recording showing the enlarged left ventricle with reduced systolic shortening fraction. Relative to the cavity size, the ventricular walls do not appear abnormal, but they are significantly thickened at about 1.5 cm.

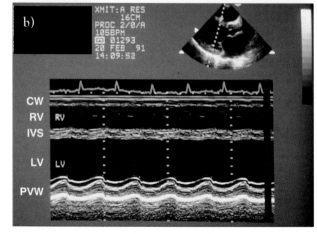

68

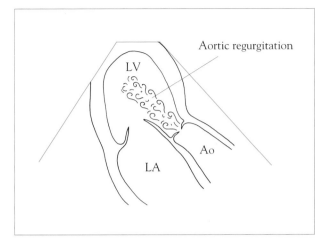
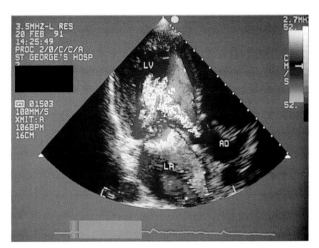

Apical long-axis view of the same patient as in [67] with color-flow Doppler showing moderately severe aortic regurgitation.

69 The isovolumic relaxation time (IVRT) is defined as the interval between aortic valve closure and mitral valve opening. It can readily be measured with pulsed Doppler. From an apical view, the sample gate is positioned between the mitral and aortic valves and lengthened to encompass flow through both valves. Sweep speed is maximized and the time interval between the respective valve motion artefacts is measured. This is normally 60–100 ms, but is longer when myocardial relaxation is impaired, as in this case from a patient with hypertension.

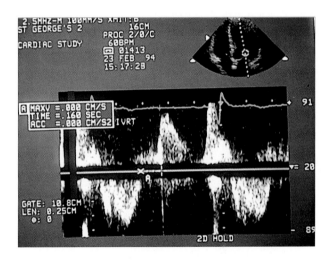

70 Normal transmitral diastolic flow pattern recorded with pulsed Doppler. Early diastolic filling accounts for the majority of ventricular filling ('e' wave) and atrial systole causes the much smaller 'a' wave. The relative filling fractions can be assessed from the areas under the two phases, and approximated from their peak amplitudes. The clinical value of this measurement is limited due to wide variation in normal values and age-related changes.

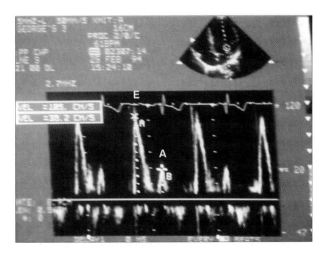

71 Very abnormal transmitral filling pattern in a patient with severe hypertension. The 'e' wave amplitude is reduced and the rate of decay very slow — comparable to that of quite severe mitral stenosis. The majority of filling occurs following atrial contraction.

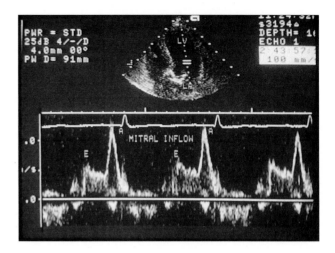

72 (a) Left ventricular hypertrophy. Coronal image through the aortic valve and left ventricle in a patient with hypertension (diastole). (b) There is severe symmetric hypertrophy with almost total obliteration of the left ventricular cavity at end-systole.

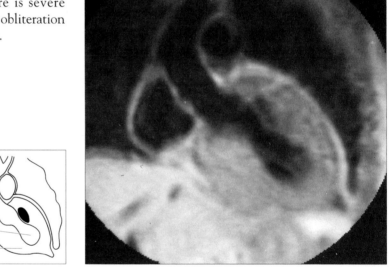

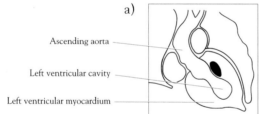

a)

Ascending aorta

Left ventricular cavity

Left ventricular myocardium

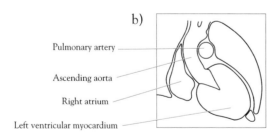

b)

Pulmonary artery

Ascending aorta

Right atrium

Left ventricular myocardium

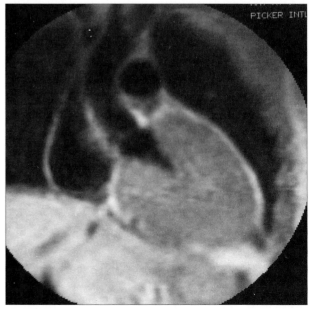

73 Normal kidneys. Coronal section through both kidneys. On the left, the distinction between cortex and medulla can be seen.

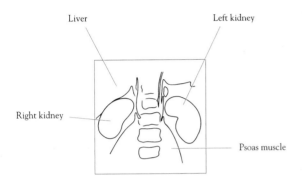

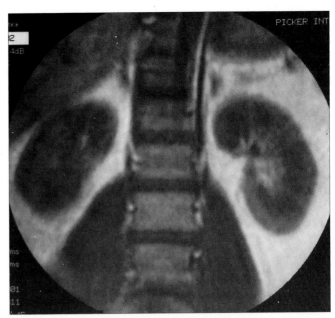

74 Renal arteries. Coronal section through the abdominal aorta showing the origins of both renal arteries. The inferior vena cava, the lower pole of the right kidney, and the right ureter are also seen.

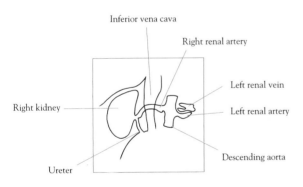

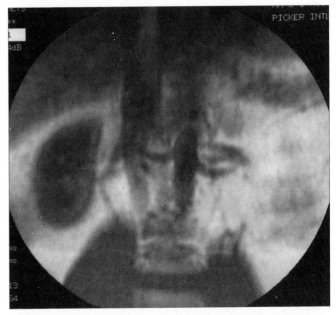

75 Coarctation. Oblique section through the aortic arch showing a coarctation just beyond the origin of the left subclavian artery.

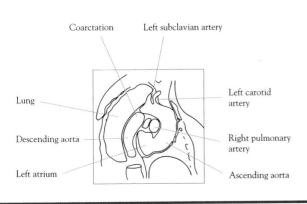

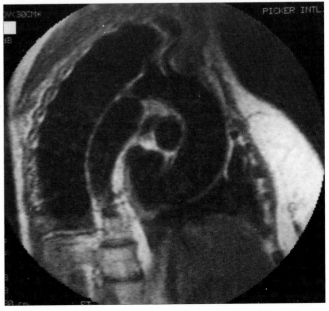

76 Dissection. Four coronal sections through the aortic arch from posterior (top left) to anterior (bottom right). There is an intimal flap dividing the lumen into true and false channels.

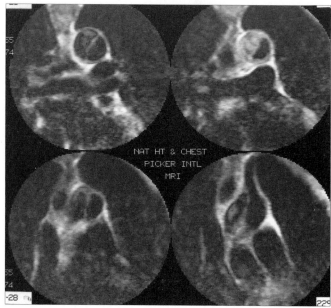

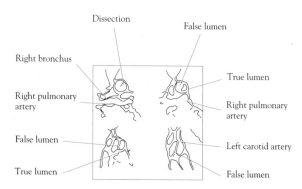

77 The management of mild hypertension.

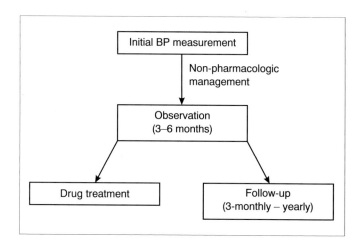

78 The non-pharmacologic management of hypertension.

- Weight reduction

- Reduction of heavy alcohol intake

- Salt restriction

- Regular exercise

CHAPTER 4
Valve Disease

MITRAL STENOSIS

MITRAL REGURGITATION

AORTIC STENOSIS

AORTIC REGURGITATION

TRICUSPID VALVE DISEASE

Abbreviations

a	Anterior leaflet	MR	Mitral regurgitation
AMVL	Anterior mitral valve leaflets	MV	Mitral valve
Ao	Aorta	MVL	Mitral valve leaflets
AV	Aortic valve	p	Posterior leaflet
AVL	Aortic valve leaflets	PAWP	Pulmonary artery wedge pressure
CW	Chest wall	PCWP	Pulmonary capillary wedge pressure
En	Endocardium	PE	Pericardial effusion
Ep	Epicardium	PMVL	Posterior mitral valve leaflets
FA	Femoral artery	PVW	Posterior ventricular wall
IVC	Inferior vena cava	RA	Right atrium
IVS	Interventricular septum	RV	Right ventricle
LA	Left atrium	SVC	Superior vena cava
LCA	Left coronary artery	TR	Tricuspid regurgitation
LV	Left ventricle	TV	Tricuspid valve
LVDP	Left ventricular diastolic pressure	TVL	Tricuspid valve leaflets
LVOT	Left ventricular outflow tract	Veg	Vegetation

The principal valve diseases encountered in adults are disorders of the mitral and aortic valves. Primary isolated tricuspid and pulmonary valve disease are very uncommon.

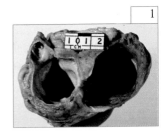

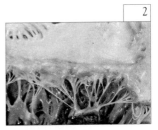

MITRAL STENOSIS

Definition

Mitral stenosis can be defined as a reduction in the effective mitral valve orifice area, which is normally 5–6 cm^2 [1]. Virtually all cases of mitral stenosis are rheumatic in etiology. Congenital abnormalities, systemic lupus erythematosus, and mucopolysaccharidosis are rare causes of mitral stenosis.

Pathology

During the acute phase of rheumatic fever, the valvular endocardium shows edema and inflammatory cell infiltration, with areas of endothelial denudation exposing subendothelial collagen and other thrombotic materials to the circulating blood. The endothelial changes are important in the genesis of the rheumatic valvular deformities. The pertinent features of rheumatic endocarditis are formation of flat vegetations, consisting largely of platelets, on the closure lines of the valve leaflets [2]. During the acute phase of rheumatic fever, edema and stiffening of the mitral valve leaflets may produce restricted valve movement. These pathologic features may be accompanied clinically by the presence of an apical low-pitched mid-diastolic murmur (Carey-Coombs murmur). Rheumatic myocarditis has a specific histologic picture typified by the presence of Aschoff bodies, which are microscopic foci of degenerate collagen surrounded by giant cells. Aschoff bodies are present in approximately 50% of patients with chronic rheumatic valvular heart disease. Rheumatic pericarditis is non-specific with an acute fibrinous exudate.

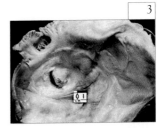

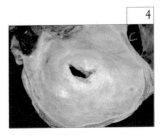

In rheumatic mitral stenosis, fusion of the anterior and posterior commissures reduces the anatomic mitral valve area to a varying degree [3]. Mild to moderate stenosis frequently gives the valve a fish-mouth appearance with relatively mobile leaflets [4]. Severe commissural fusion produces a marked narrowing of the mitral valve orifice, giving it the appearance of a buttonhole. Cusp fibrosis and calcification of the deformed valves contribute to its rigidity [5]. Chordal fibrosis, fusion, and shortening may produce subvalvular stenosis, which may be more important than orifice stenosis in some instances. The left atrium is enlarged to a variable degree and frequently contains thrombus, which may be the source of systemic emboli [6].

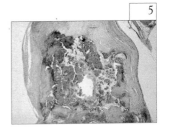

Presentation

Symptoms
The main symptom is breathlessness on exertion, which is caused by a rise in left atrial pressure with a passive increase in pulmonary venous pressure. Dyspnea develops gradually in about 50% of patients. An asymptomatic period of 20 years or longer after the episode of rheumatic fever is not uncommon. Sometimes the onset of symptoms coincides with the onset of atrial fibrillation or pregnancy. Patients with severe mitral stenosis may develop orthopnea and paroxysmal nocturnal dyspnea.

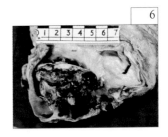

Hemoptysis, which occurs in approximately 15% of patients with mitral stenosis, usually results from pulmonary edema. Pulmonary infarction and rupture of the bronchial venous varicosities are other, less common causes of hemoptysis which almost always indicate severe mitral stenosis. Symptoms of systemic embolism include transient cerebral ischemia: this may occur in patients with paroxysmal or established atrial fibrillation. Fatigue due to low cardiac output usually occurs in patients with severe mitral stenosis and pulmonary hypertension.

Angina-like symptoms may occur in some patients with severe pulmonary hypertension in the absence of coronary artery disease, and these have been thought to represent right ventricular ischemia. Palpitation may be a presenting feature in patients with rheumatic heart disease, usually due to atrial tachyarrhythmias.

Signs

The patient may have cyanotic patches with distended venules over the cheeks — the so-called mitral facies. The arterial pulse volume and character are usually normal; the pulse volume may be decreased in patients with severe mitral stenosis with a low cardiac output. The jugular venous pressure may be elevated when secondary right ventricular failure occurs with or without secondary tricuspid regurgitation. A prominent 'a' wave in the jugular venous pulse may be present in patients with pulmonary hypertension and right ventricular hypertrophy. Tricuspid regurgitation is associated with a prominent 'v' wave and a sharp 'y' descent. The 'tapping' apex beat is due to a palpable loud first heart sound. A sustained parasternal impulse may indicate right ventricular hypertrophy. Left atrial systolic pulsation due to associated mitral regurgitation may also cause a similar left parasternal lift.

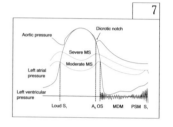

A loud first heart sound, an opening snap, followed by a low-pitched mid-diastolic murmur are the usual auscultatory findings of mitral stenosis. In the presence of sinus rhythm, a crescendo presystolic murmur is also frequently heard. The longer the duration of the mid-diastolic murmur and the shorter the aortic valve closure sound (A_2)–opening snap interval, the more severe the mitral stenosis will be [7]. However, when cardiac output is low due to associated severe pulmonary hypertension, and if the mitral valve is heavily calcified and immobile, these auscultatory findings may be markedly modified or may even be absent ('silent' mitral stenosis). Signs of pulmonary hypertension with a loud pulmonary component of the second heart sound, an early diastolic murmur due to pulmonary insufficiency (Graham-Steel murmur), a left parasternal lift, and tricuspid regurgitation may dominate the clinical picture in some patients with severe mitral stenosis.

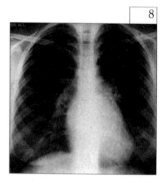

Radiology

The plain chest X-ray shows left atrial enlargement, visible as a double shadow at the right heart border, and splaying of the left bronchus [8]. Typically in mitral stenosis a prominent left atrial appendage is also seen [9]. If the pulmonary venous pressure is elevated, the upper zone vessels are dilated [10]. With higher pressures in the pulmonary veins, septal lines and pleural effusions may appear [11]. With chronic disease, the valve frequently becomes calcified [12]. In long-standing cases, hemosiderin deposits may be found in the lungs, seen as widespread mottling [13]. In patients with mixed stenosis and

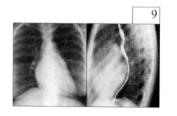

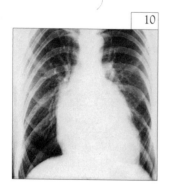

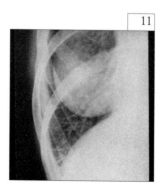

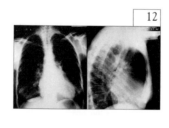

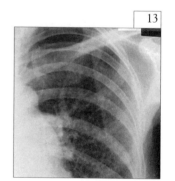

regurgitation, the left atrium may become very large and calcified [14,15]. Linear calcification of the left atrial wall may also result from calcification of mural thrombus, which almost always suggests severe mitral stenosis. Long-standing pulmonary venous hypertension gives rise to pulmonary arterial hypertension. This is reflected in a large pulmonary trunk and a greater discrepancy in size between the large upper zone and the smaller lower zone vessels [16]. In pure mitral stenosis, marked cardiomegaly is unusual. However, associated tricuspid regurgitation with right atrial and right ventricular enlargement may produce marked cardiac enlargement.

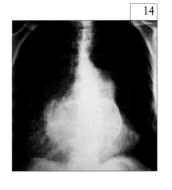

Electrocardiography
In sinus rhythm, the electrocardiogram shows P mitrale with broad notched P-waves, usually in leads II and aVF, and a prominent negative P vector in V1 [17]. Varying degrees of right ventricular hypertrophy with right axis deviation, R/S greater than 1 in V1, deep S in V6 and lead I, and small amplitude of QRS in lead V1 are seen with pulmonary hypertension. A QR pattern in V1 suggests severe right ventricular hypertrophy and a near systemic level of pulmonary vascular resistance [18]. Atrial fibrillation is common in the later stages of the disease.

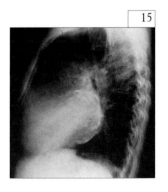

Echocardiography
Echocardiographic evaluation and Doppler studies have emerged as the most useful and essential investigations in the assessment of valvular heart disease. In mitral stenosis, commissural fusion causes abnormal movement of the mitral leaflets. On the M-mode echocardiogram, the posterior leaflet moves forward in diastole in the same direction as the anterior leaflet [19]. The 'a' wave is markedly diminished (absent with atrial fibrillation). The thickened leaflets return stronger echoes than normal, and when calcification is present, multiple dense echoes are seen.

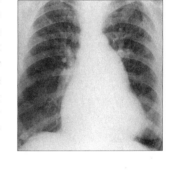

The two-dimensional echocardiogram enables visualization of the abnormal valve and its deranged movement [20]. It also allows direct measurement of the mitral valve orifice area using the parasternal short-axis view [21]. Two-dimensional echocardiography is also useful for the assessment of left and right ventricular function and of changes in the sizes of all four cardiac chambers [22]. In patients with pure or predominant mitral stenosis, left ventricular size is normal but the left atrium is enlarged. In patients with pulmonary hypertension and right heart failure, right ventricular and right atrial enlargement are seen. Left ventricular ejection fraction is usually normal, although in some patients left ventricular systolic function is depressed, with a wall-motion abnormality of the posterior basal segments of the left ventricle. Transesophageal echocardiography provides better anatomic delineation [23] and is more likely to detect left atrial thrombus [24].

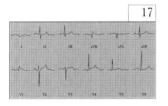 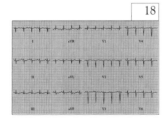 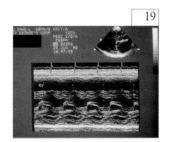 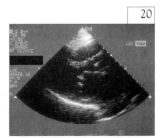

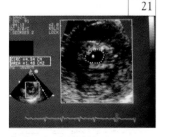 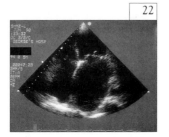 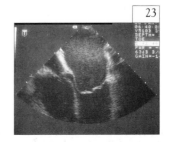 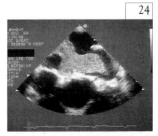

Continuous-wave Doppler is extremely useful in assessing the severity of mitral stenosis [25]. The velocity of blood flow allows the pressure gradient across the mitral valve during diastole to be determined, using the Bernoulli principle ($P_1-P_2=4V_{max}^2$). Correct alignment of the ultrasound beam with the blood jet can be ensured with the help of color Doppler [26]. The mitral valve area can also be calculated by measuring the rate of decay of the Doppler-measured maximum velocity (so-called 'pressure half-time' method) [27].

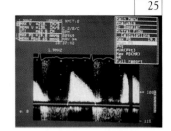

Color Doppler facilitates the diagnosis of coexisting mitral regurgitation and other valve lesions [28]. Continuous-wave Doppler is useful in assessing the degree of pulmonary hypertension in patients with mitral stenosis [29].

Magnetic Resonance Imaging (MRI) and Computed Tomography (CT)
Both cardiac MRI and CT can demonstrate chamber enlargement, mitral valve abnormalities, and changes in ventricular function. However, neither MRI nor CT provides any advantage over other imaging modalities and they are not indicated in the routine diagnosis and management of mitral stenosis.

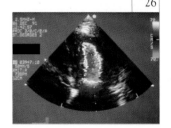

Cardiac Catheterization and Angiography
Unless information about the coronary arteries is required, cardiac catheterization is unnecessary in most cases of mitral stenosis. In the occasional patient, catheterization is performed to assess changes in pulmonary artery pressure and pulmonary capillary wedge pressure during exercise, to clarify the mechanism of exercise-induced symptoms. Assessment of the severity of associated mitral regurgitation may also require left ventriculography.

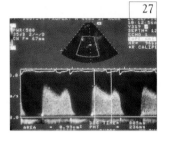

In a typical case of mitral stenosis, pulmonary capillary wedge pressure will be elevated and left ventricular diastolic pressure will be normal, demonstrating a transmitral diastolic pressure gradient [30]. The pressure gradient is proportional to the severity of mitral stenosis. Simultaneous determination of cardiac output allows measurement of mitral valve area, which in critical stenosis is 1 cm^2 or less. Pressure and cardiac output measurements also allow determination of pulmonary vascular resistance, which can be significantly elevated in some patients with long-standing severe mitral stenosis. Angiocardiography is usually carried out to assess the severity of mitral regurgitation and left ventricular function [31].

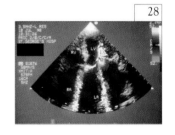

Principles of Management

Symptomatic patients with hemodynamically significant mitral stenosis require balloon-catheter valvuloplasty, surgical valvotomy, or valve replacement [32]. The results of catheter mitral valvuloplasty are comparable to those of closed or open surgical

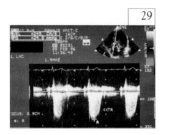

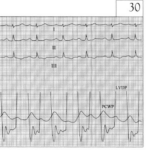

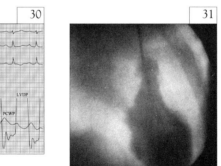

1. Symptomatic patients with hemodynamically significant mitral stenosis: catheter (valvuloplasty), surgical valvotomy, or valve replacement

2. Transesophageal echocardiography prior to catheter valvuloplasty to exclude left atrial thrombus (a contraindication to valvuloplasty)

3. Patients with a heavily calcified distorted mitral valve are more suitable for valve replacement

4. Patients with atrial fibrillation require digitalization and long-term anticoagulation

5. Antibiotic prophylaxis for bacterial endocarditis

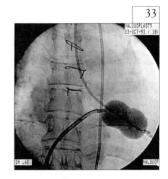

valvotomy [33–35]. Transesophageal echocardiography should be performed to exclude left atrial thrombus and severe disorganization of subvalvular structures, which are contraindications for catheter valvuloplasty. Valve replacement is more suitable for heavily calcified distorted mitral valves.

Patients with atrial fibrillation require digitalization and long-term anticoagulation in an attempt to prevent systemic embolism. Antibiotic prophylaxis is recommended for dental treatment.

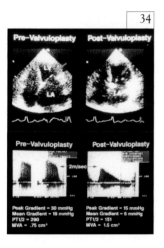

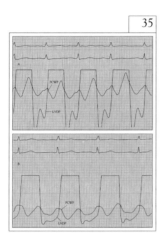

1 Fully open normal mitral and tricuspid valves viewed from left and right atria.

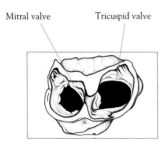

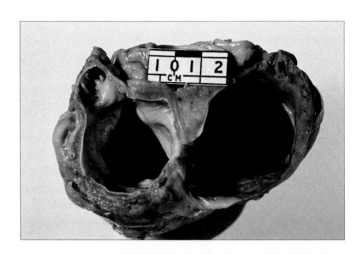

2 Mitral valve in the acute phase of rheumatic fever showing the characteristic row of small sessile vegetations along the line of closure.

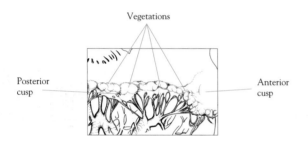

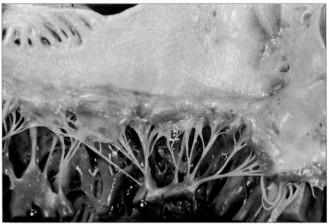

3 Rheumatic mitral stenosis viewed from left atrium. The valve orifice is a small crescentic fixed opening. The atrium is enlarged. Some calcification is present in the anterior cusp.

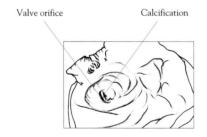

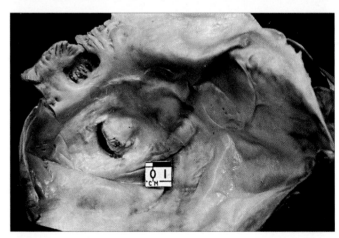

4 Mitral stenosis viewed from the left atrium. The valve orifice has a 'fish-mouth' shape. A small thrombus fills the left atrial appendage.

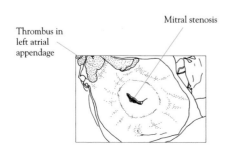

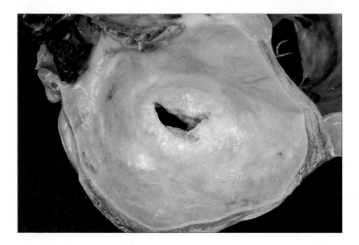

5 Histology of a rheumatic mitral valve. The valve is thickened with masses of dystrophic calcification.

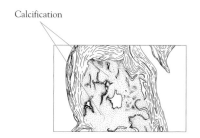

Calcification

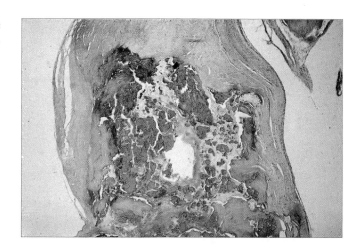

6 Typical mitral stenosis viewed from left atrium. The valve orifice is a small oval. A large mass of thrombus almost fills the atrium arising from the left atrial appendage.

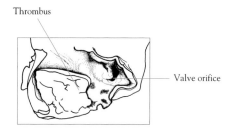

Thrombus

Valve orifice

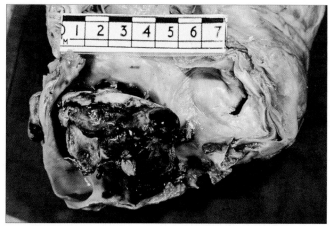

7 Diagrammatic illustration of the auscultatory findings in pure mitral stenosis. Due to mitral valve obstruction, left atrial pressure increases to maintain diastolic flow and there is a diastolic transmitral pressure gradient. The more severe the stenosis, the longer is the duration of this pressure gradient, explaining a longer duration of the mid-diastolic low-pitched murmur in more severe mitral stenosis. During left atrial systole, transmitral flow increases, explaining the pre-systolic murmur. At end-diastole, the mitral valve remains in an open position due to the pressure gradient, and thus the rate of mitral valve closure increases at the beginning of isovolumic systole, which explains the increased intensity of the first

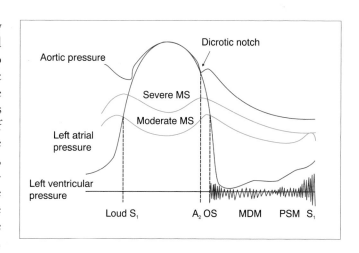

heart sound. The opening snap coincides with the opening of the mitral valve at the end of the isovolumic relaxation period, when the pressure in the left ventricle falls below the pressure in the left atrium. With increased left atrial pressure due to mitral stenosis, this pressure crossover point comes closer to the aortic dicrotic notch, which marks the time of aortic valve closure and the aortic component of the second heart sound.

With increasing severity of mitral stenosis with higher left atrial pressure, the dicrotic notch mitral valve opening interval gets shorter, explaining the inverse relation between the severity of mitral stenosis and the A_2–opening snap interval.

S_1=First heart sound; A_2=aortic component of the second heart sound; OS=opening snap; MDM=mid-diastolic murmur; PSM=presystolic murmur; MS=mitral stenosis.

8   Chest X-ray showing left atrial enlargement.

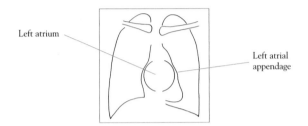

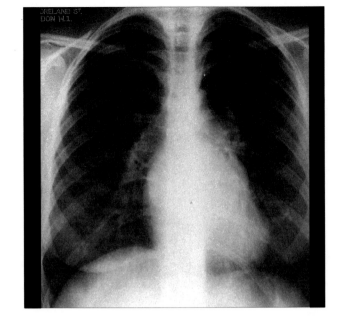

9

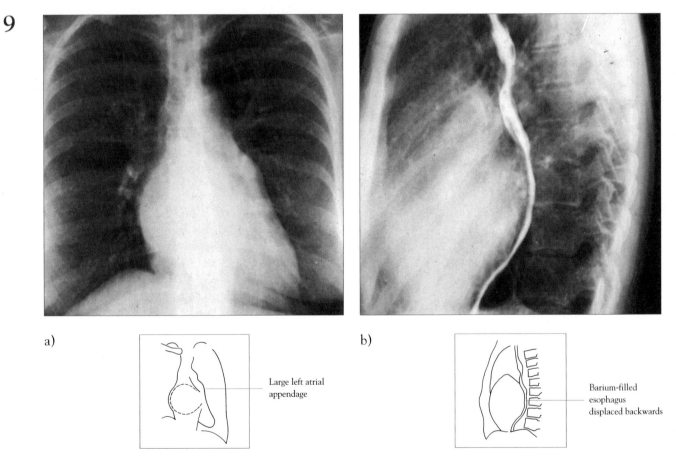

a)

b)

Frontal (a) and lateral (b) views of the chest in mitral valve disease. The double shadow of the large left atrium can be seen on the right. Note how it disappears beyond the spine going to the left. There is a localized bulge on the left upper heart border in the position of the left atrial appendage. The left bronchus is elevated. The descending thoracic aorta is slightly displaced to the left. The barium-filled esophagus, in immediate posterior relation to the left atrium, is displaced posteriorly over the length of contact with the left atrium.

10 Chest X-ray of a patient with mitral valve disease showing (1) enlargement of left atrium, (2) distended upper lobe pulmonary veins, and (3) constricted lower lobe veins.

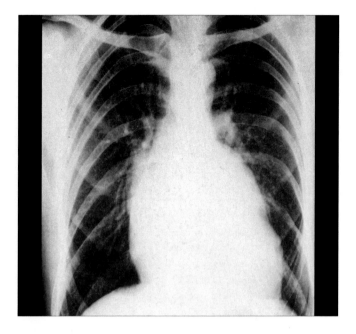

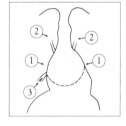

11 Detail from chest X-ray showing septal lines and pleural effusion.

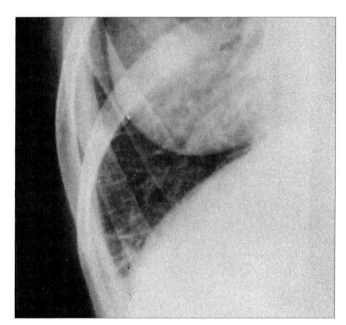

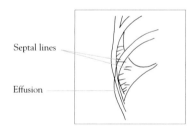

12

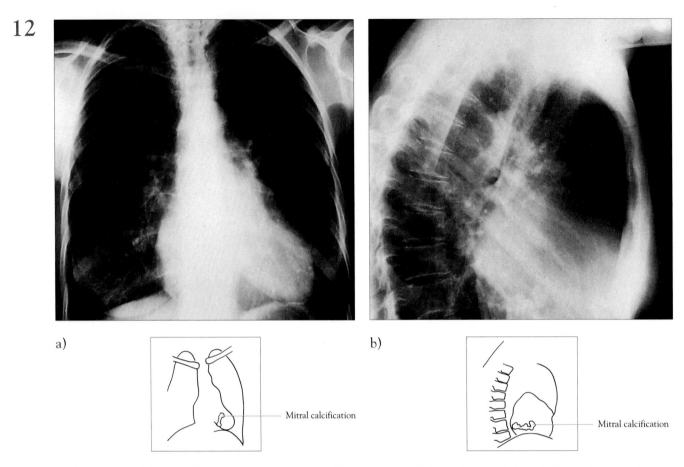

a) b)

Calcification of the mitral valve in mitral stenosis. The penetrated frontal view (a) and the right lateral view (b) show marked calcification in the position of the mitral valve. This is a particularly florid example and calcification is often difficult or impossible to see on the plain chest X-ray, particularly in the frontal view.

13 Hemosiderosis in chronic mitral valve disease. In this localized view of the lung field in a patient with mitral valve disease, the nodules of hemosiderosis can be seen.

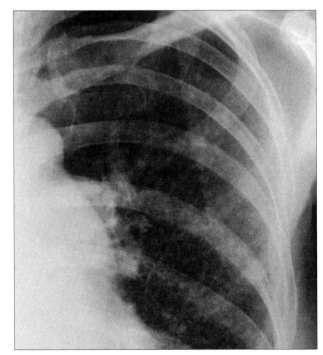

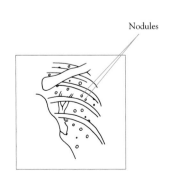

14   Chest X-ray (penetrated postero-anterior view) showing a very large, calcified left atrium.

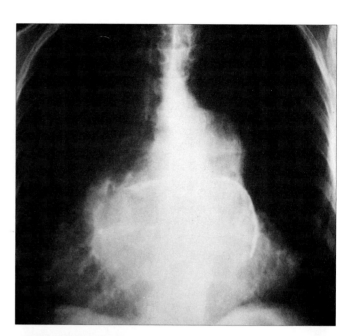

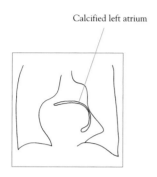

Calcified left atrium

15   Chest X-ray (lateral projection) from same patient as in [14] showing calcified left atrium.

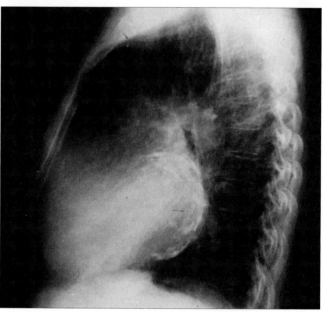

Calcified left atrium

16   Chest X-ray showing a large pulmonary trunk and upper zone vessels. Lower segmental vessels are small.

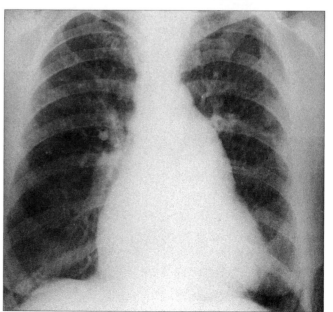

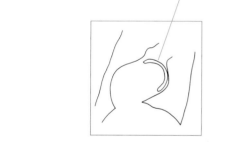

Large upper lobe vessels

Large pulmonary trunk

Small segmental vessels

17

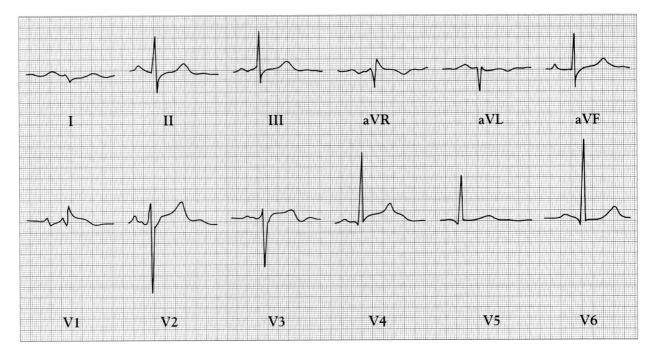

Electrocardiogram of moderately severe mitral stenosis showing the broad bifid P-wave of left atrial enlargement (P mitrale), with right ventricular hypertrophy as shown by a dominant R-wave in lead V1. Note: for V3 to V5 1 mV =0.5 cm.

18

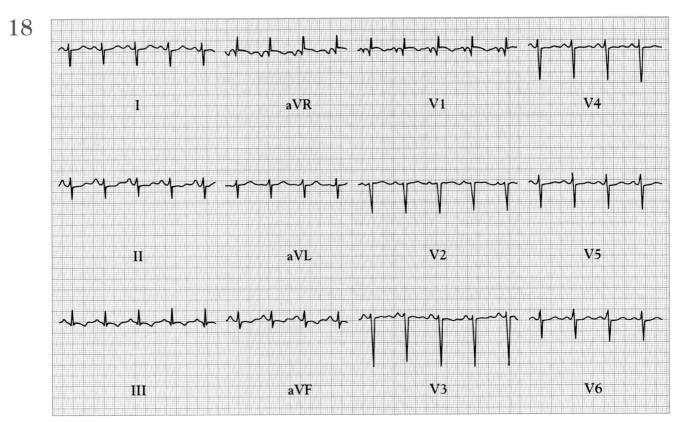

A QR pattern in V1 with right-axis deviation suggests severe right ventricular hypertrophy and marked increase in pulmonary vascular resistance.

19   M-mode recording from a patient with moderately severe mitral stenosis. The leaflets are thickened and relatively immobile. As a result of commissural fusion, the posterior leaflet moves in the same direction as the anterior during diastole. There is no mid-diastolic closure or re-opening with atrial systole, even though the patient is in sinus rhythm.

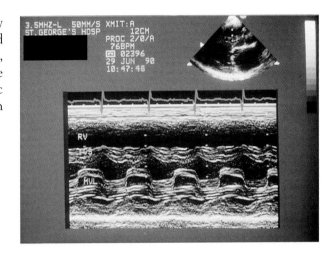

20

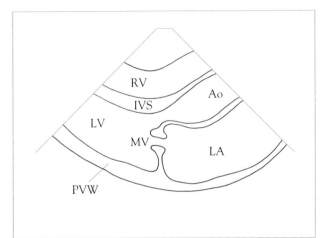

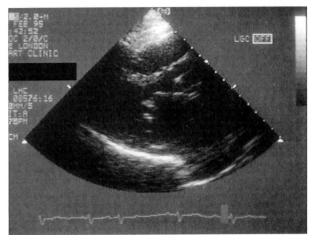

Parasternal long-axis view of mitral stenosis. The valve leaflets are thickened, with 'clubbed' tips and commissural fusion gives the anterior leaflet a characteristic 'elbow' shape. The greatly reduced valve orifice is evident. The left atrium is enlarged.

21   Magnified parasternal short-axis view of the mitral valve orifice in mitral stenosis showing measurement of the valve orifice area by planimetry.

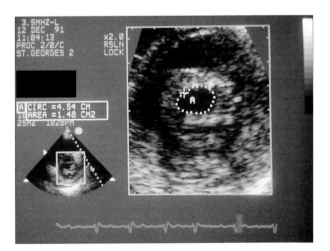

22

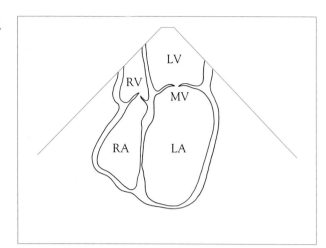

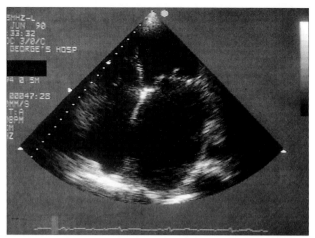

Apical four-chamber view of mitral stenosis, showing the chamber enlargement and displaced interatrial septum resulting from high left atrial pressure. Thickening of the mitral valve leaflets is evident.

23

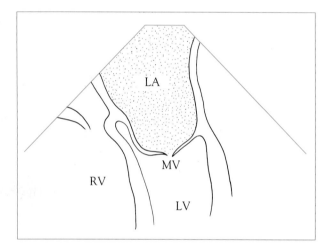

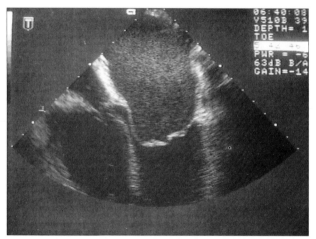

Transesophageal study in a patient with mitral stenosis being evaluated for suitability for balloon valvuloplasty. The speckled pattern in the large left atrium is 'spontaneous echo contrast' — a phenomenon arising from interaction of high-frequency ultrasound with static blood — but there is no evidence of thrombus. The mitral valve leaflets are pliable and not calcified, making the valve a good candidate for balloon dilatation.

24

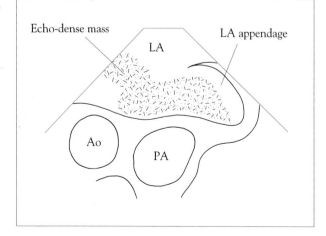

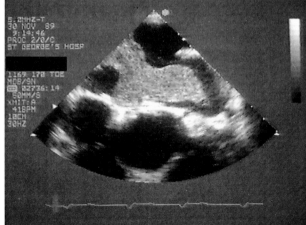

Transesophageal study showing a close-up view of the left atrial appendage. There is an echo-dense mass filling the appendage and protruding into the left atrial cavity which is probably thrombus.

25 Continuous-wave spectral Doppler recordings of the diastolic flow velocity across the stenotic mitral valve can determine peak, mean, and end-diastolic pressure gradients. The velocity spectrum is recorded from an apical view. The outline of the velocity spectrum is traced and the machine software calculates the relevant pressures. In this example, the peak transvalvular gradient is 20 mmHg and the mean is 9 mmHg indicating quite severe stenosis.

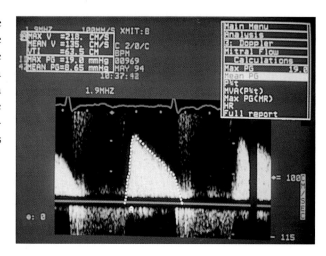

26

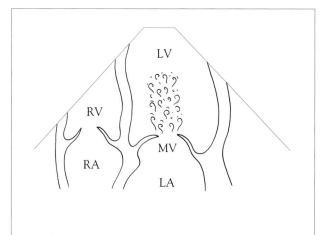

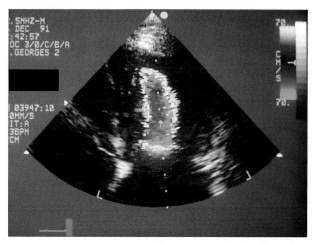

Apical four-chamber view of the left ventricle in a case of mild mitral stenosis. Color-flow Doppler indicates the width of the jet passing through the valve in diastole and its direction allows the angle of the ultrasound beam to be optimized for correct continuous-wave spectral Doppler velocity and pressure gradient measurements.

27 Continuous-wave spectral Doppler recording of transmitral diastolic flow from an apical view. The early diastolic peak velocity is over 2 m/s (normally <1 m/s) and there is a reduced rate of diastolic velocity decay. The 'pressure half-time' can be calculated from the decay slope. In this case it is a little over 200 ms, from which the mitral orifice area is calculated to be 1.1 cm^2.

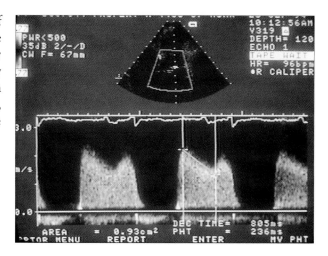

28

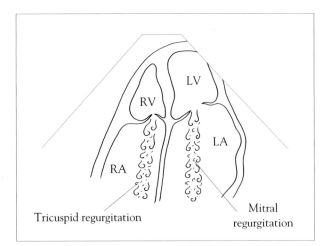

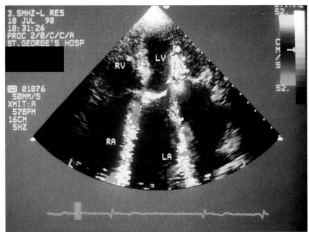

Apical four-chamber view with color-flow Doppler showing both mitral and tricuspid regurgitation in a patient with rheumatic valve disease. The mechanism of the mitral regurgitation is cusp shrinkage and retraction leading to failure of apposition and the jet direction is usually straight back towards the roof of the left atrium.

29 Continuous-wave spectral Doppler recording of tricuspid regurgitation. The jet velocity can be used to calculate pulmonary artery pressure.

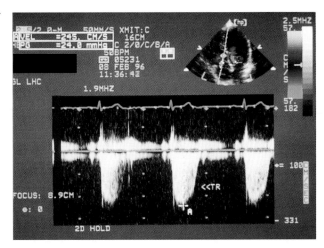

30 Simultaneous recordings of pulmonary capillary wedge and left ventricular diastolic pressures to assess the severity of mitral stenosis. The higher the transmitral diastolic pressure gradient, the more severe is the mitral stenosis. Simultaneous measurement of cardiac output also allows measurement of the mitral valve area.
PCWP=pulmonary capillary wedge pressure;
LVDP=left ventricular diastolic pressure.

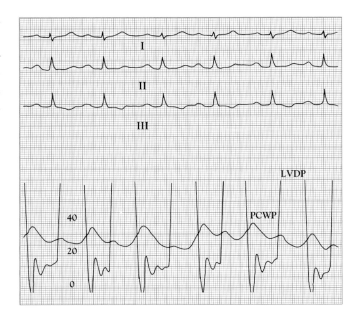

31   Left ventricular angiogram (right anterior oblique projection) showing slight mitral regurgitation through a stenotic valve.

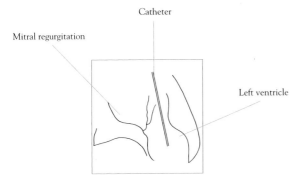

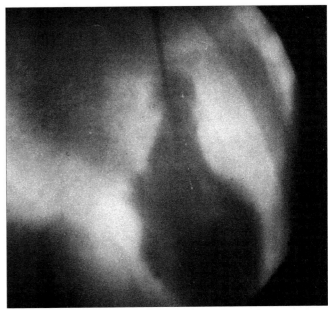

32   Principles of management of mitral stenosis.

1. Symptomatic patients with hemodynamically significant mitral stenosis: catheter (valvuloplasty), surgical valvotomy, or valve replacement

2. Transesophageal echocardiography prior to catheter valvuloplasty to exclude left atrial thrombus (a contraindication to valvuloplasty)

3. Patients with a heavily calcified distorted mitral valve are more suitable for valve replacement

4. Patients with atrial fibrillation require digitalization and long-term anticoagulation

5. Antibiotic prophylaxis for bacterial endocarditis

33   Balloon mitral valvuloplasty. The balloon catheter is placed across the stenotic valve and valvuloplasty is carried out by inflation of the balloon.

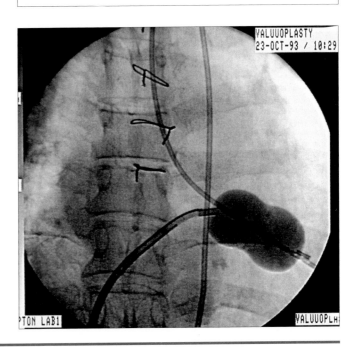

34 (a) Two-dimensional echocardiograms showing increase in mitral valve orifice size following catheter valvuloplasty in a patient with mitral stenosis. (b) Transmitral pressure gradient before and after catheter mitral valvuloplasty as determined by Doppler echocardiography. Peak and mean transvalvular gradients and pressure half-time ($PT_{1/2}$) decreased and the mitral valve area (MVA) increased.

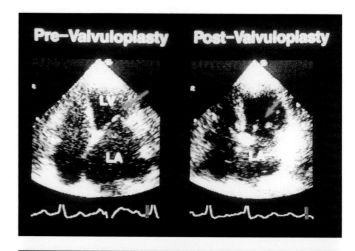

a)

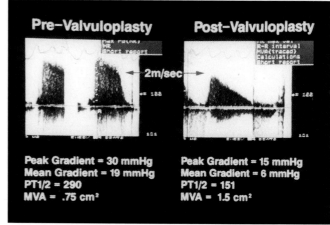

b)

35

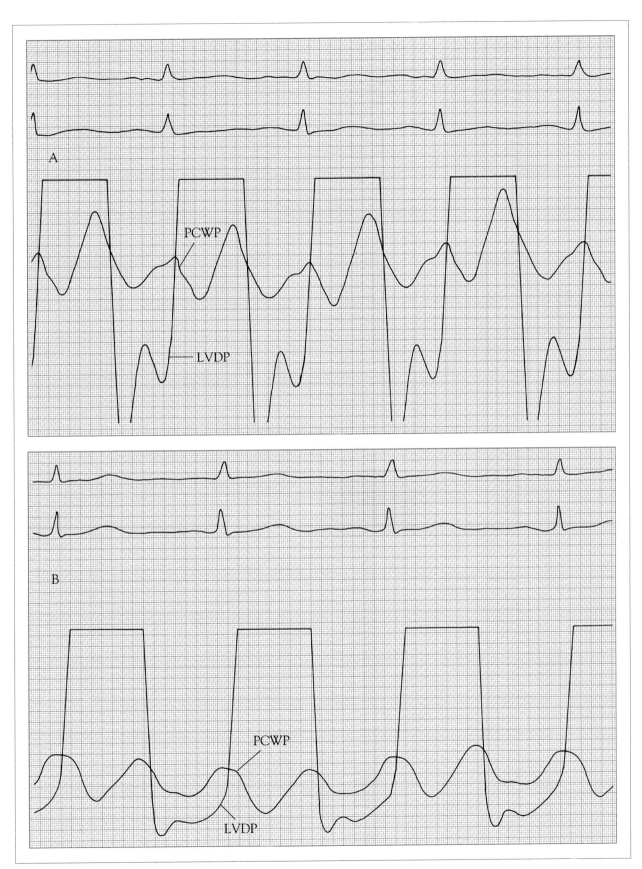

A decrease in the pressure gradient after catheter valvuloplasty is illustrated by measuring pulmonary capillary wedge and left ventricular diastolic pressures simultaneously during cardiac catheterization.
A=Pre-valvuloplasty; B=post-valvuloplasty.

MITRAL REGURGITATION

Definition

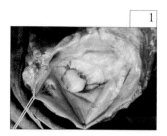

Mitral regurgitation is defined as retrograde blood flow from the left ventricle to the left atrium. Mitral regurgitation occurs usually during systole due to the ineffective closure of the mitral valve. Diastolic mitral regurgitation is rare and occurs when the left ventricular diastolic pressure exceeds left atrial pressure, allowing retrograde flow through the open mitral valve.

Pathology

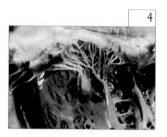

The competence of the mitral valve depends upon the normal co-ordinated function of the left atrial wall, mitral annulus, leaflets, chordae tendineae, papillary muscles, and left ventricular myocardium. Disease may affect any one or all of these structures and result in mitral regurgitation. Redundant cusp tissue and elongation of the chordae tendineae, due to myxomatous degeneration, can result in a floppy mitral valve permitting mitral regurgitation to occur [1]. More severe mitral regurgitation may develop over a long period of time or may occur acutely if there is chordal rupture spontaneously or as a result of infective endocarditis [2,3].

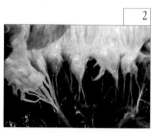

In patients with coronary artery disease, infarction involving a papillary muscle may lead to its rupture with the development of sudden severe mitral regurgitation [4,5]. Ischemia of the papillary muscles can cause long-standing disorganization of the subvalvular mitral apparatus with resultant mitral regurgitation [6]. Mitral regurgitation may also occur secondary to left ventricular dilatation and depressed left ventricular systolic function as in dilated cardiomyopathy. Lateral displacement of the papillary muscles and mitral annular dilatation appear to be the mechanism for mitral valve incompetence. Anterior displacement of the mitral valve during systole may cause significant mitral regurgitation in hypertrophic cardiomyopathy. Disorganized subvalvular structures may also produce substantial mitral regurgitation in endomyocardial fibrosis and primary restrictive cardiomyopathy.

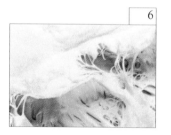

Mitral regurgitation is common in some systemic disorders such as Marfan's syndrome [7], pseudoxanthoma elasticum, Ehler–Danlos syndrome, Hurler's syndrome, and pseudohypertrophic muscular dystrophy. Mitral annular calcification in the elderly usually produces mild mitral regurgitation.

A rheumatic etiology is still common in the countries where rheumatic fever remains prevalent. Chronic rheumatic mitral valve disease usually results in mixed mitral stenosis and mitral regurgitation.

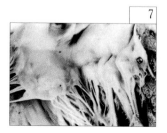

Presentation

Symptoms
Patients with mild mitral regurgitation, due for example to a floppy mitral valve, are usually asymptomatic, although patients with mitral valve prolapse may complain of atypical chest pain and palpitation due to various arrhythmias.

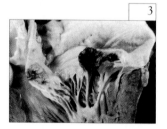

Patients with acute severe mitral regurgitation, for example due to ruptured chordae tendineae, invariably develop sudden severe dyspnea, paroxysmal nocturnal dyspnea, and orthopnea. Anginal symptoms may be present in patients with ischemic heart disease.

In chronic severe mitral regurgitation patients may remain asymptomatic for several years and the symptoms may develop gradually. Exertional dyspnea and impaired exercise tolerance are the usual presenting symptoms. Patients may complain of disturbing palpitation and dyspnea with the onset of atrial fibrillation.

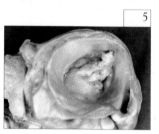

Signs
Unless mitral regurgitation is severe, the carotid pulse will be normal. With long-standing significant mitral regurgitation, atrial fibrillation may develop. The reduction of forward stroke volume in severe cases will result in a small carotid pulse with a sharp upstroke due to increased left ventricular dP/dT resulting from increased left ventricular preload. With the development of pulmonary hypertension, and the retention of sinus rhythm, the

jugular venous pulse may show abnormal dominance of the 'a' wave. In chronic moderate or severe mitral regurgitation, the apical impulse is hyperdynamic due to a normal or increased ejection fraction and a large left ventricular stroke volume.

A high-pitched pansystolic murmur over the apex radiating to the axilla is the consistent auscultatory finding in more than trivial mitral regurgitation. It is usually accompanied by a third heart sound.

In patients with very mild mitral regurgitation, for example due to mitral valve prolapse or papillary muscle dysfunction, a late systolic murmur is usually present together with mid-systolic clicks [8]. A third heart sound is usually absent in very mild mitral regurgitation.

Significant mitral regurgitation may cause wide but physiologic splitting of the second heart sound due to shortening of left ventricular ejection time. The pulmonary component will be accentuated if there is additional pulmonary hypertension.

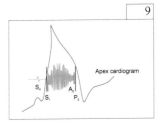

Acute or subacute primary significant mitral regurgitation due to ruptured chordae tendineae is usually associated with a small sharp carotid pulse and an elevated jugular venous pressure. A hyperdynamic left ventricular impulse is common [9]. The regurgitant murmur may be of crescendo-decrescendo type, may be early rather than pansystolic in acute severe regurgitation, and may radiate towards the base or axilla. A thrill can be palpated in many patients.

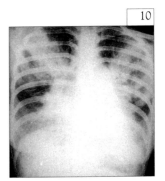

Investigations

Radiology
Acute severe mitral regurgitation due to chordal rupture results in pulmonary edema, often with little or no cardiac enlargement [10]. If mitral regurgitation is long-standing and hemodynamically significant, the chest X-ray shows cardiac enlargement with left atrial dilatation [11]. Dilatation of the upper lobe pulmonary veins will reflect elevation of pulmonary venous pressure. In the presence of a stiff ventricle, as in hypertrophic or restrictive cardiomyopathy, even significant mitral regurgitation may not produce cardiac enlargement. Mitral annular calcification, which is usually associated with mild mitral regurgitation, shows a C or J shaped appearance on plain chest X-ray [12].

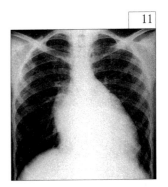

Electrocardiography
In a patient with a floppy mitral valve with only slight mitral regurgitation, the electrocardiogram may be normal or may show minor ST-T changes, particularly in the inferior leads [13]. The electrocardiogram may also be normal in patients with ruptured chordae, despite severe mitral regurgitation. In long-standing significant mitral regurgitation, evidence of eccentric left ventricular hypertrophy, i.e. increased QRS voltage with a leftward frontal plane QRS axis, may be present. Atrial fibrillation tends to occur late in the course of the disease [14]. Mitral regurgitation resulting from a papillary muscle infarct is almost always associated with electrocardiographic evidence of acute myocardial infarction, more frequently of the left ventricular inferior wall [15]. In patients with secondary mitral regurgitation from left ventricular myocardial disease, the electrocardiogram often shows left bundle branch block [16].

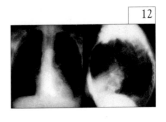

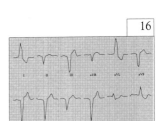

Echocardiography
Two-dimensional echocardiography, in combination with color-flow mapping, can usually determine the etiology of mitral regurgitation from the appearance of the valve and the

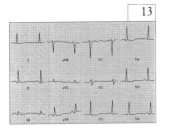

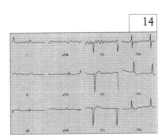

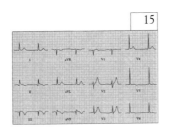

direction and pattern of the associated regurgitant jet. If clear images cannot be obtained by the transthoracic route, transesophageal studies provide unimpeded access to the mitral valve, with the enlarged left atrium ensuring good contact with the transducer.

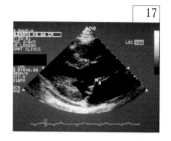

In primary mitral regurgitation due to mitral valve prolapse, either or both of the leaflets buckle towards the left atrium in systole, with part of the cusp crossing the plane of the valve annulus [17]. The jet is usually very eccentric and its direction indicates which leaflet is involved [18,19]. In many cases, the leaflets themselves have a thickened, 'myxomatous' appearance [20]. M-mode recordings do not show which leaflet is involved, but indicate whether the prolapse is present throughout or only late in systole. With superimposed color, the timing relationship between the prolapse and the regurgitation can be demonstrated [21]. Ruptured chordae may be seen, and the presence of irregular-shaped, mobile masses lends support to a clinical diagnosis of infective endocarditis [22]. Vegetations may remain for many years after the infection has been cured [23]. The absence of vegetations, even using a transesophageal study, does not exclude active infection.

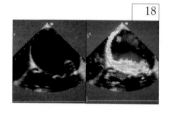

By contrast, secondary mitral regurgitation due to ischemic heart disease may cause fibrosis and retraction of either or both papillary muscles, pulling the smaller posterior mitral leaflet into the left ventricle. The resulting failure of apposition of the leaflets causes an eccentric jet of regurgitation [24]. Dilatation of the mitral annulus due to left ventricular disease results in failure of coaptation similar to that of rheumatic disease, with similar jet appearance [25].

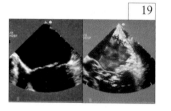

Useful data can be obtained from M-mode recordings of the left ventricular dimensions. Chronic mitral regurgitation increases left ventricular end-diastolic volume, which normally should result in vigorous contraction, further facilitated by the reduced afterload. To find obviously impaired systolic function with mild or moderate regurgitation strongly suggests that the problem lies with the myocardium, with secondary, functional regurgitation.

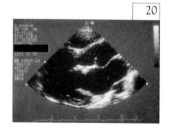

While color Doppler is a very sensitive means for detecting mitral regurgitation, techniques such as measuring the width of the jet orifice, or jet length or area, provide only a very rough indication of severity. This is especially true when the jet sweeps around the wall of the left atrium, as it may appear narrow in one dimension while being wide in the other.

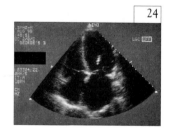

The severity of mitral regurgitation can be assessed by simultaneous phonocardiography and continuous-wave Doppler [26]. If regurgitation is severe (and particularly acute), mitral regurgitation will cease at the time of aortic valve closure, or even before it, because of left atrial and left ventricular pressure equilibration.

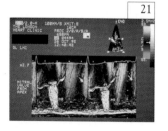
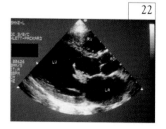
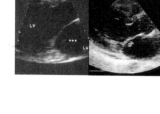
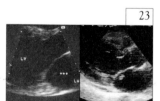

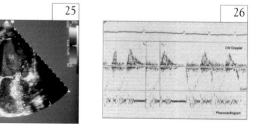

Nuclear Techniques

Gated blood pool imaging is useful, not only to assess left ventricular ejection fraction but also for quantitative assessment of the severity of mitral regurgitation [27]. The regurgitation index can be calculated from the relation: left ventricular stroke volume/right ventricular stroke volume. A ratio of 1.7 or greater indicates significant mitral regurgitation. This index, however, cannot be used in the presence of aortic or tricuspid regurgitation.

In patients with coronary artery disease, stress thallium myocardial perfusion imaging may be helpful to assess reversible myocardial ischemia as a potential cause of mitral regurgitation.

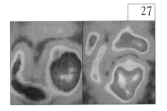

Magnetic Resonance Imaging (MRI) and Computed Tomography (CT)

Both MRI and CT have the potential to provide information regarding left ventricular function and the regurgitation fraction [28]. In addition, MRI can quantify regurgitation. However, these investigations are seldom used currently in clinical practice.

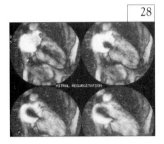

Cardiac Catheterization and Angiography

Coronary angiography is necessary preoperatively in patients with a high risk of coronary artery disease or in patients in whom coronary artery disease is suspected as the cause of mitral regurgitation. In acute or subacute severe mitral regurgitation, pulmonary capillary wedge pressure is elevated with a prominent 'v' wave [29]. Pulmonary capillary wedge pressure may also be higher than the pulmonary artery diastolic pressure. Pulmonary artery pressure is elevated and post-capillary pulmonary hypertension is also present.

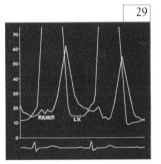

Contrast left ventriculography reveals the state of left ventricular function. Systolic function (ejection fraction) will be preserved if the cause of the regurgitation is a chordal or leaflet abnormality [30,31]; it will be impaired if the cause is left ventricular myocardial disease, which may be generalized in dilated cardiomyopathy or show regional abnormalities in coronary artery disease. It should be recognized that even in patients with primary mitral regurgitation, left ventricular systolic function may deteriorate due to chronic volume overload. Contrast ventriculography can be used to assess the severity of mitral regurgitation semiquantitatively from the rate and extent of left atrial opacification.

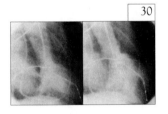

Principles of Management

Primary Mitral Regurgitation

Asymptomatic patients with a normal left ventricular ejection fraction can be followed conservatively [32]. Long-term anticoagulation is also not required in patients who remain in sinus rhythm. All symptomatic patients should be considered for surgical treatment, provided that the symptoms are attributable to mitral regurgitation. Reduced left ventricular ejection fraction is an indication for surgical therapy even in asymptomatic patients. An end-diastolic diameter approaching 75 mm and an end-systolic diameter approaching 50 mm are also indications for surgical intervention. Mitral reconstruction surgery is preferable to prosthetic valve replacement, as it results in a better postoperative left ventricular ejection fraction and long-term survival. Thus, mitral reconstruction should be considered whenever feasible, even though the risk of early reoperation for residual mitral regurgitation is 2–3%. Vasodilators, such as hydralazine, nitroprusside, and angiotensin converting enzyme inhibitors, decrease regurgitant volume, left ventricular diastolic and pulmonary capillary wedge pressures, and increase forward stroke volume and cardiac output. These agents may be useful for short-term therapy preoperatively or for patients who are not candidates for surgery. Antibiotic endocarditis prophylaxis is indicated in all patients with mitral regurgitation except when mitral regurgitation occurs secondary to left ventricular dilatation. If atrial fibrillation occurs, digitalis therapy is indicated.

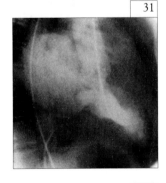

1. Patients with symptoms due to significant primary mitral regurgitation are candidates for surgical therapy
2. Resting ejection fraction of less than 55%, and end-diastolic and end-systolic diameters approaching 75 mm and 50 mm, respectively, are indications for surgery even in asymptomatic or mildly symptomatic patients
3. Mitral reconstruction surgery is preferable to prosthetic valve replacement. Mitral reconstruction provides better preservation of left ventricular function and late prognosis. Long-term anticoagulation is not required after mitral reconstruction
4. Vasodilators which decrease regurgitant volume and increase cardiac output may be used for short-term therapy preoperatively or for patients who are not surgical candidates
5. Antibiotic endocarditis prophylaxis is indicated in all patients with primary mitral regurgitation
6. Patients with secondary mitral regurgitation require vasodilator therapy and, if they remain symptomatic, cardiac transplantation

Secondary Mitral Regurgitation

Operations on the mitral valve in patients who have left ventricular myocardial disease and secondary mitral regurgitation are unlikely to be of benefit. Vasodilator therapy is indicated, and if the patient remains symptomatic, cardiac transplantation should be considered.

1   Floppy mitral valve viewed from the left atrium. A portion of the posterior cusp is domed into the atrium (prolapsed cusp).

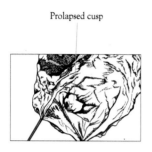

Prolapsed cusp

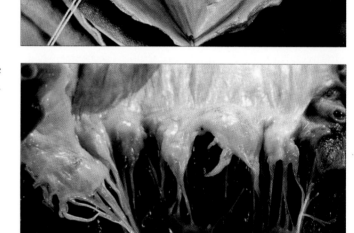

2   Floppy mitral valve with ruptured chordae. The posterior cusp is domed upward into the atrium. Stumps of ruptured chordae are present.

Atria   Posterior cusp

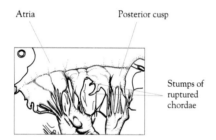

Stumps of ruptured chordae

3   Mitral valve with ruptured chordae due to infective endocarditis. The posterior cusp is covered by a mass of thrombotic vegetations. Stumps of ruptured chordae are present.

Thrombotic vegetations

Posterior cusp

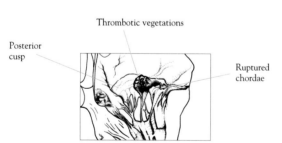

Ruptured chordae

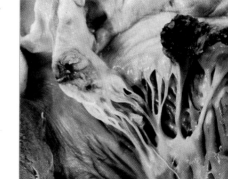

4   Partial avulsion of a papillary muscle during acute myocardial infarction producing mitral regurgitation. One head of the postero-medial papillary muscle is torn from the ventricular wall.

Anterior cusp   Posterior cusp

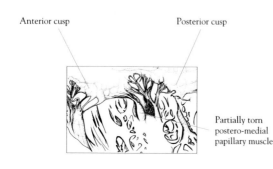

Partially torn postero-medial papillary muscle

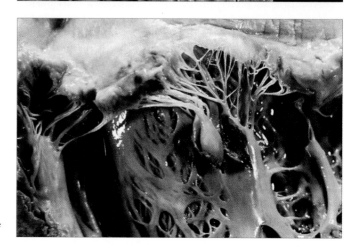

5 Mitral regurgitation secondary to acute myo-cardial infarction. The papillary muscle is infarcted and ruptured, and prolapses into the left atrium, resulting in acute mitral regurgitation

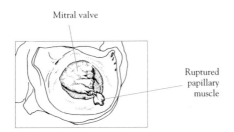

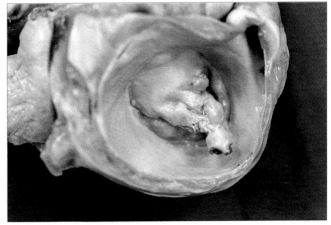

6 Fibrosis and shrinkage of the papillary muscles, resulting in mitral regurgitation following myocardial infarction. The apex of the postero-medial papillary muscle is elongated and the body of the muscle is shrunken. A small chord has avulsed from the papillary muscle.

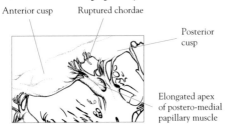

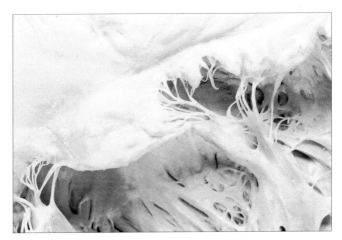

7 Mitral valve in Marfan's syndrome. Both anterior and posterior cusps are increased in area and the surface appears folded. Chordae are elongated.

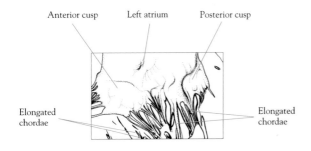

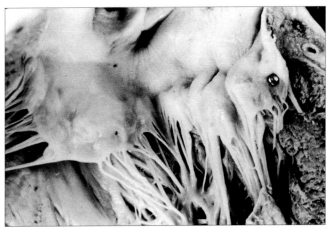

8 Schematic illustration of the auscultatory findings in mitral valve prolapse which show a mid-systolic click followed by a crescendo late systolic murmur.
S_1=First heart sound; A_2=aortic component of the second heart sound; MSC=mid-systolic click; LSM=late-systolic murmur

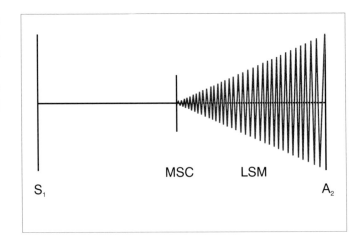

9 Chordal rupture usually produces severe mitral regurgitation and is associated with a hyper-dynamic apical impulse, a crescendo-decrescendo pansystolic murmur, a widely split second heart sound with accentuated pulmonic component, and an apical fourth heart sound.
S_4=Fourth heart sound; A_2=aortic component of second heart sound; P_2=pulmonary component of second heart sound

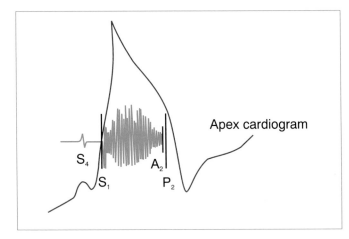

10 Chest X-ray in acute chordal rupture. The heart is normal in size but there is gross pulmonary edema.

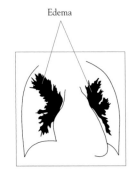

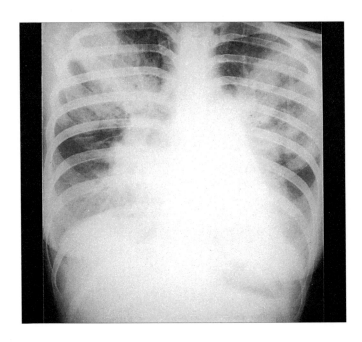

11   Chest X-ray in chronic mitral regurgitation showing cardiac enlargement, dilatation of the left atrium, and the prominent upper lobe pulmonary veins.

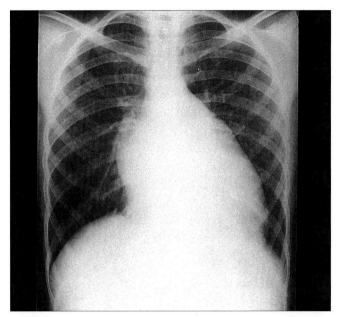

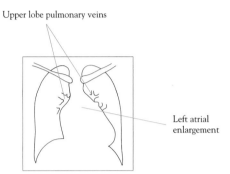

12   Calcification in the mitral valve has to be distinguished from calcification in the mitral valve ring. Valvar calcification is usually only slight or moderate in extent, and the valve leaflet can often be seen to be moving to a degree within the cardiac cycle. Calcification of the mitral valve ring has a characteristic C or J shape and can be seen in the frontal view (a) and better in the lateral view (b) in this example.

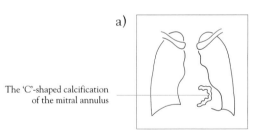

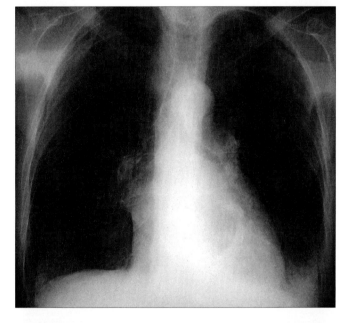

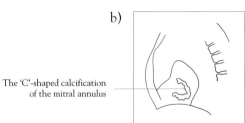

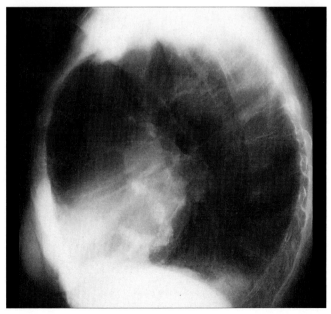

13

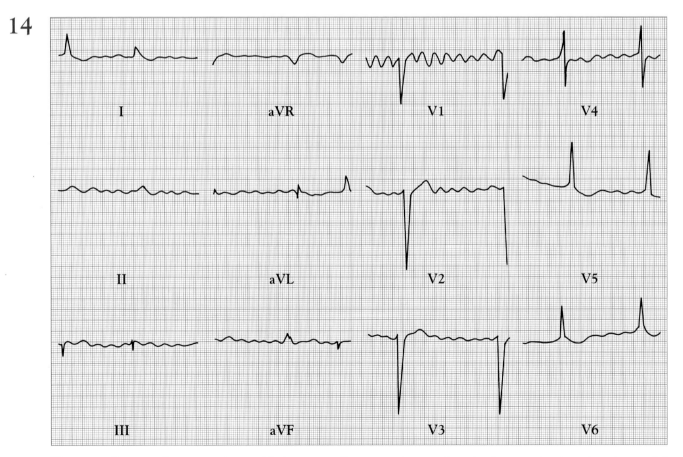

Electrocardiogram from a patient with mitral valve prolapse showing infero-lateral ST-T wave abnormalities.

14

Electrocardiogram from a patient with long-standing non-rheumatic mitral regurgitation showing atrial fibrillation and left ventricular hypertrophy.

15

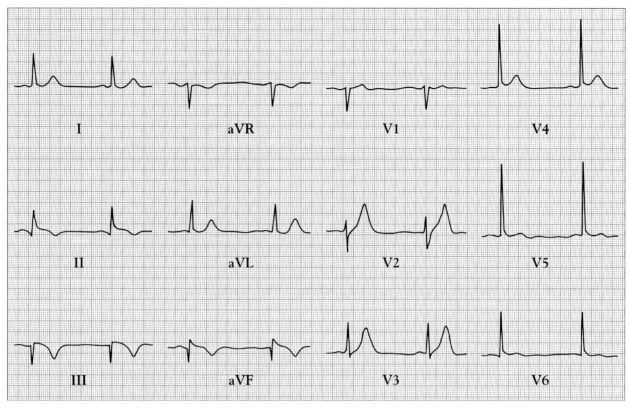

Electrocardiogram from a patient with acute papillary muscle rupture showing inferior myocardial infarction.

16

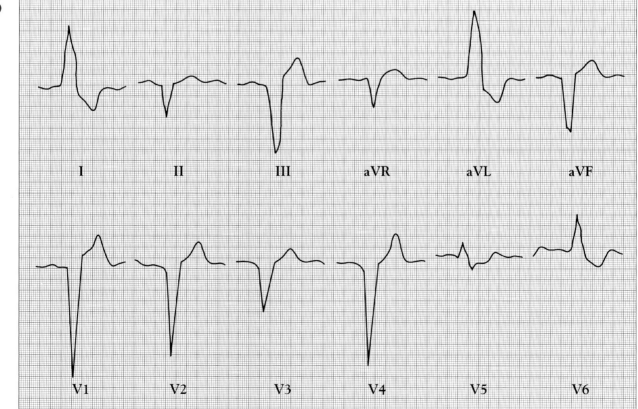

Electrocardiogram showing left bundle branch block in a patient with chronic mitral regurgitation due to dilated cardiomyopathy.

17

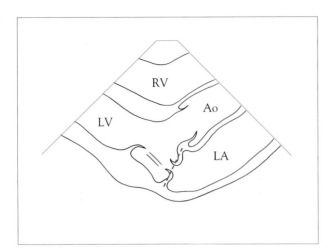
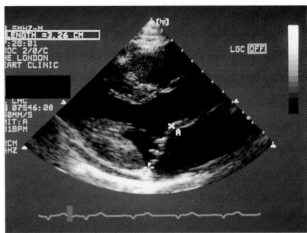

Parasternal long-axis late-systolic image of a 'floppy' mitral valve. Both leaflets show 'myxomatous' thickening and have prolapsed behind the plane of the valve annulus (dotted line).

18

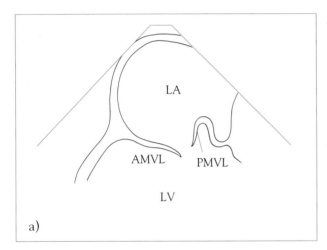
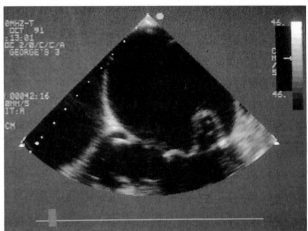

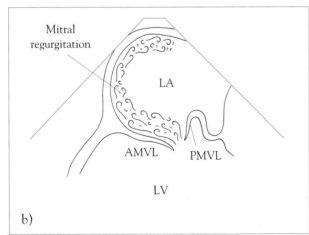
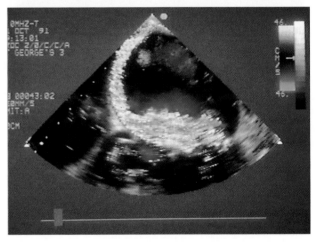

(a) Intra-operative transesophageal view showing gross prolapse of the central section of the posterior mitral valve leaflet. The left atrium is enlarged. (b) The addition of color-flow Doppler shows an eccentric jet of mitral regurgitation directed anteriorly and sweeping around the wall of the atrium.

19

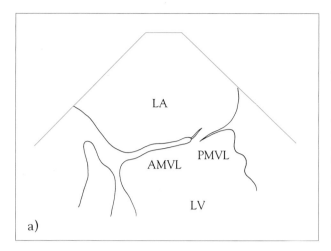

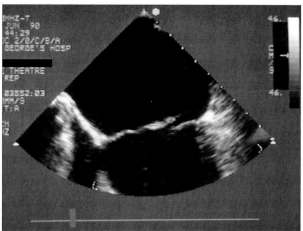

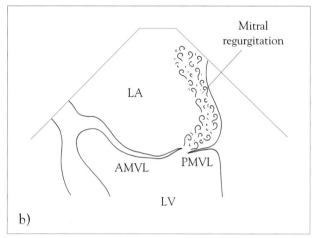

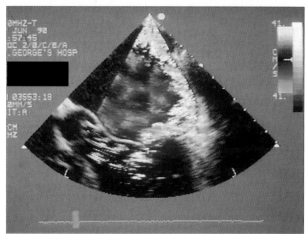

(a) Intra-operative transesophageal view showing prolapse of the anterior mitral valve leaflet. There is failure of leaflet coaptation and a ruptured chorda can be seen at the tip of the leaflet. (b) The regurgitant jet is eccentric and directed posteriorly.

20

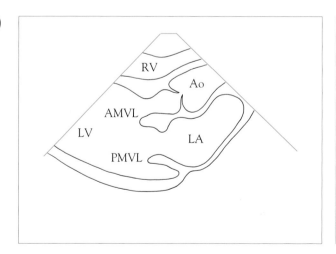

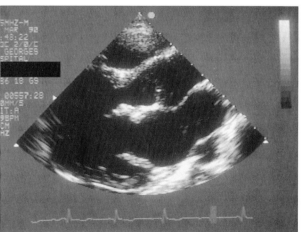

Diastolic frame in the parasternal long-axis view showing the thickened, 'shaggy' appearance of the mitral valve leaflets, often described as 'myxomatous', in a patient with mitral valve prolapse.

21   Color M-mode image taken from the apex to show the
timing of flow across the mitral valve. There is late-
systolic mitral regurgitation (predominantly blue)
caused by mitral valve prolapse.

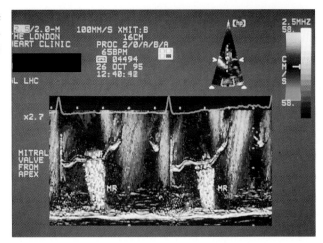

22

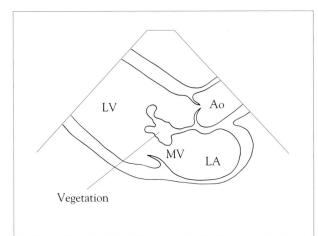

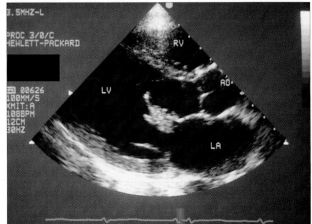

Parasternal long-axis view showing a large, irregular mass attached to the tip of the anterior mitral valve leaflet.
Its appearance and location are strongly suggestive of a vegetation.

23

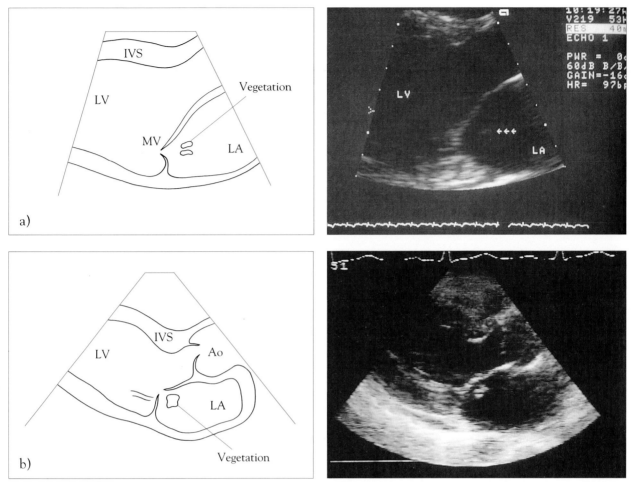

(a) Parasternal long-axis view from a study of a young woman who presented with a transient ischemic attack, mild mitral regurgitation, and clinical signs of infective endocarditis following day-case surgery. A small mobile mass is seen behind the anterior mitral leaflet. (b) The same patient 15 years later. The appearance of the vegetation is essentially identical.

24

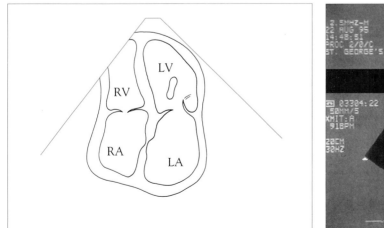
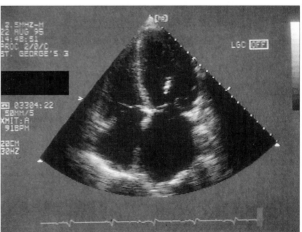

Apical four-chamber view showing 'tethering' of the posterior mitral leaflet associated with mitral regurgitation secondary to ischemic disease. There is failure both of leaflet apposition and of coaptation. Note the intense echoes from the postero-medial papillary muscle. Both the left ventricle and the left atrium are enlarged.

25

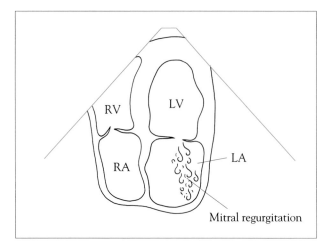
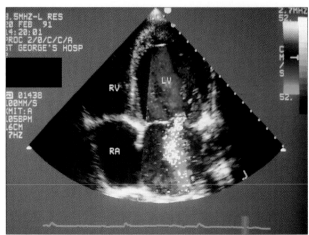

Apical four-chamber view with color-flow Doppler showing severe secondary mitral regurgitation caused by dilatation of the valve annulus in a patient with left ventricular disease.

26

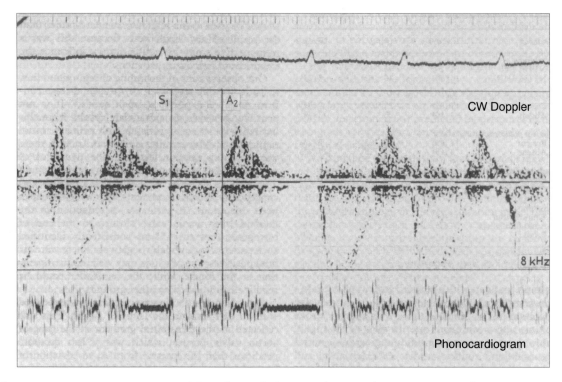

Simultaneous continuous-wave spectral Doppler and phonocardiogram from a patient with severe, acute mitral regurgitation. The onset and end of systole are marked by the heart sounds S_1 and A_2, respectively. The end of mitral regurgitant flow was synchronous with A_2. Note also cessation of regurgitant murmur in mid-systole.

Reproduced from Bradley JA and Gibson BG, *Br Heart J* 1988; 60: 134–40 with permission.

27

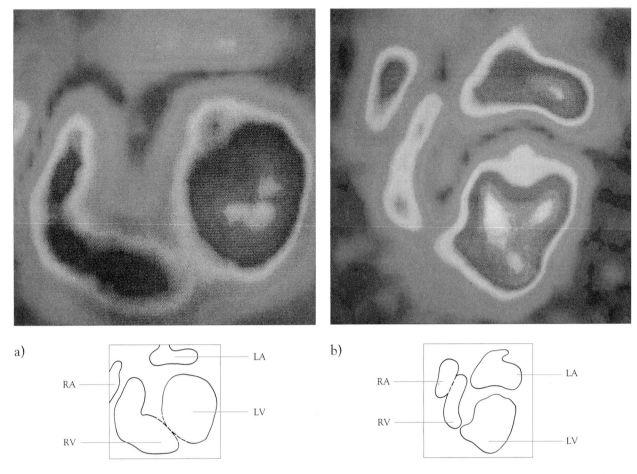

a)

b)

Blood pool imaging for estimating the severity of mitral regurgitation by determining the regurgitation index is usually performed in the best septal projection. The ratio of left ventricular stroke volume to right ventricular stroke volume is the regurgitation index, and the higher the ratio, the more severe is the mitral regurgitation. Gated blood pool imaging also allows assessment of both right and left ventricular systolic function. (a) Amplitude image of a normal subject. (b) Amplitude image in a patient with mitral regurgitation showing high values in the left atrium, and dominant values in the left ventricle compared with the right ventricle.

28 Magnetic resonance gradient echo cine imaging of mitral regurgitation. Four images at successive points in the cardiac cycle through systole in the vertical long-axis plane showing signal loss in the left atrium due to a jet of mitral regurgitation.

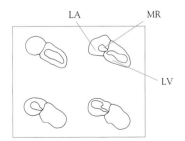

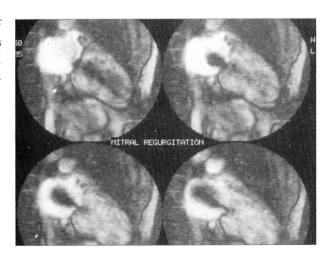

29   A prominent 'v' wave is recorded in the pulmonary capillary wedge pressure in a patient with mitral regurgitation.

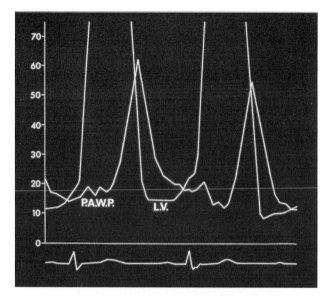

30

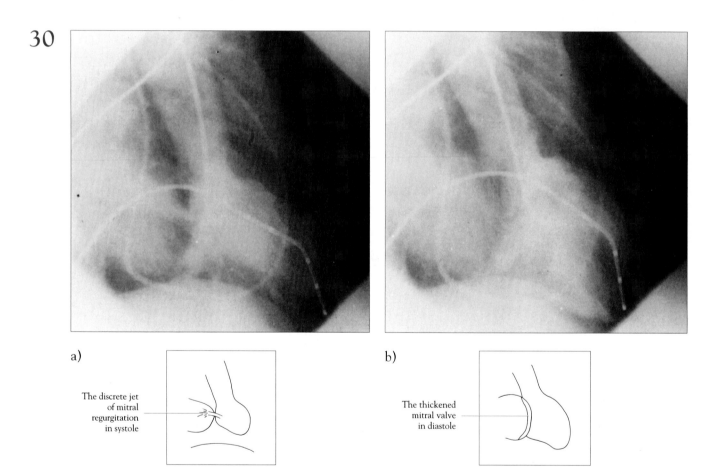

a)   The discrete jet of mitral regurgitation in systole

b)   The thickened mitral valve in diastole

Rheumatic mitral regurgitation. In systole (a), the discrete central jet of rheumatic mitral regurgitation can be seen passing from the left ventricle into the left atrium. Note the rather foreshortened and abnormally shaped ventricle with the distortion of its inferior aspect, typical of rheumatic mitral disease. In diastole (b), the thickened mitral valve is visible.

31 Non-rheumatic mitral regurgitation. This systolic left ventricular frame in the right anterior oblique view shows passage of contrast from the left ventricle to the left atrium. The explanation can be seen in the prolapse of the posterior leaflet of the mitral valve, clearly outlined by contrast medium on its ventricular aspect.

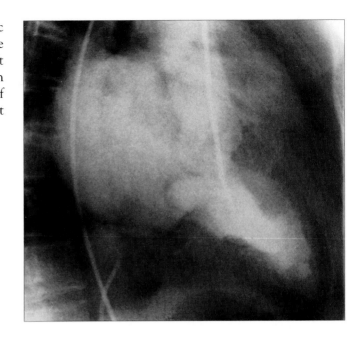

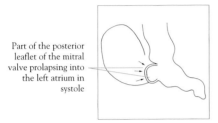

Part of the posterior leaflet of the mitral valve prolapsing into the left atrium in systole

32 The principles of management of mitral regurgitation.

1. Patients with symptoms due to significant primary mitral regurgitation are candidates for surgical therapy

2. Resting ejection fraction of less than 55%, and end-diastolic and end-systolic diameters approaching 75 mm and 50 mm, respectively, are indications for surgery even in asymptomatic or mildly symptomatic patients

3. Mitral reconstruction surgery is preferable to prosthetic valve replacement. Mitral reconstruction provides better preservation of left ventricular function and late prognosis. Long-term anticoagulation is not required after mitral reconstruction

4. Vasodilators which decrease regurgitant volume and increase cardiac output may be used for short-term therapy preoperatively or for patients who are not surgical candidates

5. Antibiotic endocarditis prophylaxis is indicated in all patients with primary mitral regurgitation

6. Patients with secondary mitral regurgitation require vasodilator therapy and, if they remain symptomatic, cardiac transplantation

AORTIC STENOSIS

Definition

Narrowing of the left ventricular outflow tract causing obstruction to systolic flow from the left ventricle to the aorta.

Pathophysiology

Fixed obstruction to left ventricular outflow can occur at three levels. Most frequently it is at valve level (aortic valve stenosis), but it may also occur above or beneath the valve (supravalvular and subvalvular aortic stenosis, respectively).

Aortic Valve Stenosis

The normal aortic valve is tricuspid, and the normal valve area is between 2.6–3.5 cm/m² [1,2]. The most common cause of isolated aortic stenosis in the adult is a congenitally bicuspid valve [3]. Dystrophic calcification of the bicuspid valve develops gradually with time and is rarely present before the age of 40 [4]. Up to 2% of the population are born with a bicuspid aortic valve, with the occurrence more frequent in males than in females. In time, the hemodynamic stresses on the slightly unequal valve leaflets produce fibrosis and dystrophic calcification of the valve.

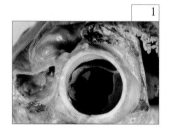

Rheumatic aortic stenosis is characterized by fusion of all three commissures to produce a central triangular aperture [5]. Leaflet vascularization and fibrosis, with or without significant calcification, are also present. Gross or microscopic evidence of involvement of the mitral valve is almost always present in patients with rheumatic aortic stenosis.

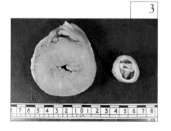

Senile calcific aortic stenosis or Monckeberg's aortic stenosis occurs as a result of dystrophic calcification in the normal tricuspid aortic valve [6]. Sometimes, lipid-laden cells are also present. The calcification may extend to the aortic root, mitral annulus, and conducting system.

The rare causes of acquired aortic valvular stenosis include familial hypercholesterolemia, rheumatoid heart disease, systemic lupus erythematosus, ochronosis, and treatment with methylsergide.

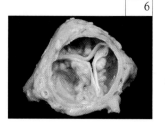

All forms of aortic valve stenosis cause obstruction to left ventricular outflow, which is associated with increased left ventricular systolic pressure, leading to concentric left ventricular hypertrophy due to a marked increase in the thickness of individual myocardial cells [7]. Although hypertrophy is beneficial in reducing left ventricular wall stress and, hence, in maintaining adequate pump function despite outflow obstruction, in the end-stage, considerable subendocardial fibrosis due to ischemia may occur. Thus, in some patients, dilatation of the left ventricular cavity, together with impaired systolic function, may develop.

Supravalvular Aortic Stenosis

Supravalvular aortic stenosis, rare in adults, can occur as a focal hour-glass constriction, a fibromuscular narrowing, or a generalized hypoplasia of the ascending aorta. It can be associated with hypercalcemia, mental retardation, characteristic facies, and multiple stenoses or coarctation of the major branches of the pulmonary artery (William's syndrome).

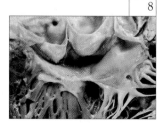

Subvalvular Aortic Stenosis

Fixed subvalvular aortic stenosis may be due to a membranous diaphragm, a fibromuscular narrowing, or a tunnel deformity. In the diaphragmatic form, the diaphragm is attached to the anterior leaflet of the mitral valve, consists of cusp-like tissue, and extends forward to insert just below the right coronary cusp of the aortic valve [8]. The fibromuscular

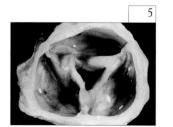

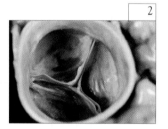

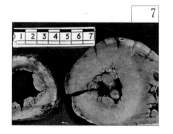

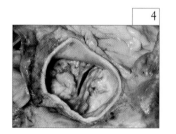

component protrudes anteriorly from the ventricular septum, opposite the anterior mitral cusp. Subvalvular aortic stenosis may be associated with a hypertrophied bulging septum and is always associated with aortic regurgitation.

Presentation

Patients with severe congenital aortic stenosis may present with heart failure soon after birth. Other patients who are asymptomatic may present at a routine clinical examination during which a cardiac murmur is heard. Furthermore, even in later life, patients with severe aortic stenosis may remain asymptomatic.

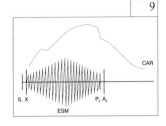

Symptoms

The major symptoms are dyspnea, angina, and syncope. Symptoms of heart failure, such as dyspnea, result from elevation of pulmonary capillary wedge pressure secondary to elevated left ventricular diastolic pressure, primarily due to left ventricular diastolic dysfunction associated with left ventricular hypertrophy. Angina may occur in the absence of coronary artery disease, due to myocardial ischemia resulting from an increased myocardial oxygen requirement and impaired myocardial perfusion. Syncope, or near syncope, may be exertional or spontaneous. Exertional syncope may occur as a result of impaired cerebral perfusion due to an inappropriate increase in cardiac output in the presence of metabolically mediated peripheral vasodilatation. Reflex peripheral vaso-dilatation originating from the walls of the left ventricle may also be contributory. Spontaneous syncope probably results from ventricular tachyarrhythmia or heart block. In general, the onset of any of the classical triad of symptoms (heart failure, angina, and syncope) is ominous and the five-year mortality rate is about 50%. The risk of sudden death in otherwise asymptomatic patients is approximately 2% per year.

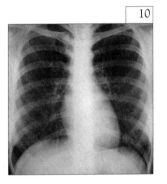

Signs

Significant aortic valve or subvalvular stenosis is associated with a slow rise in the aortic pressure pulse, which can be detected clinically as a slow rise in the carotid pulse. An anacrotic shoulder, a delayed peak, and a thrill in the carotid pulse are also frequently noted. In supravalvular aortic stenosis, the arterial pulses in the neck are usually asymmetric, with the right carotid having a sharp upstroke while the left is slow-rising due to preferential propagation of the high velocity jet into the innominate artery.

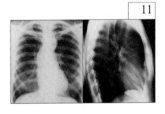

In significant aortic stenosis, a systolic thrill may be palpated over the right second interspace. The apical impulse is sustained due to left ventricular hypertrophy. A pre-systolic wave (palpable S_4) may be present, resulting in a 'double' impulse, indicating decreased compliance of the left ventricle with elevated end-diastolic pressure. A low-pitched harsh ejection systolic murmur with a delayed peak and reversed splitting of the second heart sound (in the absence of left bundle branch block), indicating a prolonged left ventricular ejection time, usually indicates significant aortic stenosis [9]. The intensity of the aortic component of the second heart sound is decreased due to decreased aortic diastolic pressure and restricted valve movement. An aortic ejection sound may be present if the valve remains pliable; this sound is absent in supra- and subvalvular aortic stenosis. An early high-pitched diastolic murmur indicates associated aortic regurgitation. The intensity of the first heart sound may be diminished; this is usually due to increased left ventricular diastolic pressure. A third heart sound is absent until the left ventricle is dilated.

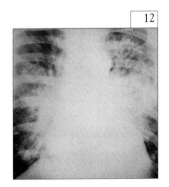

Investigations

Radiology

In uncomplicated aortic stenosis, the heart size remains within normal limits [10], although a prominent left border is frequently present. The ascending aorta may appear prominent due to post-stenotic dilatation [11]. In the later stages, left ventricular dilatation may occur in some patients with radiographic evidence of cardiac enlargement and evidence of raised pulmonary venous pressure [12]. Aortic valve calcification can also be seen, although this is better detected by fluoroscopy [13]. In adults, absence of valve calcification suggests insignificant stenosis.

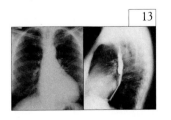

In supravalvular aortic stenosis, the chest X-ray shows a normal-sized heart with an inconspicuous aorta [14]. There may also be evidence of associated pulmonary artery stenosis [15]. In subvalvular aortic stenosis, the chest X-ray is usually normal, although occasionally post-stenotic dilatation of the aorta may be present.

Electrocardiography
Evidence of left ventricular hypertrophy with ST-T abnormalities of left ventricular strain is present in most patients with significant aortic stenosis. The frontal plane QRS axis is usually normal, suggesting concentric hypertrophy [16]. In some patients, a poor R-wave progression in the precordial leads (pseudo-infarction) may be present, due either to severe left ventricular hypertrophy or to left bundle branch block [17]. The electro-cardiogram is normal in about 10% of patients. Ventricular arrhythmias are detected by ambulatory electrocardiography in 20–25% of patients.

Echocardiography
A non-stenotic bicuspid aortic valve is recognized by 'doming' of the valve in systole in the two-dimensional long-axis view, and by the shape of the orifice on the short-axis view [18,19]. An M-mode echocardiogram may show a markedly eccentric closure line [20], but in some cases appears normal. Where stenosis develops, thickening and calcification progressively obliterate detail of the valve structure and motion [21–23].

In an adult patient, important stenosis is unlikely if the valve cusps are seen clearly to separate in systole, and if there is no evidence of left ventricular hypertrophy. Echocardiography also allows assessment of the degree of left ventricular hypertrophy [24], and of systolic [25] and diastolic function.

The ability to measure aortic valve pressure gradients by continuous-wave Doppler permits accurate assessment of the severity of the lesion and is a major contribution of Doppler to clinical cardiology. Recordings of peak and mean velocity are made from apical, right parasternal, and, if possible, suprasternal sites [26]. The corresponding pressure gradients are calculated using the Bernoulli equation (gradient = $4V_{max}^2$) [27]. Concurrent measurement of left ventricular stroke volume by echocardiography allows

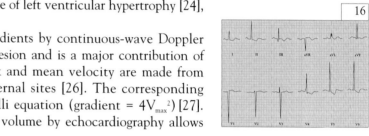

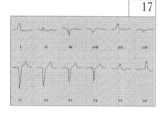
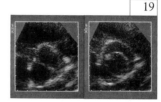
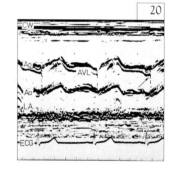

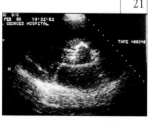
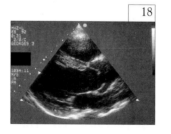
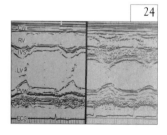

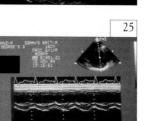
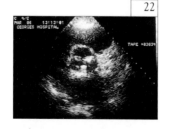
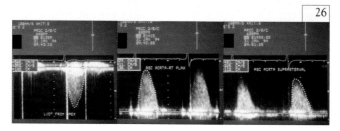
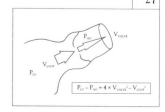

calculation of the aortic valve area. This is important in patients with impaired systolic function, when the pressure gradient does not reflect the severity of the lesion. Combined use of imaging with color Doppler, either transthoracic or transesophageal, locates the anatomic site of left ventricular outflow obstruction and identifies other associated abnormalities.

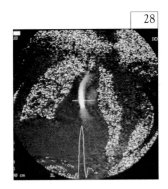

Nuclear Techniques
Gated blood pool imaging, which can detect changes in left ventricular volumes and function, is seldom employed in clinical practice.

Magnetic Resonance Imaging (MRI) and Computed Tomography (CT)
Both MRI and CT have been used to evaluate left ventricular function and left ventricular mass in patients with aortic stenosis. MRI can also be used to measure aortic flow and transvascular gradient [28]. However, these imaging techniques are only needed for management of selected patients with aortic stenosis.

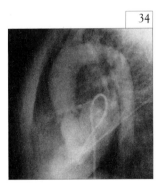

Cardiac Catheterization and Angiography
Coronary arteriography is indicated preoperatively in patients with aortic stenosis with or without angina. Cardiac catheterization is also indicated when the severity of aortic stenosis cannot be determined non-invasively. In valvular aortic stenosis, there is a systolic pressure difference across the valve [29], while in supravalvular stenosis, the pressure difference is between the supravalvular chamber and the aorta [30], and in subvalvular stenosis it is within the left ventricle [31]. In patients with significant aortic stenosis with left ventricular hypertrophy and abnormal left ventricular diastolic function, the left ventricular diastolic pressure is elevated. Secondary pulmonary hypertension and evidence of right heart failure are uncommon.

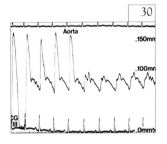

Left ventricular hypertrophy may be seen by contrast left ventriculography [32] which, however, is rarely required if echocardiographic evaluation is adequate. In valvular aortic stenosis, angiography may also reveal the thickening of the valve cusps with systolic doming and a central ejection jet [33–35].

In supravalvular stenosis, angiography shows the obstructive lesion above the sinuses of Valsalva [36,37]. If additional pulmonary artery stenoses are present they can be seen on a

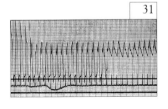
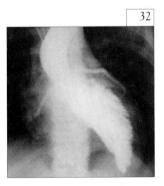
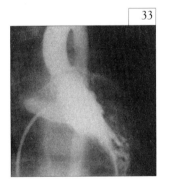
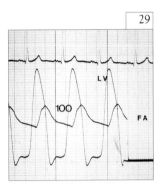

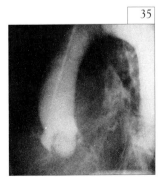
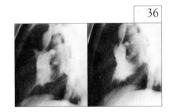
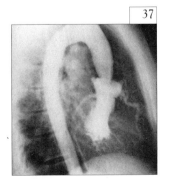

right ventricular angiogram [38]. In subvalvular aortic stenosis, the left ventricular angiogram shows the subvalvular obstruction [39] or a more diffuse fibromuscular lesion [40]. Associated aortic regurgitation can be demonstrated by aortography.

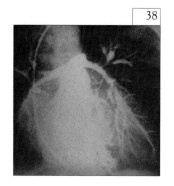

Principles of Management

Symptomatic patients with significant aortic stenosis should always be considered for valve replacement, irrespective of the status of left ventricular function [41]. In some high-risk patients, catheter aortic valvuloplasty can be performed initially to improve clinical status and left ventricular function prior to surgery [42]. Valvuloplasty is also suitable for patients in whom surgery is contraindicated, although the risk of restenosis within six months is 60–70%. In patients with mild to moderately severe aortic stenosis with heart failure, vasodilators such as hydralazine may increase cardiac output and may be of benefit. Vasodilators are contraindicated in patients with severe aortic stenosis. Atrial fibrillation should be treated with digitalis, and maintenance of sinus rhythm should be attempted with antiarrhythmic drugs. Antibiotic endocarditis prophylaxis is always indicated.

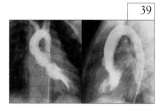

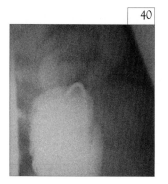

1. Symptomatic patients with significant aortic stenosis require valve replacement irrespective of the status of left ventricular function

2. Catheter balloon valvuloplasty is indicated only as a temporary and rescue procedure

3. Arteriolar vasodilators can improve symptoms and left ventricular function in patients with mild to moderately severe aortic stenosis. Vasodilators are contraindicated in severe aortic stenosis

4. Maintenance of sinus rhythm is beneficial

5. Antibiotic endocarditis prophylaxis is always indicated

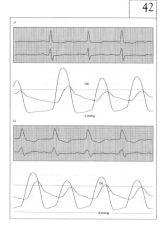

1   Fully open normal aortic valve. The cusps fold back into the aortic sinuses to leave a large central opening.

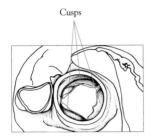

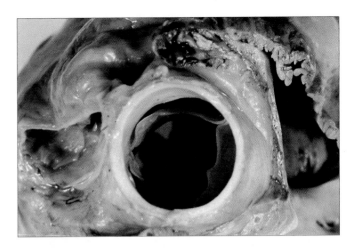

2   Fully closed normal aortic valve. The cusps meet and overlap providing support for each other in the closed position.

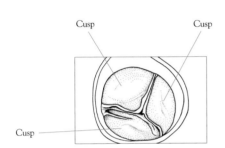

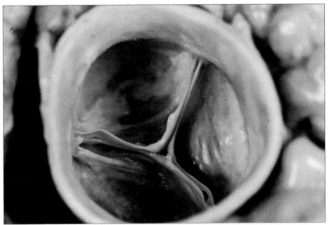

3   Bicuspid aortic valve resulting in severe left ventricular hypertrophy. The transverse section of the ventricles shows marked concentric left ventricular hypertrophy and a nearly virtual obliteration of the left ventricular cavity.

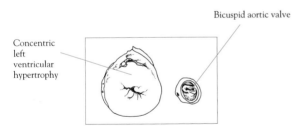

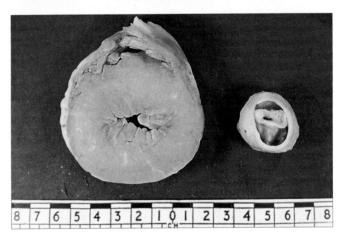

4   Calcific bicuspid aortic stenosis. The aperture of the valve is a transverse slit across the aortic root between two cusps. Masses of calcium bulge from each cusp.

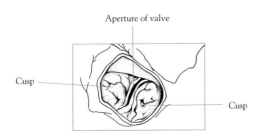

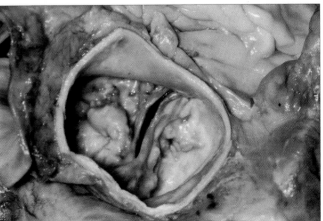

5   Rheumatic aortic stenosis in a patient with coexistent mitral disease. The aortic valve aperture is triangular due to fusion of all three commissures.

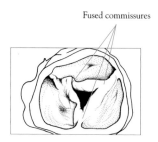

Fused commissures

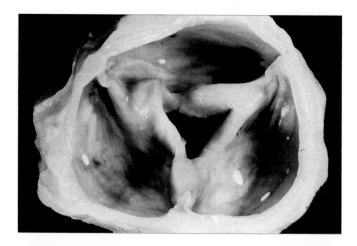

6   'Senile' aortic stenosis in a tricuspid aortic valve due to extreme age-related dystrophic calcification in the cusps.

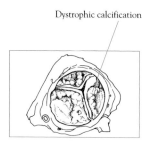

Dystrophic calcification

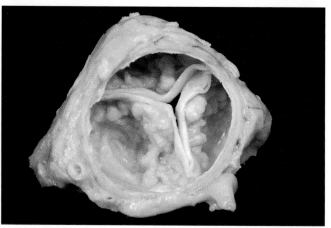

7   Transverse slice of left ventricle from a patient with a normal heart compared with a patient with aortic stenosis. In aortic stenosis the ventricular wall is thick and the cavity is small.

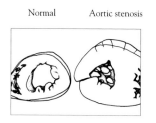

Normal   Aortic stenosis

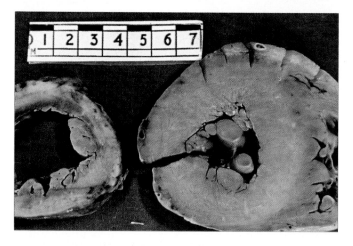

8   The aortic outflow tract in a case with sub-valvular aortic stenosis. A membrane joins the anterior cusp of the mitral valve to the interventricular septum beneath the aortic valve.

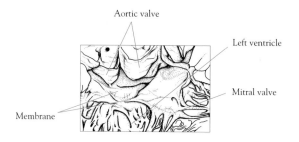

Aortic valve

Left ventricle

Mitral valve

Membrane

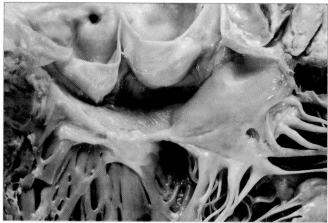

9   Schematic illustration of the physical findings that suggest significant aortic stenosis. Slow-rising, delayed-peaking carotid pulse with anacrotic shoulder, ejection systolic murmur, and reversed splitting of the second heart sound are illustrated.

S_1=First heart sound; P_2=pulmonic component of the second heart sound; A_2=aortic component of the second heart sound; ESM=ejection systolic murmur; CAR=carotid pulse; X=ejection sound.

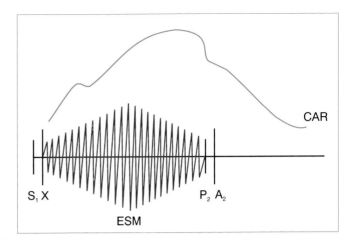

10   Chest X-ray of uncomplicated aortic valve stenosis, showing normal heart size.

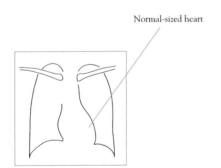

Normal-sized heart

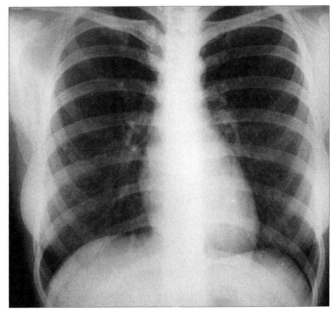

11 Congenital aortic valve stenosis in a young adult. The frontal chest X-ray (a) shows a normal-sized heart but a prominent ascending aorta and aortic arch, which would be quite abnormal for a 20-year-old woman. The lateral view (b) shows the left ventricle bulging posteriorly to the right atrium, marked by the inferior vena cava.

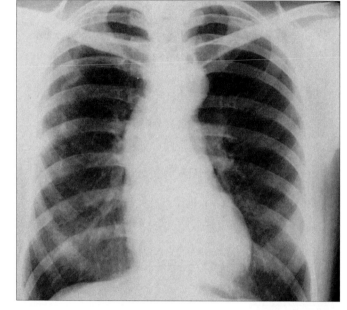

a)

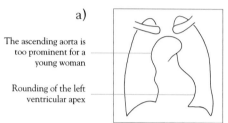

The ascending aorta is too prominent for a young woman

Rounding of the left ventricular apex

b)

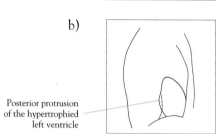

Posterior protrusion of the hypertrophied left ventricle

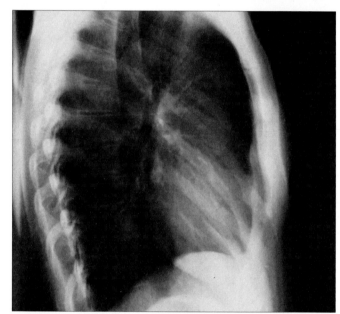

12 Chest X-ray of aortic valve stenosis showing pulmonary edema.

Edema

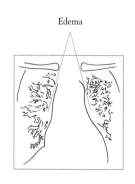

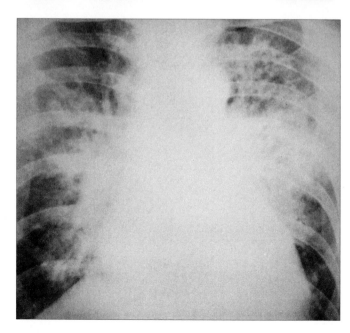

13 Calcific aortic valve stenosis in an adult. The frontal view (a) shows left ventricular hypertrophy as rounding of the cardiac apex, and dilatation as enlargement to the left. The ascending aorta is unremarkable. The lateral view (b) shows dense calcification in the position of the aortic valve. Post-stenotic dilatation of the aorta is much more common in younger than in older patients.

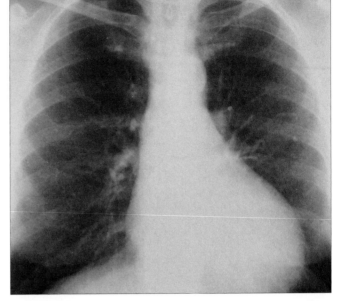

a)

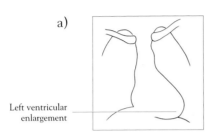

Left ventricular enlargement

b)

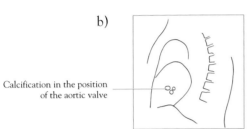

Calcification in the position of the aortic valve

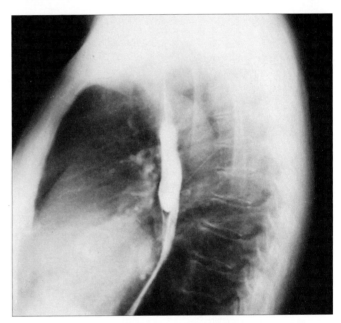

14 Chest X-ray in supravalvular stenosis. The heart size is normal and the ascending aorta inconspicuous.

Aorta

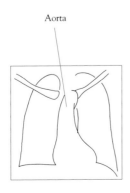

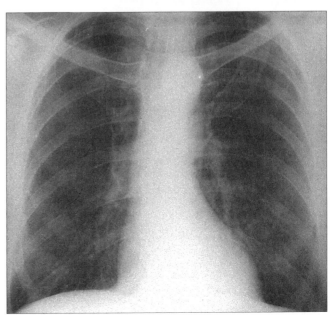

15 Chest X-ray in supravalvular aortic stenosis associated with central pulmonary artery stenosis. The aortic arch is inconspicuous; there is post-stenotic dilatation of the pulmonary arteries.

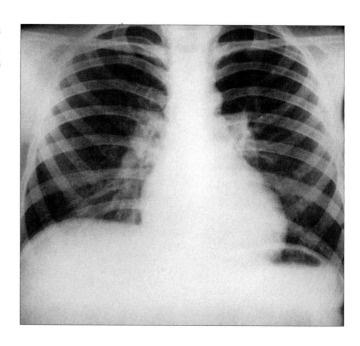

Post-stenotic dilatation

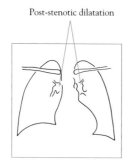

16

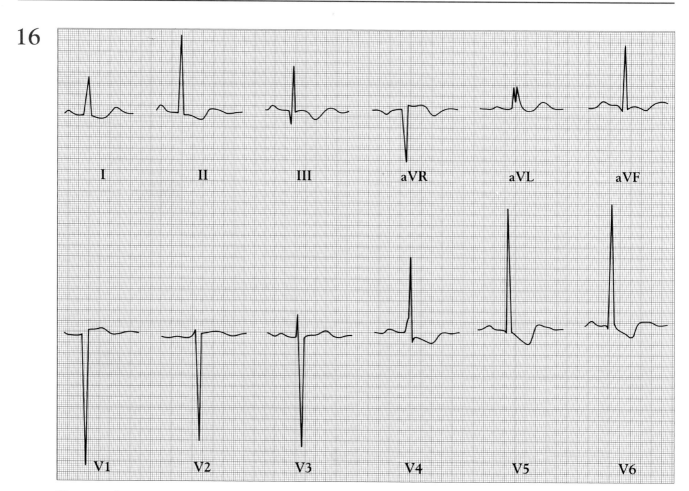

Electrocardiogram in severe aortic stenosis showing deep S-wave in V1 and tall R-wave in V5, with ST- and T-wave changes indicating left ventricular hypertrophy.

17

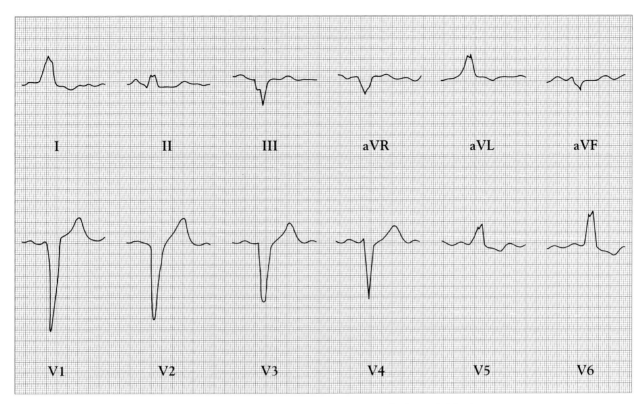

Electrocardiogram in a patient with aortic stenosis showing left bundle branch block.

18

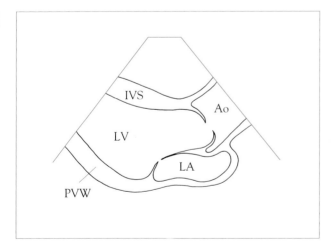 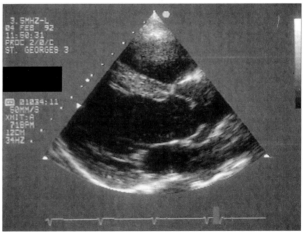

Parasternal long-axis view of a patient with a congenitally bicuspid aortic valve. The cusps are slightly thickened and show a characteristic 'doming' action in systole. There is mild enlargement of the proximal ascending aorta.

19

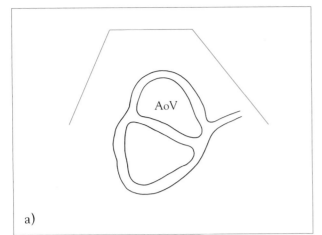

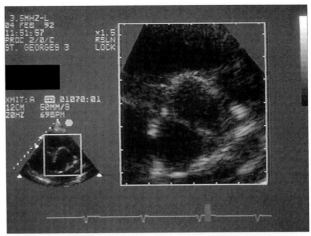

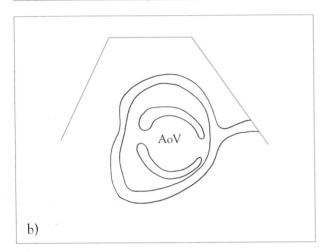

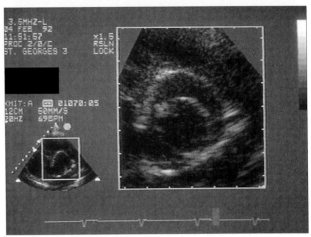

Parasternal short-axis views of a congenitally bicuspid aortic valve (a) in diastole showing a diagonal closure line and (b) in systole showing the open valve orifice as a 'lemon' shape rather than the normal triangle.

20   M-mode echocardiogram of a patient with a bicuspid aortic valve showing anterior displacement of the diastolic closure line (arrowed).

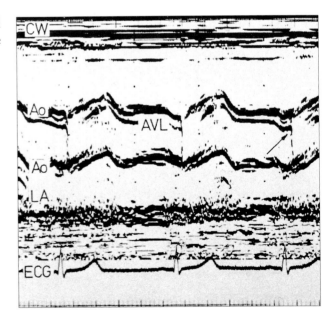

21

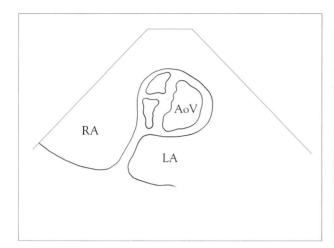
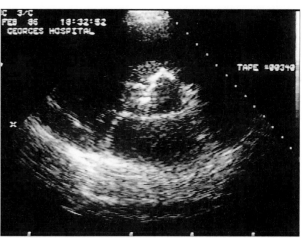

Parasternal short-axis section in a case of aortic stenosis. The distribution of the calcification can sometimes give a clue as to etiology: in this case a diagonal bar suggests a congenitally bicuspid valve.

22

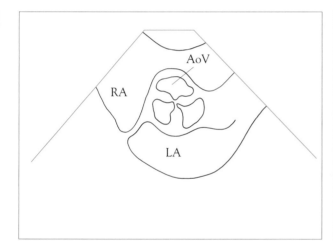
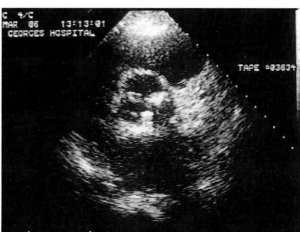

Parasternal short-axis section from a patient with aortic stenosis of rheumatic etiology. Calcification in the fused commissures of a three-cusp aortic valve is seen.

23 Magnified parasternal short-axis view showing a heavily calcified aortic valve. In advanced disease there is such dense calcification that the cusp structure cannot be determined, obscuring the etiology.

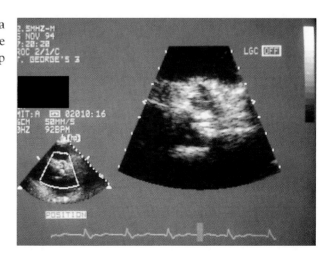

24

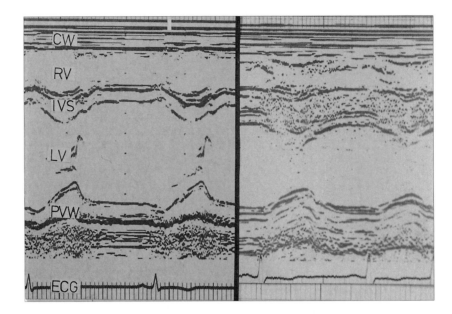

M-mode echocardiograms showing (left) a normal left ventricle and (right) a case of aortic stenosis with severe concentric hypertrophy and a greatly reduced rate of early filling. The filling dynamics are equivalent to those of mitral stenosis.

25 M-mode echocardiogram from a patient with long-standing, severe aortic stenosis resulting in impairment of both systolic and diastolic ventricular function. The left ventricle is enlarged and hypertrophied. Systolic shortening fraction is under 30% and diastolic filling rate reduced.

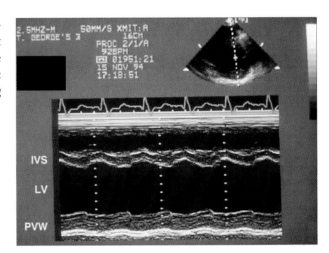

26 Continuous-wave spectral Doppler recordings taken from the apex (top), right upper parasternal border (middle), and suprasternal notch (bottom) in a young man discovered to have a loud systolic murmur. Peak gradient is over 130 mmHg, with essentially identical values obtained from the apex and right parasternal edge. This indicates that the two beam directions are essentially conjugates and confirms that the recordings are technically correct.

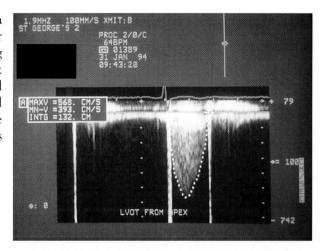

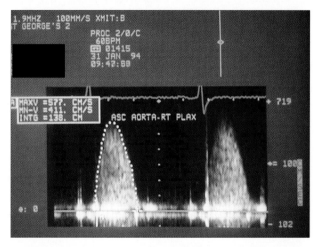

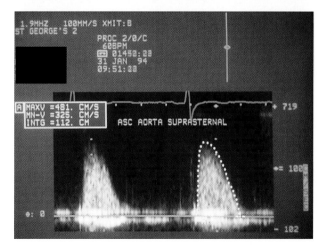

27 Diagram showing the theory of measurement of transvalvular gradients from inlet jet velocities using Bernoulli's equation.
P_{LV} = Pressure in the left ventricle; P_{AO} = pressure in the aorta; V_{VALVE} = velocity in the valve; V_{LVOT} = velocity in the left ventricular outflow tract

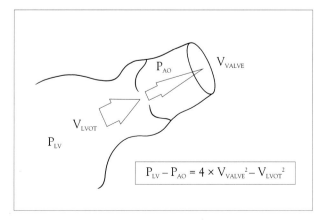

$$P_{LV} - P_{AO} = 4 \times V_{VALVE}^2 - V_{LVOT}^2$$

28   Magnetic resonance velocity mapping of aortic stenosis. The imaging plane has been turned obliquely to show the jet vertically in the frame. Measurement of the peak aortic jet velocity was shown to be nearly 4 m/sec which is equivalent to 64 mmHg pressure gradient.

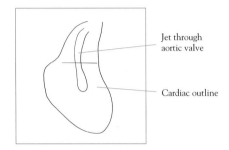

Jet through aortic valve

Cardiac outline

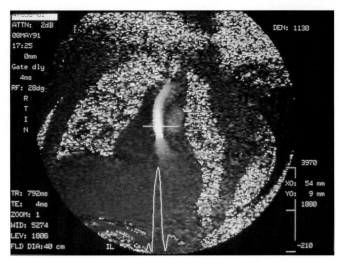

29   Pressure tracing showing gradient across the aortic valve.

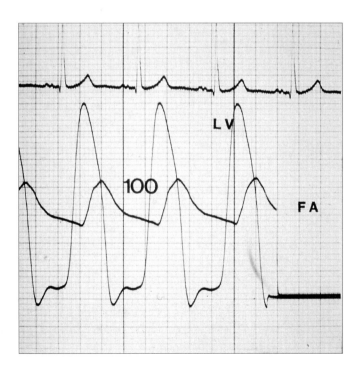

30

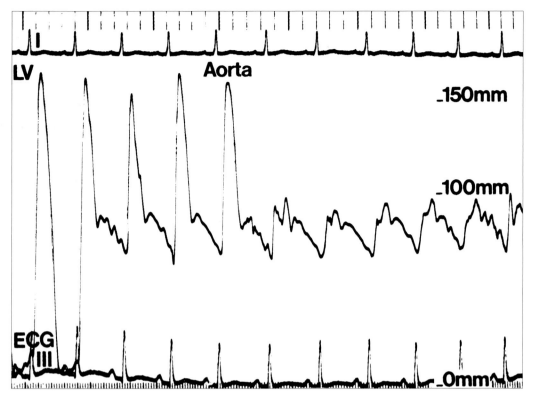

Withdrawal pressure tracing showing gradient across a supravalvular stenosis.

31

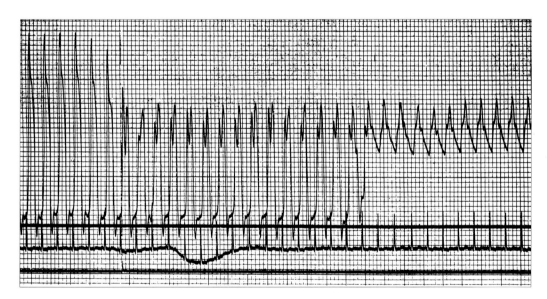

Withdrawal pressure tracing showing gradient across a subvalvular stenosis.

32 Left ventricular angiogram (right anterior oblique projection) in aortic valve stenosis showing gross left ventricular hypertrophy.

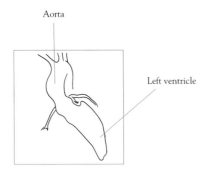

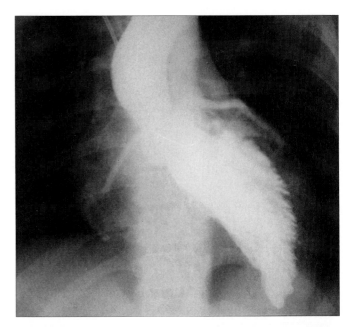

33 Systolic frame from the same patient as in [32] showing a thick domed valve.

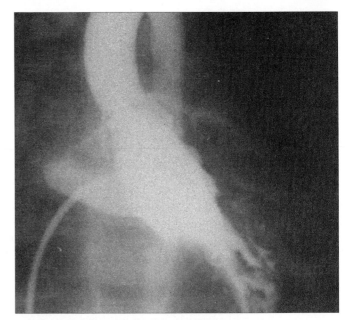

34 Lateral view of a ventricular angiogram in aortic stenosis showing a thick domed valve with post-stenotic dilatation of the aorta.

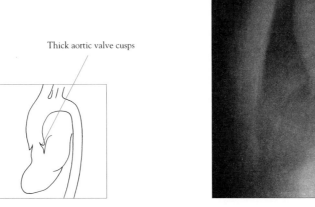

35 Lateral view of an aortogram in aortic stenosis, showing thick irregular rigid cusps of the aortic valve.

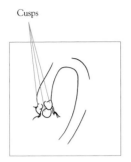

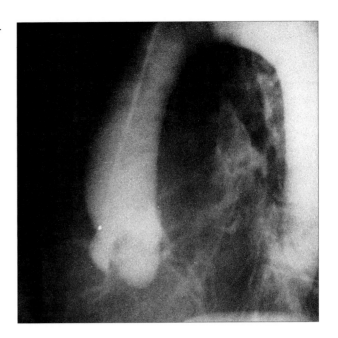

36

a)

b)

Lateral aortogram in supravalvular aortic stenosis. In systole (a), the stenosis is clearly visible just above the aortic valve, where the cusps can be seen to be almost occluding the coronary arteries. In diastole (b), the coronary cusps have moved away from the obviously dilated coronary arteries which sit in the high pressure zone between the valve and the supravalvular stenosis.

37   Left ventricular angiogram in the lateral view showing supravalvular stenosis and left ventricular hypertrophy.

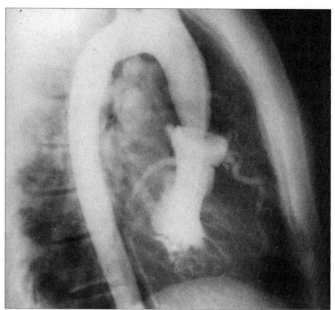

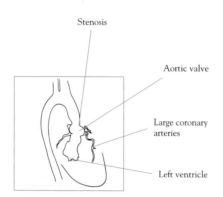

38   Right ventricular angiogram (antero-posterior projection) in the same patient as in [37] showing pulmonary artery stenosis.

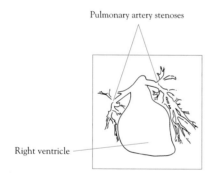

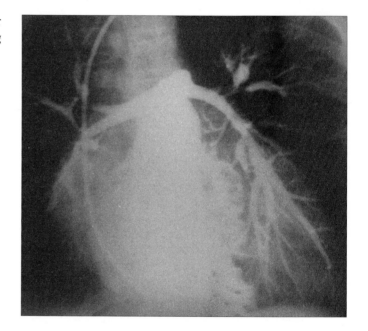

39

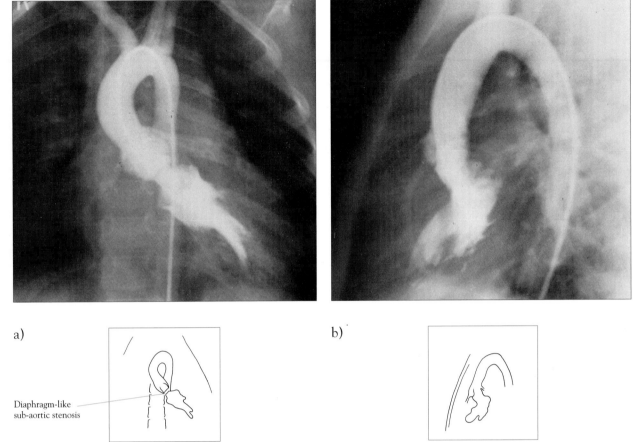

a)

Diaphragm-like
sub-aortic stenosis

b)

Left ventriculography in subaortic stenosis. In the frontal view (a), the line of the diaphragm-like subaortic stenosis can be seen lying just below the level of the aortic cusps. Note the muscular impressions on the ventricular cavity indicative of severe left ventricular hypertrophy. In the lateral view (b), although the hypertrophy can be seen, no diaphragm can be identified. The visualization of the diaphragm of subaortic stenosis is best achieved by echocardiography. Its recognition at ventriculography is very dependent on the projection chosen.

40   Left ventricular angiogram (lateral projection) with tunnel subvalvular aortic stenosis.

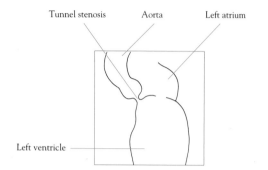

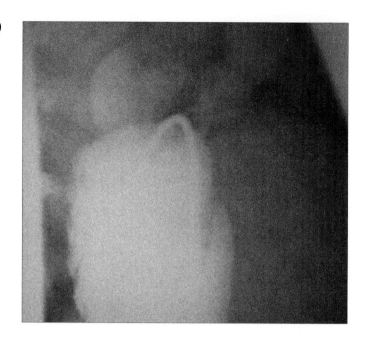

41   The principles of management of aortic stenosis.

1. Symptomatic patients with significant aortic stenosis require valve replacement irrespective of the status of left ventricular function

2. Catheter balloon valvuloplasty is indicated only as a temporary and rescue procedure

3. Arteriolar vasodilators can improve symptoms and left ventricular function in patients with mild to moderately severe aortic stenosis. Vasodilators are contraindicated in severe aortic stenosis

4. Maintenance of sinus rhythm is beneficial

5. Antibiotic endocarditis prophylaxis is always indicated

42

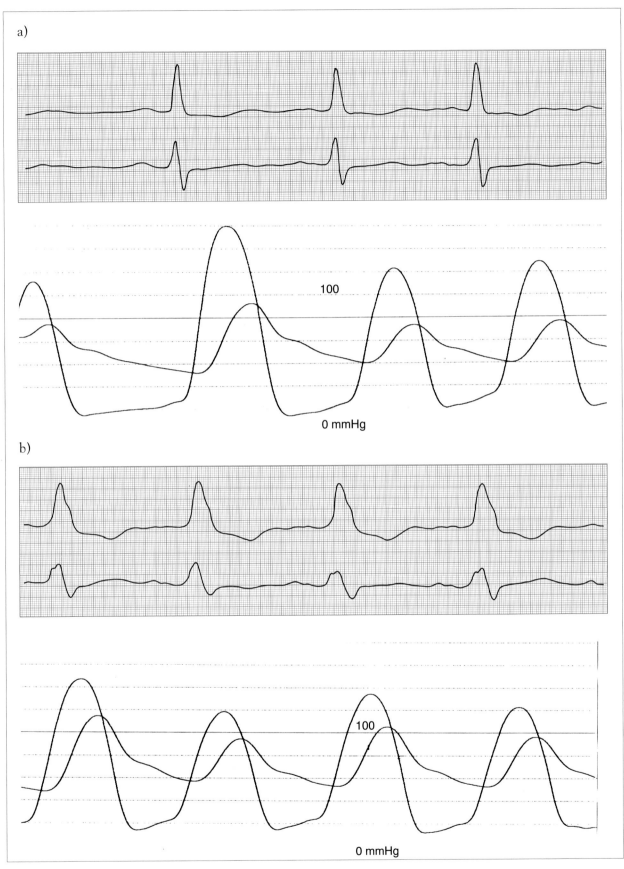

Catheter balloon valvuloplasty in a patient with aortic stenosis which produced a substantial decrease in the pressure gradient. Pre-valvuloplasty (a), the peak systolic pressure gradient between the left ventricle and aorta was between 55–70 mmHg, which decreased to about 30 mmHg after valvuloplasty (b).

AORTIC REGURGITATION

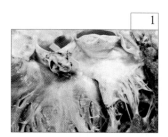

Definition

Retrograde flow from the aorta to the left ventricle in diastole.

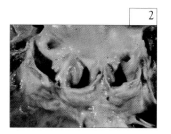

Pathology

Aortic regurgitation can result from intrinsic abnormalities of the valve leaflets, aortic annulus, or aortic root. Pathologic processes affecting the leaflets include infective endocarditis involving either the bicuspid or tricuspid aortic valve. This may result in perforation of a cusp and consequent acute aortic regurgitation [1]. Rheumatic heart disease can involve the aortic valve leaflets and remains a common cause of chronic aortic regurgitation [2]. Acute inflammatory disorders, such as rheumatic fever, may also cause, albeit mild, aortic regurgitation. Progressive degenerative changes of a congenitally bicuspid valve with shrinkage and retraction can also cause chronic aortic insufficiency [3].

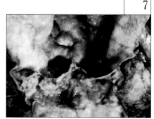

Abnormalities of the aortic root [4] and annulus can cause significant aortic regurgitation and these conditions include annulo-aortic ectasia, Marfan's syndrome [5,6], and cystic medial necrosis without other features of Marfan's syndrome. Acute aortic regurgitation from aortic dissection is usually due to cystic medial necrosis of the aortic root. Rheumatoid arthritis, ankylosing spondylitis [7], Behçet's disease, Reiter's disease, and syphilis [8] produce chronic inflammation of the proximal aorta and may cause chronic aortic regurgitation.

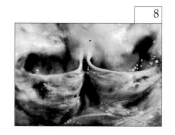

Aortic disease associated with pseudoxanthoma elasticum, Ehlers-Danlos syndrome, Hurler's and Hunter's syndromes, and osteogenesis imperfecta may also cause mild chronic aortic regurgitation. Systemic lupus erythematosus, radiation, aortic root masses and mixed connective tissue disease, and cardiolipin syndrome may be associated with aortic regurgitation. Aortic dilatation and aortic regurgitation can also result from long-standing hypertension.

Chronic aortic regurgitation leads to left ventricular dilatation and eccentric hypertrophy due to replication of the sarcomeres in series. There may be a considerable increase in left ventricular preload and afterload (systolic wall stress) which may eventually cause myocardial dysfunction. Myocardial ischemia causing fibrosis may result from impaired myocardial perfusion and increased myocardial oxygen demand. The regurgitant jet may hit the interventricular septum [4] or the ventricular aspect of the anterior cusp of the mitral valve, producing patches of endocardial thickening.

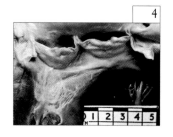

Aortic regurgitation associated with congenital anomalies, such as ventricular septal defect, and due to prosthetic valve malfunction, including paraprosthetic leak, may produce similar pathophysiologic changes and hemodynamic abnormalities.

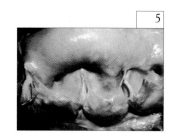

Presentation

Symptoms
Patients with slight aortic regurgitation may present following the discovery of a cardiac murmur at routine medical examination. Symptoms occur in patients with chronic, usually severe, aortic regurgitation after several years of a latent asymptomatic period. Dyspnea, resulting from increased pulmonary venous pressure secondary to

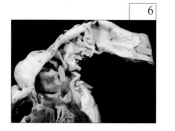

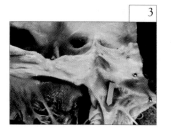

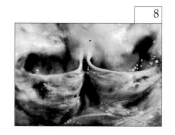

increased left ventricular diastolic pressure, is the most common presenting symptom. Palpitation and a pounding sensation in the chest is also quite common, reflecting the large left ventricular stroke volume. Angina occurs in about 20% of patients, usually with severe aortic regurgitation. Coronary atheromatous disease is found in about 20% of patients. Coronary artery ostial stenosis associated with aortitis may also cause angina. However, angina may occur with no detectable abnormality in the coronary arteries due to an imbalance between myocardial oxygen supply and demand. Abdominal pain due to splanchnic ischemia may be a rare presenting symptom.

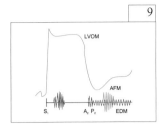

Acute severe aortic regurgitation, due to a ruptured cusp from infective endocarditis or aortic dissection, is poorly tolerated. Pulmonary edema develops rapidly due to a rapid increase in left ventricular diastolic and pulmonary venous pressures. Clinical manifestations of impaired organ perfusion due to decreased effective forward cardiac output may also be present.

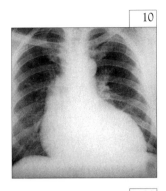

Signs

The constant physical sign of aortic regurgitation is the presence of an early diastolic murmur. An ejection systolic murmur may also occur, due either to an increased stroke volume through a normal aortic valve or, more likely, to the development of turbulence around a leaflet or an aortic wall abnormality. An ejection sound due either to a bicuspid aortic valve or to aortic root dilatation may be present.

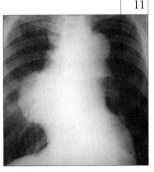

In mild chronic aortic regurgitation, the physical findings reflecting chronic volume overload are absent. In moderate or severe chronic aortic regurgitation, a wide pulse pressure with a rapid upstroke and downstroke in the arterial pulse is present (Corrigan's pulse). A pulse-synchronous movement of the head (Musset's sign), the uvula (Muller's sign), and the larynx (Oliver–Cardarelli's sign), along with capillary pulsations, usually indicates severe chronic aortic regurgitation. A pistol-shot sound heard over the brachial artery almost always indicates severe aortic regurgitation. A systolic-diastolic murmur heard over the femoral artery (Durosier's sign) indicates significant diastolic backflow. The apical impulse is hyperdynamic, reflecting the increased left ventricular stroke volume with a preserved ejection fraction. The early diastolic murmur is usually long and is occasionally musical ('seagull' or 'dove-coo' murmur). The presence of mid-diastolic murmur in the mitral area (Austin–Flint murmur) usually, but not invariably, indicates severe aortic regurgitation [9]. This murmur is due to the anterior leaflet of the mitral valve being displaced by the aortic regurgitation and partially impeding the left atrial–left ventricular blood flow.

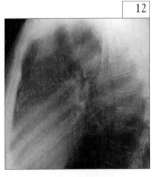

In acute severe aortic regurgitation, the pulse pressure is not wide, and the findings of altered arterial compliance and peripheral run-off are absent. The early diastolic and Austin–Flint murmurs are of shorter duration and may be difficult to hear when there is an invariable sinus tachycardia. The first heart sound may be soft, and indicates an increased left ventricular diastolic pressure. An absent first heart sound always indicates severe aortic regurgitation and a very rapid rise in left ventricular diastolic pressure causing premature closure of the mitral valve.

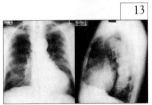

Investigations

Radiology

If aortic regurgitation is due to abnormalities of the aortic wall, the ascending aorta may be seen to be enlarged on the chest X-ray. Usually there is generalized dilatation in annulo-aortic ectasia [10] but in syphilis and Marfan's syndrome a localized aneurysm of the ascending aorta may be seen [11]. Linear calcification, along with dilatation of the ascending aorta, is very suggestive, but not diagnostic, of syphilitic aneurysm [12].

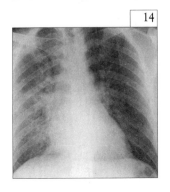

In long-standing significant aortic regurgitation, the left ventricle dilates producing cardiac enlargement in the chest X-ray [13]. In acute severe aortic regurgitation there may be pulmonary edema but the cardiac silhouette remains normal [14].

Electrocardiogram

The electrocardiogram may be normal in both acute aortic and mild chronic aortic regurgitation. Evidence of left ventricular hypertrophy by voltage criteria [15], usually with a leftward shift of the frontal plane QRS axis, is seen in patients with chronic hemodynamically significant aortic regurgitation. ST-T changes of a 'strain' pattern suggest a worse prognosis [16]. QS complexes in the anterior precordial leads probably indicate eccentric hypertrophy with a horizontal rotation. Left bundle branch block, prolonged P-R interval, and ventricular arrhythmias are also seen in some patients with aortic regurgitation.

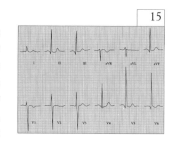

Echocardiography

The etiology of aortic regurgitation (aortic leaflet abnormalities or aortic root disease) can usually be identified by M-mode and two-dimensional echocardiography using long-axis and short-axis views [17–20]. In aortic dissection, a transthoracic study may suggest the presence of an intimal flap but the sensitivity is only about 50%. In contrast, a transesophageal echocardiogram, which allows both the ascending and descending limbs of the thoracic aorta to be visualized very clearly, is highly sensitive and specific for this diagnosis [21].

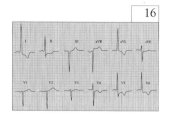

A clue to the presence of aortic regurgitation can be obtained from an M-mode recording showing diastolic fluttering of the anterior mitral valve leaflet, its chordae, or sometimes the endocardial surface of the interventricular septum [22]. This is quite a sensitive sign, but is unrelated to the severity of the regurgitation. Premature closure of the mitral valve resulting from equalization of left ventricular and left atrial pressures indicates acute, severe aortic regurgitation and suggests the need for urgent surgical intervention [23].

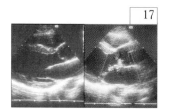

Both M-mode and two-dimensional echocardiography can be used to assess left ventricular stroke volume and ejection fraction. Dilatation of the left ventricle occurs as a consequence of increased regurgitant and, hence, stroke volume [24]. Disproportionate increase of the end-systolic dimension indicates impaired systolic function.

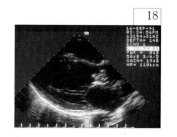

Doppler echocardiography is highly sensitive for detecting aortic regurgitation. Using color-flow mapping, the width of the jet at its origin, and the distance from the aortic valve to which the reflux penetrates into the left ventricle provide qualitative assessment of the severity of aortic regurgitation [25]. Since the velocity of the jet is determined by the driving pressure, continuous-wave Doppler allows the diastolic pressure gradient between the aorta and left ventricle to be measured. In mild aortic regurgitation, aortic pressure remains relatively high, and the Doppler signal has a relatively shallow slope

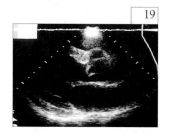
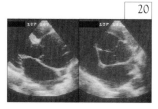
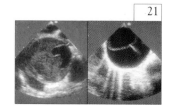
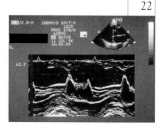

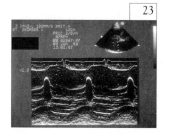
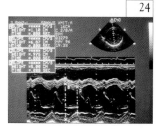
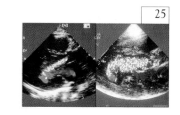

[26a]. By contrast, in severe regurgitation the combination of falling aortic pressure and rising left ventricular pressure results in a rapidly decreasing pressure gradient, shown as a steep slope on the Doppler recording [26b]. In extreme cases, where the two pressures equalize, the velocity falls to zero [27].

It is important to recognize that Doppler recordings may show trivial, clinically insignificant aortic regurgitation in normal individuals.

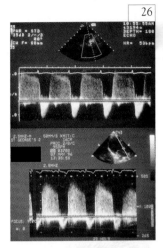

Nuclear Techniques

Gated blood pool imaging is useful in assessing left ventricular volume and function. In chronic aortic regurgitation, left ventricular end-diastolic volume is increased and ejection fraction is maintained for a long period. A decrease in resting ejection fraction is an indication for surgical intervention. Regurgitation index can also be calculated from the ratio of left ventricular stroke volume to right ventricular stroke volume [28]. This index, however, cannot be calculated in the presence of mitral or tricuspid regurgitation. Gated blood pool imaging can also be used to assess changes in left ventricular ejection fraction during exercise. Failure of ejection fraction to increase during exercise may indicate left ventricular dysfunction.

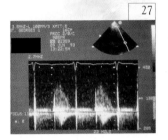

Magnetic Resonance Imaging (MRI) and Computed Tomography (CT)

Both MRI and CT can be used to assess left ventricular function, mass, and regurgitation index [29]. MRI is also capable of directly measuring the absolute volume of aortic regurgitation using velocity mapping. The importance of this technique remains to be defined. However, both MRI and CT are highly sensitive and specific techniques for the diagnosis of aortic dissection and should be considered when aortic regurgitation is suspected due to aortic dissection [30,31]. MRI is also useful for the diagnosis of aortic root disease, such as aortic aneurysm and annulo-aortic ectasia [32,33].

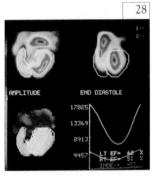

Cardiac Catheterization and Angiography

Cardiac catheterization is sometimes indicated preoperatively to assess coronary artery disease. In symptomatic patients with chronic aortic regurgitation, left ventricular diastolic pressure is usually elevated, although cardiac output may remain normal [34]. In acute severe aortic regurgitation, however, cardiac output may be low, along with a marked increase in left ventricular end-diastolic pressure. Angiography can be used for qualitative assessment of the severity of aortic regurgitation, for quantitative measurement of regurgitation fraction (total stroke volume − forward stroke volume/total

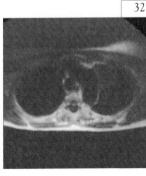

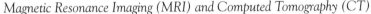

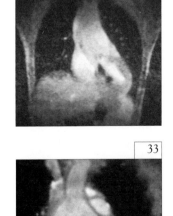

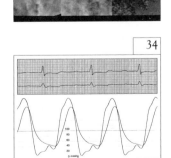

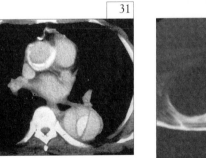

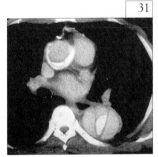

stroke volume), and for evaluation of left ventricular volumes and function. Aortography can be used for the diagnosis of aortic root disease and aortic dissection [35,36].

Principles of Management

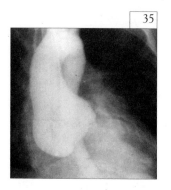

Acute hemodynamically significant aortic regurgitation is an indication for urgent surgery [37]. Such patients will usually have pulmonary edema and premature mitral valve closure. Acute aortic dissection with even mild aortic regurgitation is also an indication for immediate surgery. Symptomatic patients with chronic severe aortic regurgitation also require aortic valve replacement, irrespective of the status of left ventricular function. Decreased ejection fraction is an indication for surgical intervention, even in mildly symptomatic or asymptomatic patients. An increase in left ventricular volume is also used as an indication for operation in asymptomatic patients.

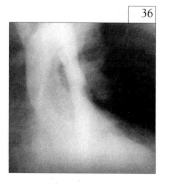

Arteriolar vasodilators and angiotensin converting enzyme inhibitors have been shown to decrease left ventricular volume and mass and to increase ejection fraction. These agents should be used in patients who are not surgical candidates or when surgery needs to be deferred. Antibiotic endocarditis prophylaxis is indicated in all patients.

37

1. Acute severe aortic regurgitation and thoracic aortic dissection including aortic regurgitation require urgent surgery

2. Symptomatic patients with chronic severe aortic regurgitation require valve replacement, irrespective of the status of left ventricular function

3. Decreased rest ejection fraction or significantly increased left ventricular volumes are indications for surgery, even in mildly symptomatic or asymptomatic patients

4. Arteriolar vasodilators or angiotensin converting enzyme inhibitors, which improve left ventricular function, should be considered in patients who are not surgical candidates or when surgery needs to be deferred

5. Antibiotic prophylaxis for endocarditis is always indicated

1   Infective endocarditis of the aortic valve with perforation of a cusp (arrowed) producing regurgitation. Vegetation present on the valve.

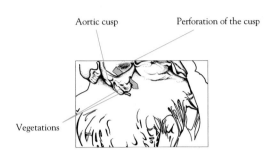

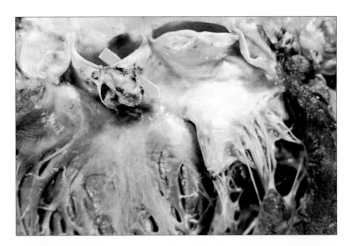

2   Rheumatic aortic regurgitation: all three cusps are fibrotic and retracted. Note the coexistent thickening of mitral chordae.

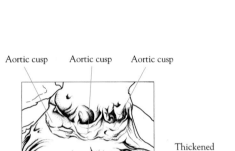

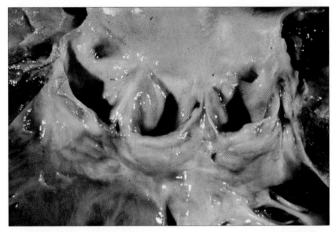

3   Bicuspid aortic valve with a cleft in the largest cusp producing mild aortic regurgitation. Jet lesion on the ventricular surface of the anterior cusp of the mitral valve (arrow).

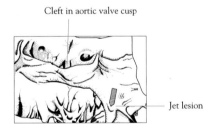

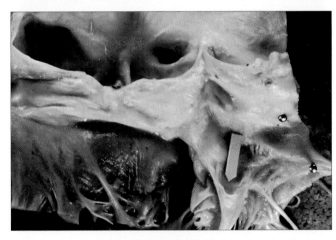

4   Aortic root dilatation with a patch of endocardial thickening on the ventricular septum due to impingement of a regurgitant jet.

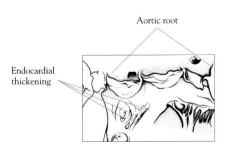

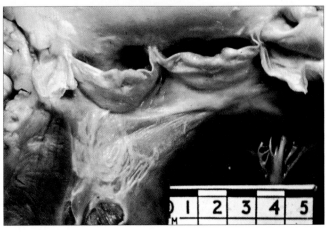

5 Dilated aortic root with ballooned thin aortic cusps producing aortic regurgitation in Marfan's syndrome.

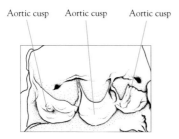

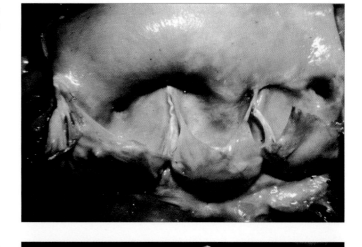

6 Aorta in Marfan's syndrome. The aortic root is dilated and there are two healed dissection tears (arrowed).

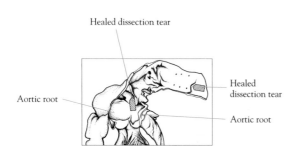

7 Ankylosing spondylitis with aortic regurgitation. The aortic root is dilated, the intima wrinkled; the valve cusps are distorted and shrunken.

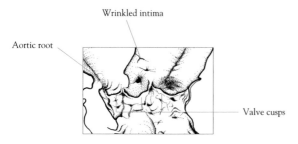

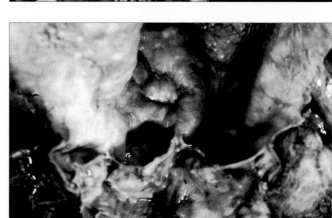

8 Mild syphilitic aortic valve disease. The commissure is widened, the two cusps not meeting. The ascending aorta shows pearly yellow flat plaques.

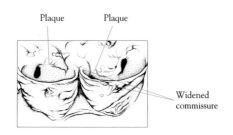

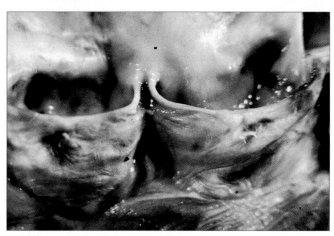

9   Schematic illustrations of the physical findings that suggest chronic moderate to severe aortic regurgitation. A hyperdynamic left ventricular apical impulse occurs as a result of chronic volume overload. A reduced intensity first heart sound indicates increased left ventricular diastolic pressure and often premature closing of the mitral valve. An Austin–Flint murmur also indicates severe aortic regurgitation.

LVOM=apical impulse; S_1=first heart sound; A_2=aortic component of the second heart sound; P_2=pulmonary component of the second heart sound; AFM=Austin–Flint murmur; EDM=early diastolic murmur.

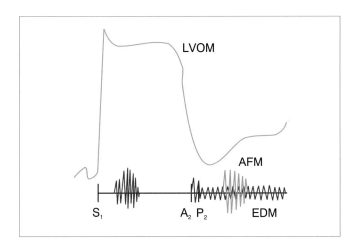

10   Chest X-ray showing dilatation of the ascending aorta with cardiac enlargement from resultant aortic regurgitation.

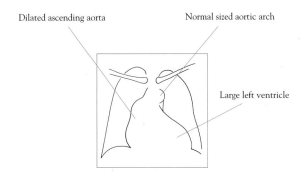

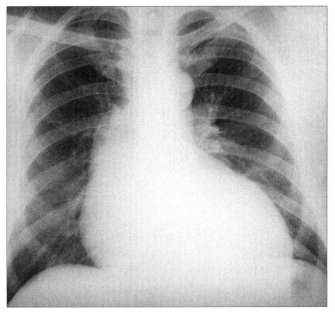

11 Chest X-ray showing a localized aneurysm of the ascending aorta due to syphilis.

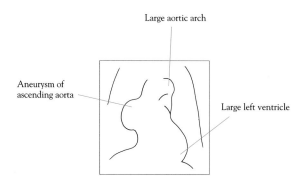

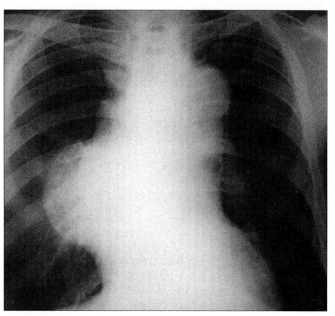

12 Lateral view showing calcification in an ascending aortic root aneurysm.

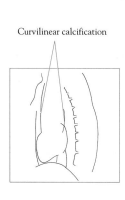

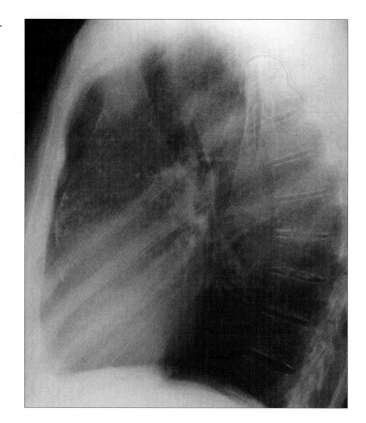

13

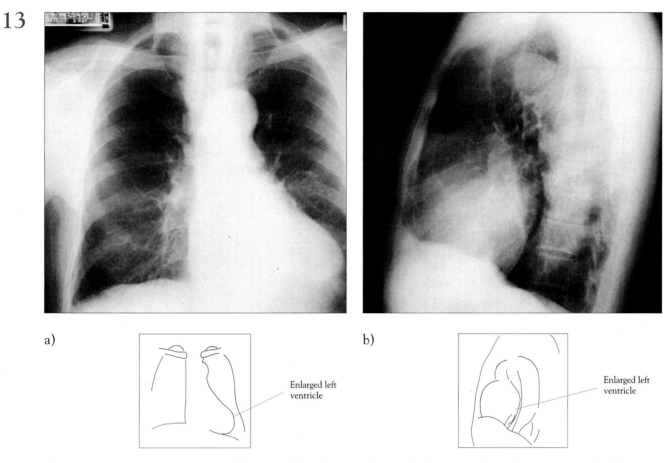

a)

b)

Rheumatic aortic incompetence. (a) Frontal chest X-ray showing left ventricular enlargement to the left, compatible with the degree of regurgitation. The ascending aorta is unremarkable. (b) The lateral view confirms the evidence of left ventricular enlargement. The ascending aorta appears normal.

14 Chest X-ray showing pulmonary edema with normal heart size due to acute aortic regurgitation from a ruptured cusp.

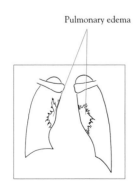

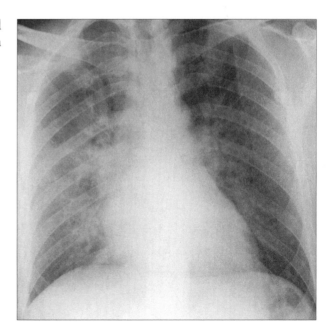

15

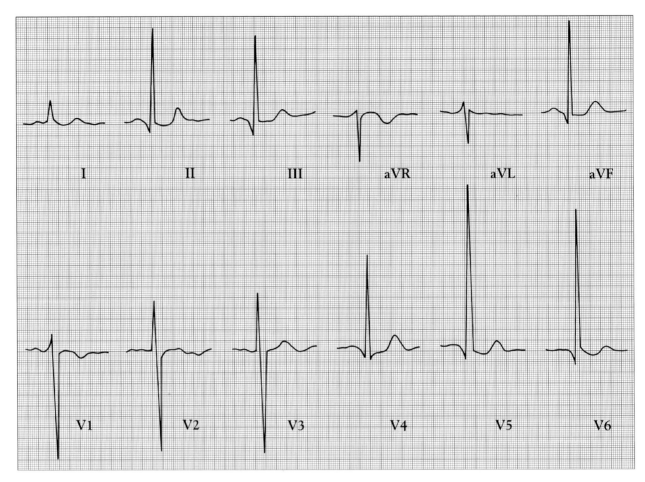

The electrocardiogram in chronic aortic regurgitation showing increased left ventricular voltage (deep S-wave V1, tall R-wave V6).

16

The electrocardiogram in chronic aortic regurgitation showing severe left ventricular hypertrophy (i.e. increased voltage and ST-T wave abnormalities in the lateral leads) with ST-T abnormalities of left ventricular strain. The frontal plane QRS axis is oriented leftward.

17

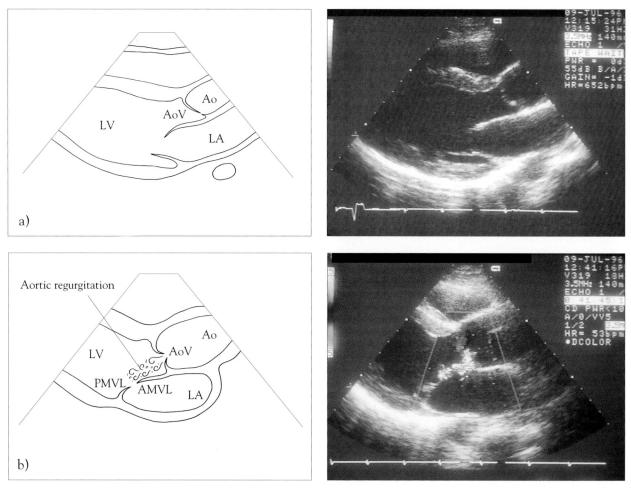

Parasternal long-axis views of a patient with aortic regurgitation caused by a congenitally bicuspid aortic valve. (a) The valve closure line is markedly eccentric, with prolapse of the anterior cusp; the proximal ascending aorta is also mildly dilated. (b) Using color-flow Doppler, a jet of aortic regurgitation passes across the face of the anterior mitral leaflet.

18

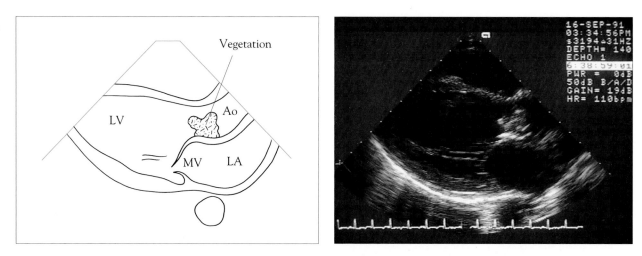

Parasternal long-axis view of severe aortic regurgitation associated with infective endocarditis. A large, irregular shaped mass of vegetations prolapses into the left ventricular outflow tract during diastole.

19

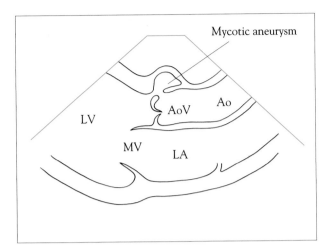 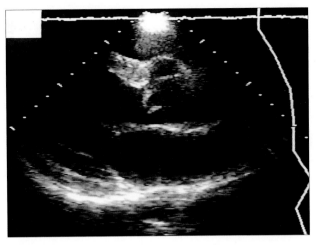

Parasternal long-axis view showing a large mycotic aneurysm in the aortic root. The presence of cusp perforation and communication between the aorta and the aneurysm at the cusp base were confirmed at surgery.

20

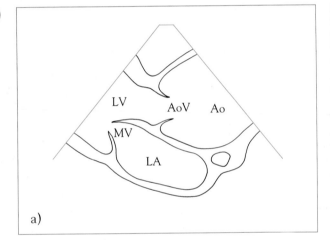 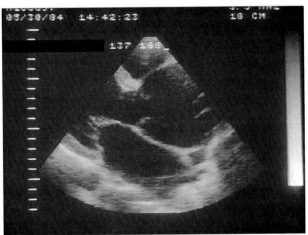

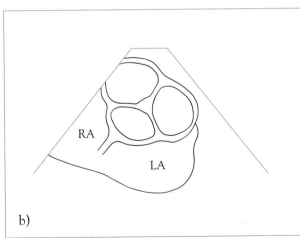 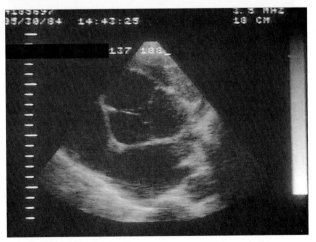

(a) Parasternal long-axis view of a patient with aneurysmal dilatation of the aortic root associated with Marfan's syndrome. There is complete loss of integrity of the supravalvular ridge (sino-tubular junction) and the proximal ascending aorta is over 8 cm in diameter. (b) The parasternal short-axis section shows a three-cusp valve with failure of apposition of the cusp margins.

21

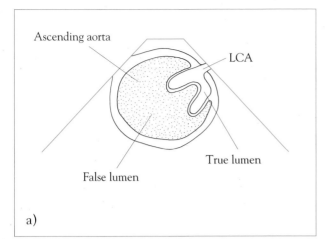

a)

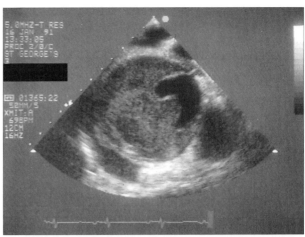

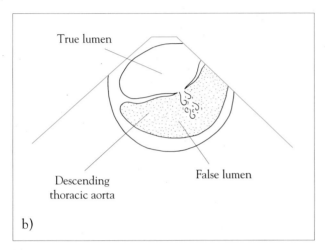

b)

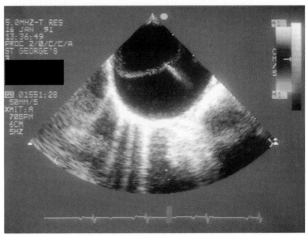

Transesophageal study of a case of aortic dissection. (a) A transverse section just above the valve cusps shows a greatly dilated aorta with the intima dissected over about 80% of the circumference. The dissection apparently has been limited by the orifice of the left coronary artery. The much larger, false lumen is filled with spontaneous echo contrast. (b) A transverse section in the same patient showing the dissection extending into the descending thoracic aorta. It is normal for color-flow Doppler to show several small jets entering the false lumen. These do not represent the primary intimal tear, but arise from perforations at the origins of small branch arteries.

22 Magnified M-mode recording of the mitral valve showing the classical fine fluttering on the anterior leaflet (sometimes seen on the septal endocardium, depending on the jet direction) associated with aortic regurgitation.

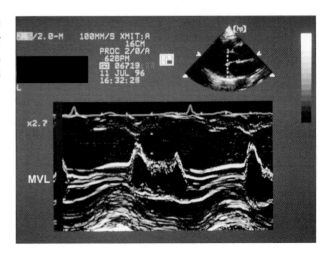

23 M-mode recording of a case of acute, severe aortic regurgitation. The regurgitant flow has elevated diastolic pressure in the left ventricle sufficiently to close the mitral valve well before even the P-wave of the next cycle.

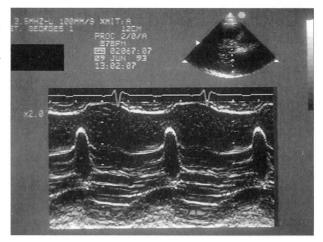

24 M-mode recording from a parasternal short-axis section of the left ventricle in a case of severe aortic regurgitation. The chamber is enlarged and contraction is hyperdynamic with a shortening fraction of 45%.

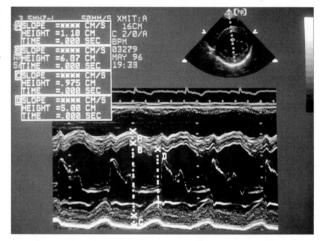

25

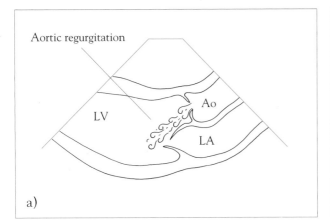

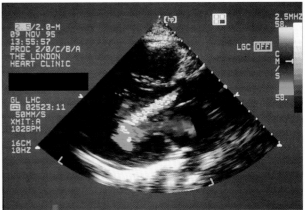

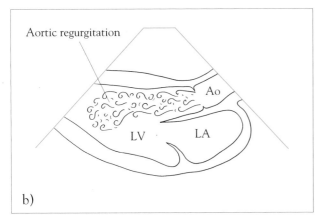

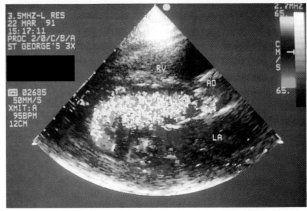

Color-flow Doppler assessment of severity of aortic regurgitation. (a) With relatively mild regurgitation, the jet is narrow, particularly at its origin, and penetration into the ventricle is limited. (b) In very severe aortic regurgitation, the jet fills the left ventricular outflow tract and penetrates right to the apex. While it is possible to distinguish such extremes, color-flow Doppler is at best a semi-quantitative tool and greatly dependent on flow angles, machine gain settings, and operator technique.

26

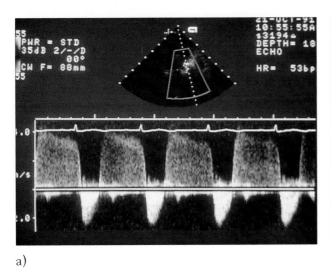

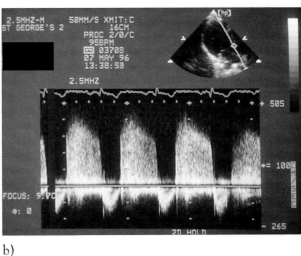

a)   b)

Continuous-wave spectral Doppler offers insights into the hemodynamics of aortic regurgitation, since the velocity of the regurgitant jet indicates the difference between aortic and left ventricular pressures. Thus, the slope of the top of the spectral display is a measure of the rate at which this pressure difference reduces as aortic pressure falls and left ventricular pressure rises. (a) Mild aortic regurgitation. Aortic diastolic pressure falls normally and there is little increase in left ventricular pressure, so a relatively large pressure difference is maintained throughout diastole. (b) Moderately severe aortic regurgitation. The slope is steeper, reflecting a rapid decay of aortic pressure and rising left ventricular pressure.

27   Very severe aortic regurgitation. The slope is very steep and the velocity falls to zero, indicating that aortic and left ventricular pressures have equalized.

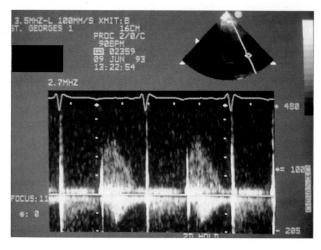

28   Gated blood pool imaging at rest in a patient with chronic severe aortic regurgitation. The left ventricle is dilated, with delayed contraction on the phase image and abnormal amplitude values in the upper septum. The regurgitant index of 4.53 is highly elevated (normal 1–1.7).

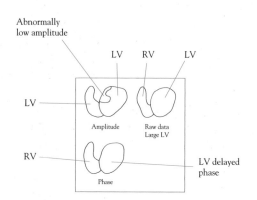

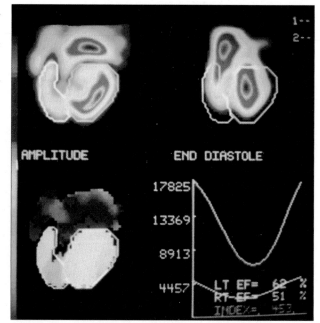

29 Magnetic resonance gradient echo imaging of aortic regurgitation. Intense signal loss is seen proximal to the aortic valve in diastole due to aortic regurgitation.

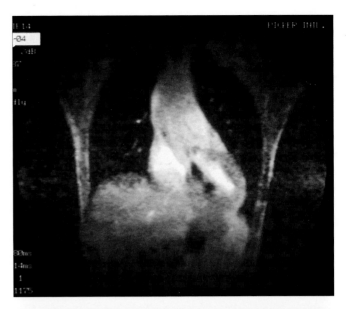

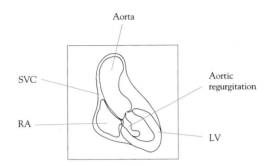

30 Magnetic resonance imaging of aortic dissection in the ascending aorta, in the transaxial plane. The left-hand panel shows a spin echo image, in which there is high intraluminal signal medially, suggestive of thrombus or slow flow. The middle panel is a gradient echo image which shows blood as high signal; the intimal flap is clearly seen. The right-hand panel shows a velocity-encoded gradient echo image (velocity map) with white signal indicating increasing velocities towards the head. High signal is seen in the pulmonary artery and the lateral portion of the aorta. In the medial portion of the aorta there is low signal due to low flow in the false lumen.

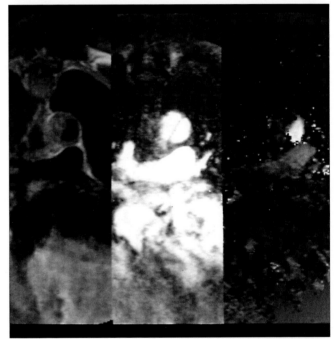

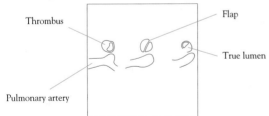

31 Computed tomography of aortic dissection in the transaxial plane. There is a complex dissection involving both the descending and the ascending aorta. Intravenous contrast agent has been given, which appears in the true lumen, forms a rim in the ascending aorta, but is centralized in the descending aorta.

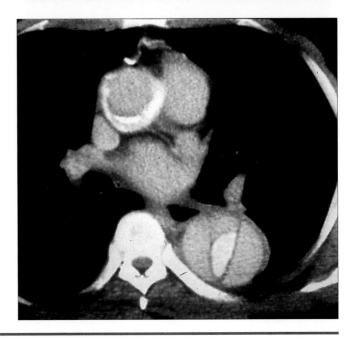

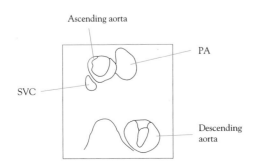

32 Magnetic resonance imaging in the transaxial plane of an aortic arch aneurysm.

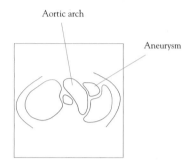

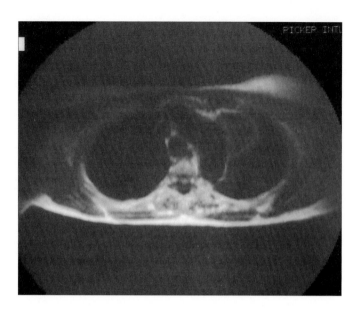

33 Sagittal ECG-gated cine MR through the ascending aorta demonstrating an ectatic pear-shaped ascending aorta measuring 7 cm in diameter in a patient with Marfan's syndrome.

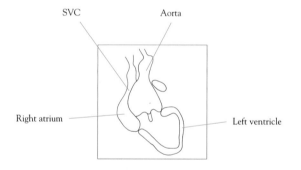

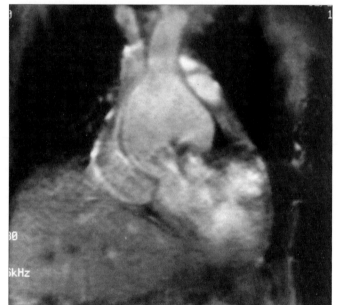

34

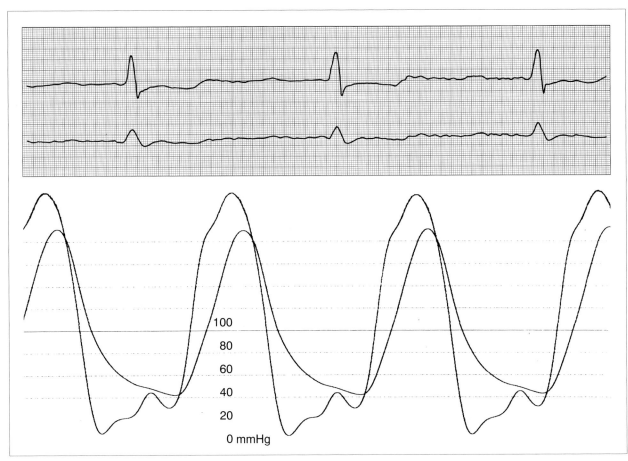

Simultaneous recording of aortic and left ventricular pressures in a patient with significant chronic aortic regurgitation showing elevated left ventricular end-diastolic pressure and low aortic diastolic pressure.

35   Aortogram (antero-posterior projection) showing aortic root dilatation in Marfan's syndrome.

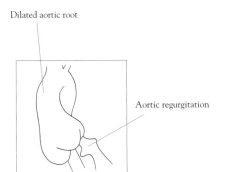

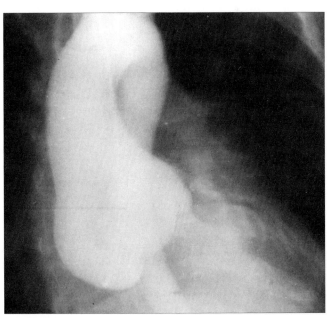

36 Aortogram (antero-posterior projection) of aortic dissection. The true lumen is compressed by the non-opaque false lumen.

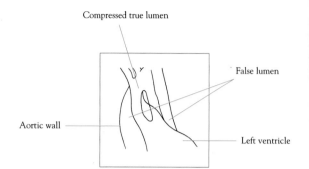

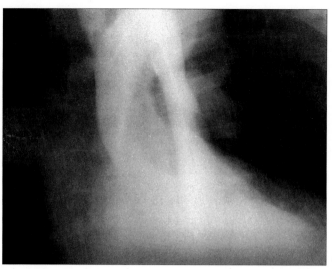

37 Principles of management of aortic regurgitation.

1. Acute severe aortic regurgitation and thoracic aortic dissection including aortic regurgitation require urgent surgery

2. Symptomatic patients with chronic severe aortic regurgitation require valve replacement, irrespective of the status of left ventricular function

3. Decreased rest ejection fraction or significantly increased left ventricular volumes are indications for surgery, even in mildly symptomatic or asymptomatic patients

4. Arteriolar vasodilators or angiotensin converting enzyme inhibitors, which improve left ventricular function, should be considered in patients who are not surgical candidates or when surgery needs to be deferred

5. Antibiotic prophylaxis for endocarditis is always indicated

TRICUSPID VALVE DISEASE

Although there are several congenital malformations that can involve the tricuspid valve, only Ebstein's anomaly and acquired tricuspid valve disease will be considered here.

Pathology

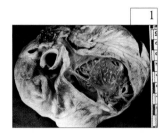

In Ebstein's anomaly the tricuspid valve leaflets are dysplastic, malformed, fused, and displaced into the right ventricular cavity [1]. The leaflets are attached in part to the annulus and in part to the right ventricular wall below the annulus. The part of the right ventricular wall above the leaflets attachment is thinned and incorporated into the right atrium (atrialized). The right atrium is enlarged, and an incompetent or patent foramen ovale or atrial septal defect is present in the majority of patients.

The most common acquired tricuspid valve disease is tricuspid regurgitation associated with right heart failure secondary to pulmonary hypertension. Right ventricular dilatation is accompanied by dilatation and malfunction of the tricuspid annulus (a thin structure), which is the principal cause of secondary tricuspid regurgitation.

Right ventricular infarction, associated with papillary muscle ischemia or infarction, may cause primary tricuspid regurgitation. Isolated tricuspid endocarditis, which occurs in about 40% of intravenous drug abusers, can also cause primary tricuspid regurgitation. Penetrating or non-penetrating trauma can result in tricuspid regurgitation from the rupture of the leaflets, chordae tendineae, or papillary muscle. Tricuspid valve prolapse, which may also be associated with tricuspid regurgitation, rarely occurs as an isolated abnormality but occurs in a minority of patients with mitral valve prolapse.

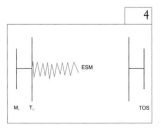

Rheumatic tricuspid valve disease producing both stenosis and regurgitation occurs almost exclusively in association with mitral and aortic valve disease. Commissural fusion analogous to mitral valve disease is seen [2]. Carcinoid heart disease may also involve the tricuspid valve and produce both stenosis and regurgitation [3]. Right atrial myxoma is another rare cause of tricuspid stenosis and regurgitation. Other rare causes of acquired tricuspid valve disease include fibroelastosis, endomyocardial fibrosis, systemic lupus erythematosus, scleroderma, hyperthyroidism, metastatic tumors, and catheter or pacemaker-induced valve disruption.

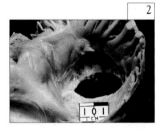

Presentation

Symptoms

All gradations of severity of Ebstein's anomaly exist and a relatively long and active asymptomatic life is compatible with milder forms. When symptoms do appear, dyspnea, fatigue, and weakness are the most common. Palpitation is usually due to atrial arrhythmias. Heart failure, severe hypoxia, and intractable dysrhythmias are the usual causes of death.

Patients with rheumatic tricuspid valve disease usually present with symptoms of related associated mitral or aortic valve disease. However, in patients with severe tricuspid valve disease, symptoms of right heart failure may predominate (fatigue, neck pulsation, right upper quadrant abdominal discomfort, abdominal distention, and peripheral edema).

Signs

In mild Ebstein's anomaly, a widely split first heart sound due to delayed closure of the abnormal tricuspid valve may be the only abnormal finding. The tricuspid closure sound usually has a scratchy quality ('sail sound'). Delayed opening of the abnormal tricuspid valve may also produce a scratchy early diastolic opening snap. An early, late, or pan-systolic murmur along the lower left sternal border is observed if tricuspid regurgitation is present [4]. In severe cases, central cyanosis, clubbing, and manifestations of severe tricuspid regurgitation and right heart failure including elevated jugular venous pressure with a prominent 'v' wave and a sharp 'y' descent, hepatomegaly with systolic pulsation, ascites, and dependent edema may be present.

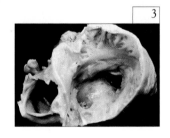

The murmur of tricuspid regurgitation, irrespective of its cause, tends to radiate to the right side of the sternum and to the epigastrium over the liver. The intensity of the murmur usually increases with inspiration (Carvallo's sign). A right ventricular third heart sound is frequently present. The secondary manifestations of severe tricuspid regurgitation are similar, irrespective of its etiology. The signs of pulmonary hypertension (loud P_2, palpable right ventricular hypertrophy) are also present in patients with secondary tricuspid regurgitation. Tricuspid stenosis offers increased resistance to right ventricular filling, and thus is associated with a prominent 'a' wave and a slow 'y' descent in the jugular venous pulse. Occasionally, a presystolic hepatic pulsation is felt. This condition is also characterized by a mid-diastolic crescendo-decrescendo murmur, usually without presystolic accentuation, but often preceded by a tricuspid opening snap. There is increased intensity of the murmur during inspiration [5].

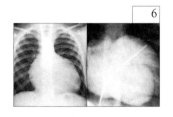

Investigations

Radiology

In Ebstein's anomaly, a large globular heart, occasionally with a bulge on the left heart border due to displacement of the right ventricular outflow tract, may be seen [6]. The right heart border may also be prominent and the lung fields may be oligemic [7].

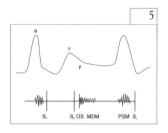

In rheumatic tricuspid valve disease, the radiographic features of mitral valve disease may be modified; the upper lobe pulmonary venous dilatation may be less obvious in the presence of tricuspid valve disease [8].

Severe long-standing tricuspid regurgitation can produce considerable cardiac enlargement due to right atrial and right ventricular dilatation. In tricuspid stenosis, right atrial enlargement causing a prominent right border of the heart and also inconspicuous pulmonary arteries are often observed [9].

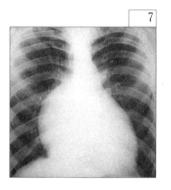

Electrocardiography

In Ebstein's anomaly, right atrial enlargement with right bundle branch block are the most frequent abnormalities [10]. Pre-excitation (Wolff–Parkinson–White) syndrome, with the accessory pathway connecting the right ventricle, occurs in 20–25% of patients [11]. Prolonged P-R interval, paroxysmal supraventricular tachycardia, and other atrial dysrhythmias occur frequently. In primary tricuspid stenosis or regurgitation, a prominent P-wave, due to right atrial enlargement, may be present. In secondary tricuspid regurgitation, findings of right ventricular hypertrophy may occasionally be present.

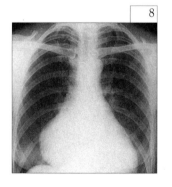
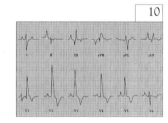
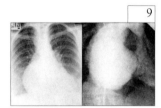
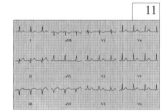

Echocardiography

Rheumatic heart disease affects the tricuspid valve only rarely. It results in thickening and retraction of the leaflets, but almost never in frank calcification. The echocardiographic and Doppler features are thus similar to those of mitral stenosis, but less pronounced. Peak and mean diastolic pressure gradients can be measured by continuous-wave Doppler, although even severe disease generates gradients only of the order of 2–8 mmHg [12]. Direct planimetry of the valve orifice is not normally possible, as the correct cross-sectional view cannot be obtained. Inflow obstruction causes the rate of decay of the pressure gradient to reduce and this can be expressed in terms of the 'pressure half-time'. However, a quantitative relationship between pressure half-time and tricuspid valve orifice area has not been established.

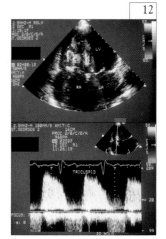

Tricuspid regurgitation may be functional, secondary to dilatation of the valve annulus or shrinkage of the cusps. It may also be caused by infective endocarditis or from instrumentation such as pacing leads [13]. Elevated right heart pressures, as in pulmonary hypertension or pulmonary stenosis, do not normally cause significant tricuspid regurgitation unless there is right ventricular enlargement.

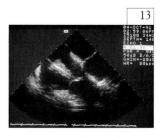

Color Doppler provides an extremely sensitive method for detecting a regurgitant jet in the right atrium, and severity can be assessed qualitatively [14]. In severe cases, the inferior vena cava is enlarged and systolic flow reversal into the engorged hepatic veins can be demonstrated [15].

Tricuspid regurgitation can also be demonstrated by injection of contrast microbubbles into a vein. The bubbles are very stable and sometimes can still be seen passing to and fro between ventricle and atrium many minutes after injection.

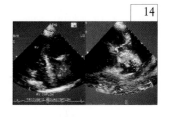

Continuous-wave Doppler allows the flow waveform to be analyzed and peak velocity to be measured. The peak velocity of the regurgitant jet is determined by the right ventricle–right atrium pressure gradient. Provided there is no outflow obstruction, systolic pressure in the right ventricle equals that in the pulmonary arteries. Thus, the jet velocity allows pulmonary systolic pressure to be related directly to right atrial pressure, and if the latter is known from manometry or inspection of the jugular venous pulse, pulmonary pressure can be stated in absolute values of mmHg [16].

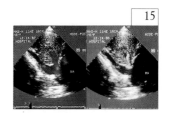

As with mitral regurgitation, the flow profile reflects increasing right atrial pressure, and very severe regurgitation can result in equalization of right atrial and right ventricular pressures.

Tricuspid regurgitation is one cause of right ventricular volume overload. The increased chamber size and hyperdynamic contraction result in so-called 'paradoxical' septal motion and can be seen on an M-mode recording.

Two-dimensional echocardiography shows anatomic abnormalities of the tricuspid valve. Ebstein's anomaly is characterized by a very large tricuspid valve, abnormally displaced into the right ventricle. This is best demonstrated in the apical four-chamber view [17]. In carcinoid disease, the tricuspid valve leaflets are characteristically thickened and retracted so that they appear fixed in a partially open position. Right atrial masses causing right ventricular inflow obstruction or tricuspid regurgitation can also be detected.

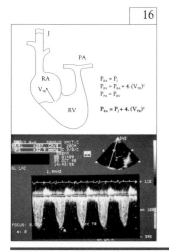

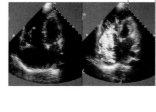

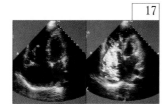

Nuclear Techniques
Gated blood pool imaging has been used to assess the severity of tricuspid regurgitation by measuring the ratio of left and right ventricular stroke volume, which is markedly reduced in severe tricuspid regurgitation. However, this investigation is seldom necessary in clinical practice.

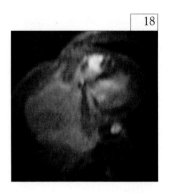

Magnetic Resonance Imaging (MRI) and Computed Tomography (CT)
MRI can be used for the diagnosis and quantification of tricuspid regurgitation and associated changes in right atrial and right ventricular size [18]. MRI is often used for the diagnosis of congenital heart disease, including Ebstein's anomaly. MRI and CT have also been used to assess right ventricular function.

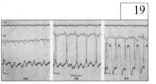

Cardiac Catheterization and Angiography
In Ebstein's anomaly, it may be evident at cardiac catheterization that a right atrial pressure trace is obtained in a position when an endocardial electrocardiogram shows characteristics of right ventricular morphology [19]. Severe tricuspid regurgitation and right-to-left atrial shunt can also be detected by a right ventriculogram.

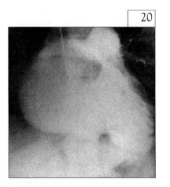

The displacement of the effective right atrioventricular orifice into the cavity of the right ventricle, with atrialization of the ventricular inlet portion, can also be demonstrated by angiography [20,21].

In severe tricuspid regurgitation, the right atrial pressure is elevated with a prominent 'v' wave. Occasionally, ventricularization of the atrial pressure tracing is recognized [22]. Equalization of the right and left ventricular diastolic pressures, due to the constraining effect of the pericardium, is also observed in some patients.

In tricuspid stenosis, simultaneous recording of right atrial and right ventricular pressures demonstrates a diastolic transvalvular pressure gradient [23]. In severe tricuspid regurgitation, right ventricular contrast angiography shows a dilated right atrium and right ventricle, and almost instantaneous opacification of the right atrium during systole.

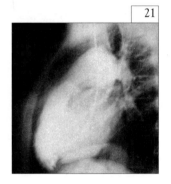

Principles of Management

Treatment of secondary tricuspid regurgitation consists of treatment of right heart failure with diuretics and sometimes digitalis, and correction of the cause of the pulmonary hypertension such as operation of mitral valve disease [24]. Tricuspid annuloplasty may be required in intractable severe primary tricuspid regurgitation. Severe tricuspid stenosis is sometimes amenable to catheter valvuloplasty. Severe Ebstein's anomaly with arterial desaturation due to atrial right-to-left shunt requires surgical correction, although operative mortality is high and the postoperative results may be less than satisfactory.

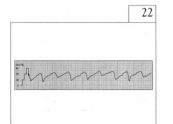

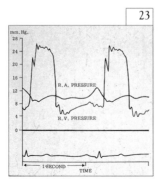

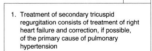

1. Treatment of secondary tricuspid regurgitation consists of treatment of right heart failure and correction, if possible, of the primary cause of pulmonary hypertension

2. Severe tricuspid stenosis is sometimes treated by catheter valvuloplasty

3. In patients with severe Ebstein's anomaly with a marked arterial desaturation, surgical correction should be considered

1   Heart with Ebstein's anomaly of the tricuspid valve viewed from the outlet portion of the right ventricle. The valve is a fenestrated curtain which is attached in such a way as to separate the inlet and outlet portions of the right ventricle. The cavity of the inlet portion (atrialized right ventricle) is behind the valve.

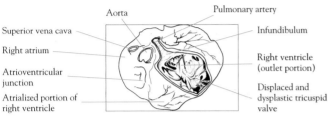

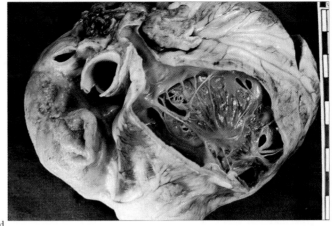

2   Heart viewed from the right atrium with tricuspid stenosis and incompetence due to rheumatic involvement of the valve cusps.

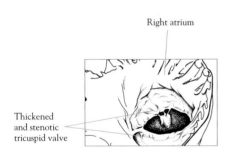

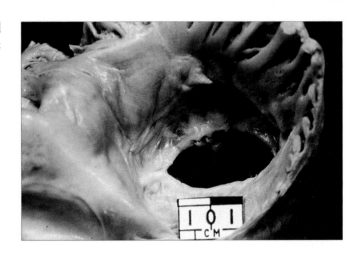

3   Heart in carcinoid disease showing fibrous thickening of the tricuspid valve.

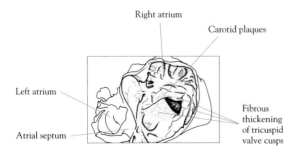

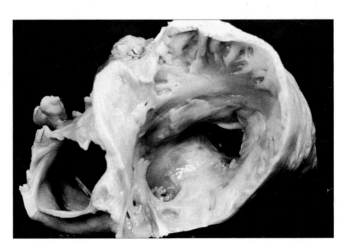

4 The auscultatory findings of Ebstein's anomaly complicated by tricuspid regurgitation are illustrated. The delayed tricuspid closure sound usually has a scratchy quality ('sail sound').
M_1=Mitral valve closure sound; T_1=tricuspid valve closure sound; ESM=early systolic murmur of tricuspid regurgitation; TOS=tricuspid opening sound.

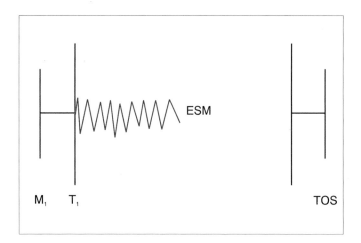

5 Schematic illustration of the important physical findings in tricuspid stenosis. A prominent 'a' wave, a slow 'y' descent, and a crescendo-decrescendo diastolic murmur, which increases in intensity during inspiration, are important findings in tricuspid stenosis. An opening snap and a pre-systolic murmur may also be present.
a=Prominent 'a' wave; v=normal 'v' wave in jugular venous pulse; y=slow 'y' descent due to tricuspid stenosis; S_1=first heart sound; S_2=second heart sound; OS=opening snap; MDM=mid-diastolic murmur; PSM=presystolic murmur.

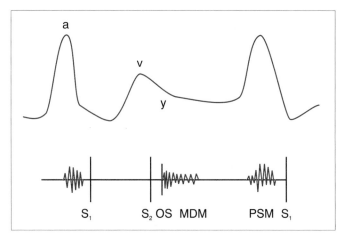

6

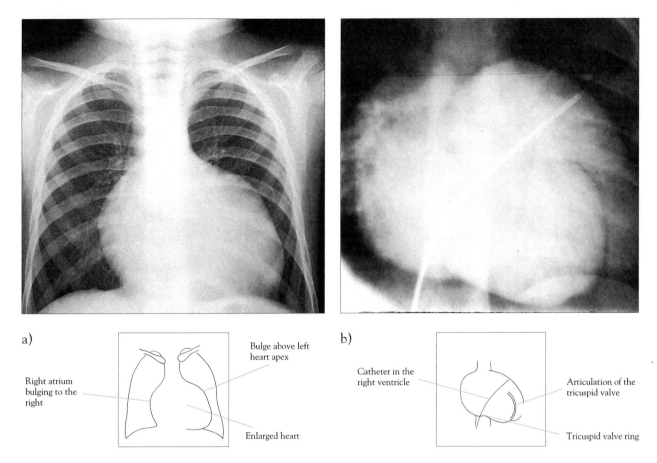

a)

Right atrium bulging to the right

Bulge above left heart apex

Enlarged heart

b)

Catheter in the right ventricle

Articulation of the tricuspid valve

Tricuspid valve ring

Ebstein's anomaly of the tricuspid valve. The septal leaflet articulates within the right ventricle, reducing its effective size and increasing the functional capacity of the right atrium. (a) The frontal chest X-ray usually shows an enlarged heart which may have the characteristic 'box-like configuration' with the right atrium bulging to the right and a small right ventricle causing a bulge above the left heart apex. The lungs are oligemic. (b) The accompanying angiogram shows the site of the tricuspid valve ring, identified by a notch at the site of articulation of the tricuspid valve within the right ventricle.

7   Chest X-ray in Ebstein's anomaly showing pulmonary oligemia and a prominent right atrial border.

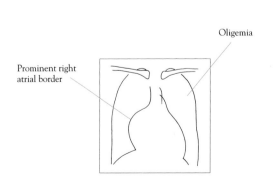

Prominent right atrial border

Oligemia

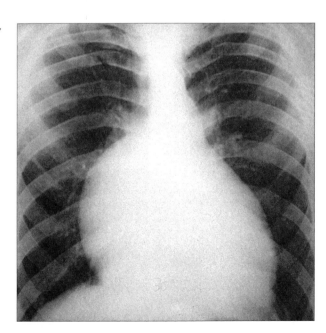

8   Chest X-ray in rheumatic tricuspid and mitral valve disease showing a large right atrium. Upper lobe blood diversion is inconspicuous.

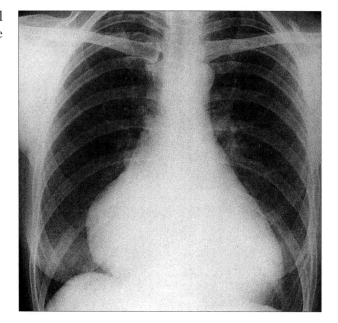

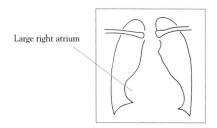

9

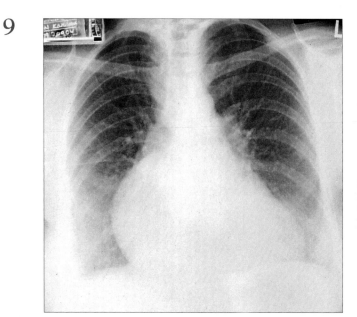

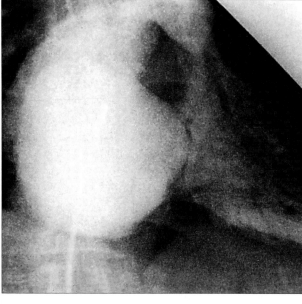

a)

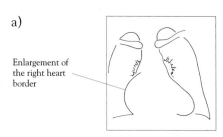

b)

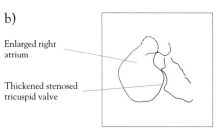

Chest X-ray in tricuspid stenosis. (a) The frontal chest X-ray shows the enlargement of the right heart border and its bulge to the right. (b) The accompanying right atrial angiogram in slight right anterior oblique projection shows the large right atrium and its appendage, and also the thickened and stenosed tricuspid valve.

10

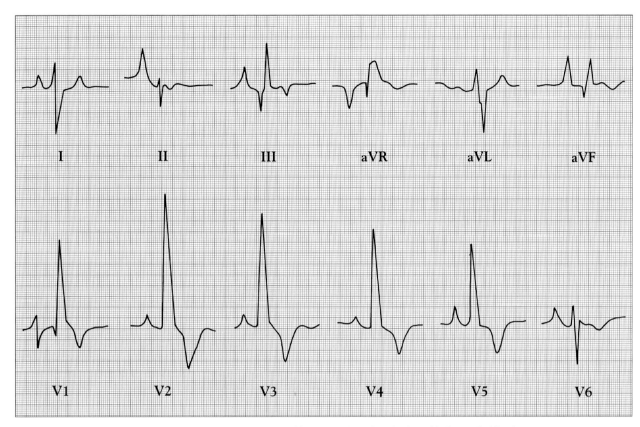

Electrocardiogram in Ebstein's anomaly showing tall P-waves and right bundle branch block.

11

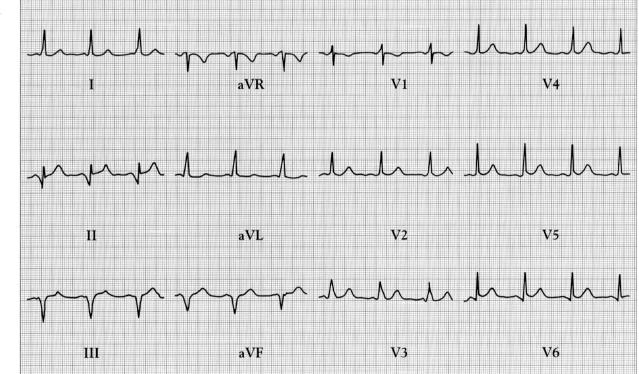

Pre-excitation syndrome is present in approximately 20–25% of patients with Ebstein's anomaly. The electrocardiogram may show a short P-R interval and right ventricular pre-excitation.

12

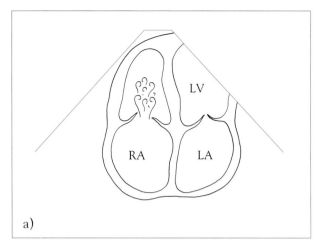

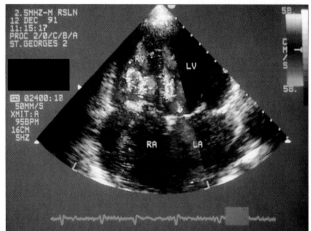

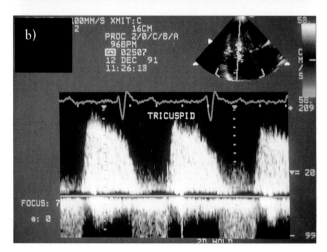

(a) Apical four-chamber view with color-flow Doppler in a case of tricuspid stenosis. The reduced orifice area is indicated by the width of the color jet and there is some aliasing indicating increased inflow velocity. (b) Continuous-wave spectral Doppler from the same patient: peak inflow velocity is 1.8 m/s with a slow rate of velocity decay.

13

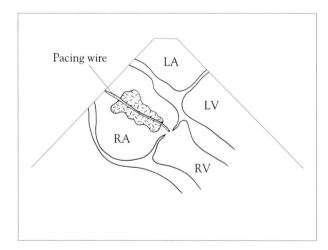

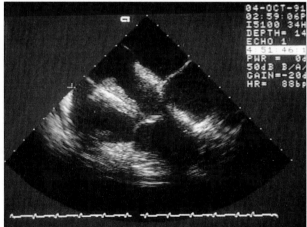

Transesophageal study showing a large vegetation in the right atrium growing around a pacing wire.

14

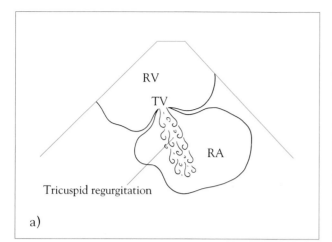

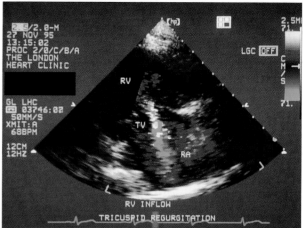

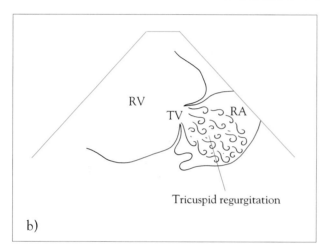

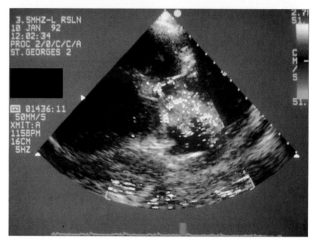

Color-flow Doppler studies of tricuspid regurgitation employing a tilted parasternal view to show the right ventricular inflow tract. (a) Mild regurgitation, with a narrow origin to the jet. (b) Very severe regurgitation with free flow backwards and forwards between the atrium and the ventricle.

15

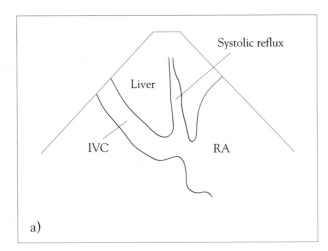

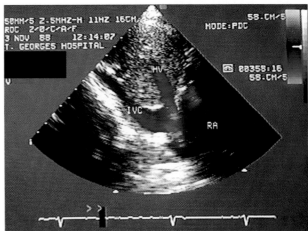

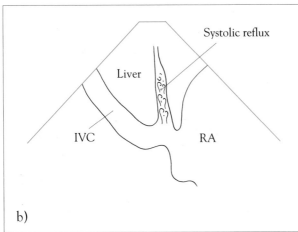

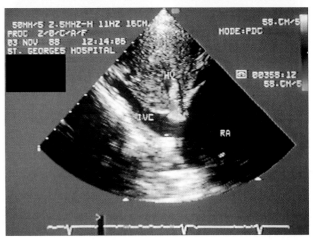

In severe tricuspid regurgitation, color-flow Doppler can be used to demonstrate systolic reflux into the hepatic veins. (a) Diastolic frame showing flow away from the transducer (blue) as blood flows from the liver into the inferior vena cava (IVC). (b) Systolic frame showing reflux towards the transducer (red) from the IVC into the enlarged hepatic veins.

16

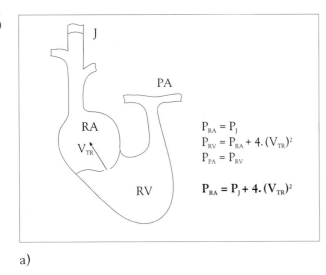

$$P_{RA} = P_J$$
$$P_{RV} = P_{RA} + 4 \cdot (V_{TR})^2$$
$$P_{PA} = P_{RV}$$

$$P_{RA} = P_J + 4 \cdot (V_{TR})^2$$

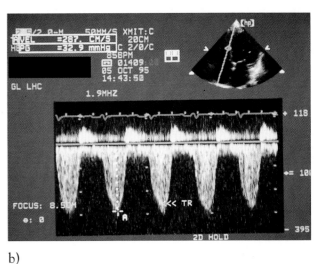

a)   b)

(a) Diagram showing the basis for assessment of pulmonary hypertension using continuous-wave spectral Doppler. Pressure in the right atrium can be determined from inspection of the jugular venous pulse. If any tricuspid regurgitation is present, the Bernoulli equation ($\Delta P = 4 \times V^2$) allows the (RV-RA) pressure gradient to be calculated from the velocity of the jet. Systolic pressure in the right ventricle equals that in the pulmonary arteries as long as there is no right ventricular outflow obstruction. (b) Continuous-wave spectral Doppler of tricuspid regurgitation. The peak jet velocity is 2.8 m/s, corresponding to a (RV-RA) gradient of 31 mmHg. Pulmonary artery pressure is thus equal to (RA pressure + 31) mmHg.

17

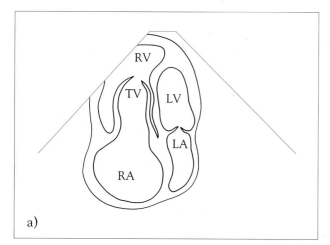

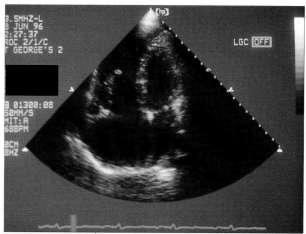

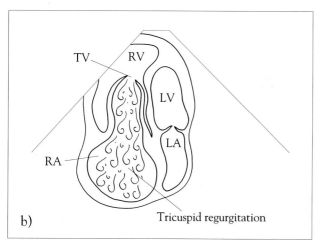

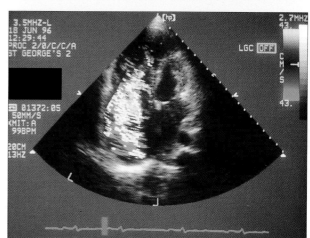

Ebstein's anomaly. (a) Apical four-chamber view showing the enlarged right heart chambers with huge, sail-like tricuspid valve leaflets. Much of the septal leaflet is adherent to the interventricular septum, and the valve orifice is displaced well towards the apex. (b) Color-flow Doppler shows severe associated tricuspid regurgitation.

18 Magnetic resonance gradient echo imaging in the transaxial plane. There is signal loss occurring from the tricuspid valve into a huge right atrium (tricuspid regurgitation).

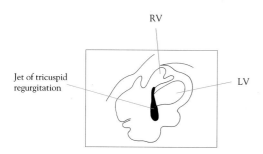

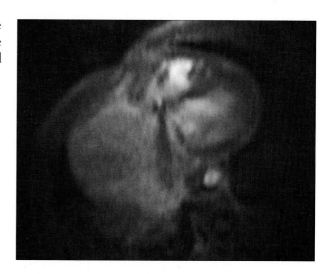

19

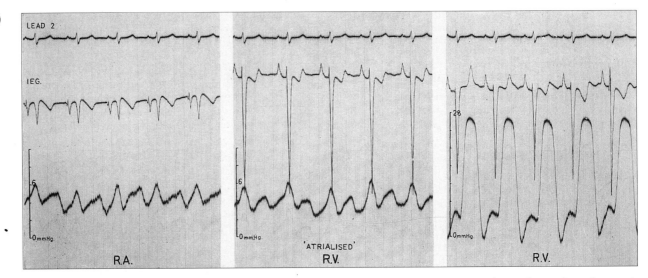

The type of tracings obtained in Ebstein's anomaly during cardiac catheterization with an electrode catheter. A ventricular intracardiac electrocardiogram (IEG) may be recorded simultaneously with an atrial pressure pulse in the 'atrialized' portion of the right ventricle.

[From: Ebstein's anomaly of the tricuspid valve. In: *Pediatric Cardiology*. Watson H (Editor). London: Lloyd-Luke (Medical Books) Ltd., 1968; First Edition: p.445].

20   Right ventricular angiogram (antero-posterior projection) in Ebstein's anomaly. The injection is in the outlet portion. Both the true atrioventricular annulus and the effective orifice are outlined by regurgitation through the downwardly displaced tricuspid valve. The right atrium is dilated. In this patient there was additional pulmonary valve stenosis.

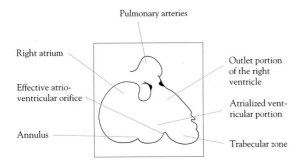

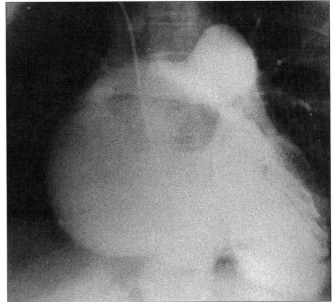

21 Lateral projection: the effective orifice of the tricuspid valve is seen between the inlet and outlet portions of the right ventricle. A thickened pulmonary valve is also seen.

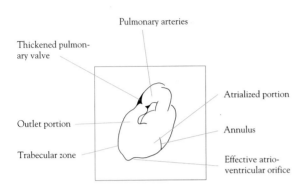

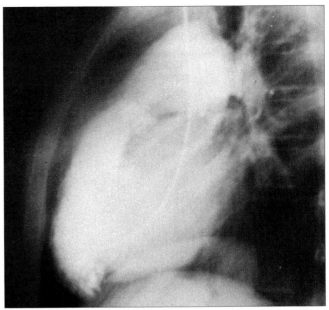

22

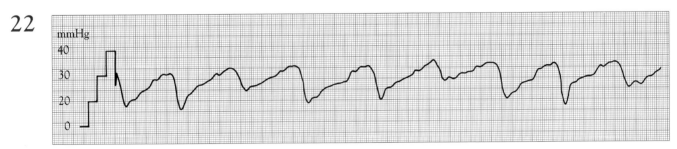

Severe tricuspid regurgitation is associated with elevated right atrial pressure with occasional ventricularization of the right atrial pressure tracing.

23 Pressure tracings from a patient with tricuspid stenosis showing a diastolic gradient between right atrium and right ventricle.

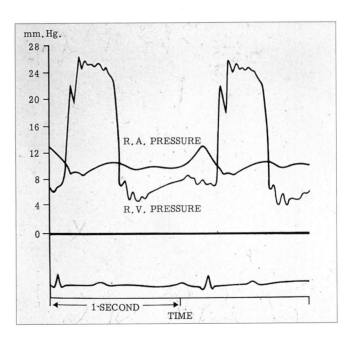

24 Principles of management of tricuspid valve disease.

1. Treatment of secondary tricuspid regurgitation consists of treatment of right heart failure and correction, if possible, of the primary cause of pulmonary hypertension

2. Severe tricuspid stenosis is sometimes treated by catheter valvuloplasty

3. In patients with severe Ebstein's anomaly with a marked arterial desaturation, surgical correction should be considered

CHAPTER 5
Congenital Heart Disease in Adults

ATRIAL SEPTAL DEFECT

VENTRICULAR SEPTAL DEFECT

PERSISTENT DUCTUS ARTERIOSUS

PULMONARY STENOSIS

FALLOT'S TETRALOGY

COARCTATION OF THE AORTA

Abbreviations

AMVL	Anterior mitral valve leaflet	LV	Left ventricle
Ao	Aorta	LVOT	Left ventricular outflow tract
AoV	Aortic valve	MPA	Main pulmonary artery
Acs Ao	Ascending aorta	MV	Mitral valve
ASD	Atrial septal defect	MVL	Mitral valve leaflet
AV	Aortic valve	PA	Pulmonary artery
CW	Chest wall	PDA	Persistent ductus arteriosus
Desc Ao	Descending aorta	PT	Pulmonary trunk
En	Endocardium	PV	Pulmonary valve
Ep	Epicardium	PVL	Pulmonary valve leaflet
Inn	Innominate artery	PVW	Posterior ventricular wall
IS	Infundibular stenosis	RA	Right atrium
IST	Isthmus	RAVL	Right atrioventricular valve leaflet
IV	Inferior vena cava	RPA	Right pulmonary artery
IVS	Interventricular septum	RV	Right ventricle
LA	Left atrium	RVOT	Right ventricular outflow tract
LAVL	Left atrioventricular valve leaflet	S	Septum
LCCA	Left common carotid artery	SVC	Superior vena cava
LPA	Left pulmonary artery	TV	Tricuspid valve
LSCA	Left subclavian artery	VSD	Ventricular septal defect

ATRIAL SEPTAL DEFECT

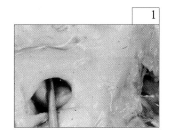

Pathophysiology

In up to 25% of all normal hearts there is a patent foramen ovale [1]. However, a shunt from left atrium to right atrium is prevented by a flap valve, and a right-to-left shunt will only occur if the right atrial pressure is raised. A secundum atrial septal defect results from a deficiency of the flap valve of the foramen ovale [2]. Other types of atrial septal defect include a 'sinus venosus' defect which lies superior to the fossa ovalis; this is usually associated with partial anomalous pulmonary venous return either into the superior vena cava or into the right atrium [3]. Rarely, a defect in the postero-inferior portion of the atrium results in the inferior vena cava draining directly into the left atrium. The ostium primum atrial septal defect, usually presenting in childhood, involves the lowermost part of the atrial septum [4] and is characteristically associated with a defect of the ventricular septum and cleft in the atrioventricular valves [5].

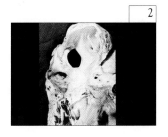

In the majority of patients with atrial septal defects, pulmonary vascular resistance is normal and lower than systemic vascular resistance, allowing a left-to-right shunt with pulmonary flow exceeding systemic flow. As the shunt occurs at atrial level, the left ventricle is spared from volume overload but left atrial, right atrial, and right ventricular sizes increase from increased volume load. When pulmonary vascular resistance increases, the left-to-right shunt decreases and when pulmonary vascular resistance is equal to or exceeds systemic vascular resistance, right-to-left shunting occurs with hypoxia and cyanosis (Eisenmenger syndrome).

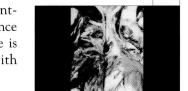

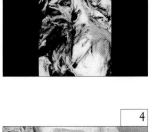

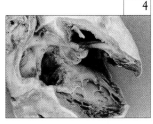

Presentation

Symptoms

Whereas most children with an atrial septal defect are asymptomatic, patients presenting over the age of 40 will often complain of breathlessness on exertion, palpitation, or fatigue. Rarely, the elderly patient presents not only in atrial fibrillation but with frank heart failure. At any age, the lesion may initially be discovered by routine chest X-ray.

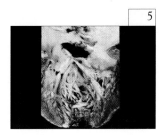

Signs

The diagnostic hallmark of an atrial septal defect is the fixed wide splitting of the second heart sound, virtually always associated with an ejection systolic murmur in the pulmonary area [6]. Irrespective of the level of the pulmonary artery pressure or the direction of the shunt, pulmonary valve closure is as loud, or louder, than aortic valve closure. With a large left-to-right shunt at atrial level there may be an additional mid-diastolic murmur increased by inspiration at the left sternal edge. This results from increased flow through the normal tricuspid valve. A pansystolic murmur due to mitral valve regurgitation may suggest an ostium primum defect, although the electrocardiogram showing left axis deviation will be more helpful. A mid-systolic click and a late systolic murmur suggest mitral valve prolapse; this sometimes occurs with a secundum atrial septal defect.

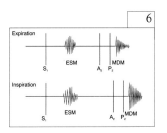

In an atrial septal defect with the Eisenmenger syndrome, central cyanosis may be present. The auscultatory signs are similar to those of a secundum atrial septal defect with a large left-to-right shunt, except that a pulmonary ejection sound is frequently heard, pulmonary valve closure is very loud, and a tricuspid flow murmur is not present.

The quality of the arterial pulse in an atrial septal defect is usually normal but the jugular venous pulse is frequently visible with a normal wave form unless there is additional tricuspid regurgitation. There may be a hyperdynamic impulse at the left sternal edge due to increased right ventricular stroke volume but this finding is often absent in the older patient.

Investigations

Radiology

Both the central and peripheral pulmonary vessels in a left-to-right shunting atrial septal defect are dilated due to increased pulmonary blood flow (pulmonary plethora) [7]. The aortic knuckle is usually small. Most adults also show cardiac enlargement as a result of right ventricular and right atrial dilatation [8]. If there is marked pulmonary hypertension with a left-to-right shunt, all these features become more obvious [9]. If the Eisenmenger reaction has occurred, the central pulmonary arteries may become very large while the distal vessels are reduced in caliber [10]. There may be calcified atheroma in the pulmonary artery. The presence of partial anomalous pulmonary venous drainage may be indicated by the anomalous veins lying in an abnormal anatomic position [11]. Although the chest X-ray of an ostium primum atrial septal defect may be indistinguishable from that of a secundum defect, upper zone vessel dilatation and left atrial enlargement may be apparent, reflecting mitral regurgitation [12].

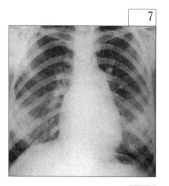

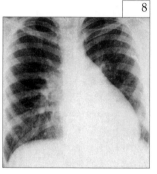

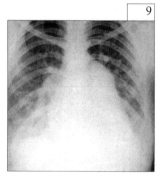

Electrocardiography

The typical ECG of a secundum atrial septal defect shows a normal QRS axis with complete or incomplete right bundle branch block [13].

In an atrial septal defect with severe pulmonary hypertension, there may be frank right ventricular hypertrophy recognized from the ECG. Left axis deviation in the ECG suggests that the atrial septal defect is of the ostium primum variety [14].

Echocardiography

Almost all cases of atrial septal defect in children can be assessed fully by echocardiography and Doppler. The subcostal four-chamber view is best for imaging the lesion. An ostium secundum defect lies within the fossa ovalis and is bounded superiorly and inferiorly by atrial septal tissue. The atrioventricular septum is intact, with separation of the insertion of the mitral and tricuspid valve leaflets [15]. In contrast, in an ostium primum defect, both valve leaflets insert into the crest of the ventricular septum at the same level and there is normally an associated cleft in the anterior mitral valve leaflet [16,17]. The location of sinus venosus defects, right at the top of the interatrial septum

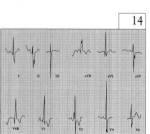

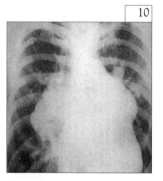

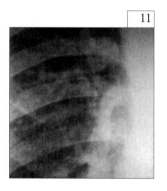

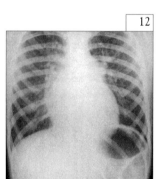

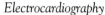

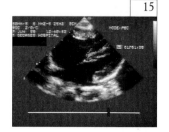

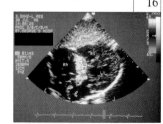

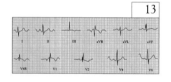

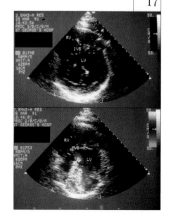

at the entry of the superior vena cava, makes them hard to visualize by transthoracic imaging in older children and adults, but this is readily accomplished by transesophageal echocardiography [18].

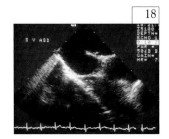

Doppler is used to confirm the presence of a shunt and to quantify shunt volume. Color Doppler can show flow passing from enlarged pulmonary veins, across the defect, and thence through the tricuspid valve [19]. A qualitative estimate of shunt size can be obtained from color or pulse-wave assessment of flows across the mitral and tricuspid valves [20].

Tracing the outline of a spectral Doppler recording of flow in a blood vessel gives the velocity–time integral or 'stroke distance'; when multiplied by the vessel cross-sectional area, this gives volumetric flow. This technique can be used in the aorta to measure systemic flow volume (Qs), and in the main pulmonary artery to measure pulmonary flow volume (Qp). Hence, the pulmonary/systemic flow ratio (Qp/Qs) can be determined. This method can be applied to all atrial and ventricular septal defects, except when there is significant aortic or pulmonary regurgitation.

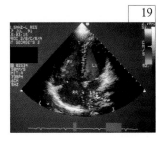

If there is a significant left-to-right shunt, the resulting volume overload causes hyperdynamic right ventricular contraction and this is reflected in reversed or 'paradoxical' motion of the interventricular septum seen on M-mode recordings [21]. However, in cases where raised pulmonary vascular resistance causes partial reversal of the shunt, the Doppler signs described above may be attenuated, or absent. In such cases, a microbubble contrast injection is invaluable as it shows the right-to-left component of the shunt [22].

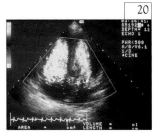

Nuclear Techniques
Although the presence, location, and the magnitude of the left-to-right shunt can be determined by radionuclide studies, such investigations are not often used in clinical practice.

Magnetic Resonance Imaging (MRI)
MRI can be used for precise delineation of the location and the anatomic size of the atrial septal defect [23,24]. Assessment of the pulmonary/systemic flow ratio (Qp/Qs) can be made by MRI, which is fast and very accurate [25].

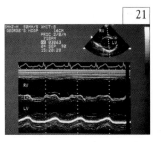

Cardiac Catheterization and Angiography
If cardiac catheterization is carried out in patients with atrial septal defects, the size of the shunt and its direction will be identified. The level of the pulmonary artery pressure and pulmonary vascular resistance can be measured.

Additional anomalous pulmonary venous drainage can be demonstrated by pulmonary arteriography. In an ostium primum atrial septal defect, left ventricular angiography shows

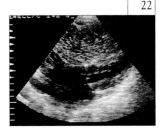
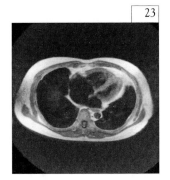
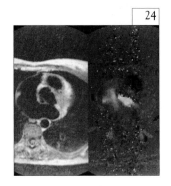
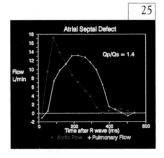

a characteristic abnormality in the left ventricular outflow tract. This is the 'goose-neck' deformity due to the abnormal position of the mitral valve [26].

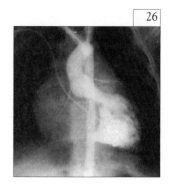

Principles of Management

Catheter or surgical closure of the defects is usually carried out in young patients with more than a trivial atrial septal defect. There is still no information concerning whether closure in childhood alters the normal natural history of problems (atrial arrhythmias and heart failure) occurring in the fifth or sixth decades of adult life. Closure of atrial septal defects first discovered in elderly adult life almost certainly does not alter the natural history (apart from preventing paradoxical embolism). Cardiopulmonary transplant is the only effective treatment in patients with the Eisenmenger syndrome.

1   The foramen ovale. The probe is passed between the flap valve and the limbus. When the probe is removed the flap valve will close the defect.

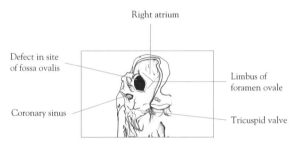

Septum primum (flap valve)   Superior limbus

Tricuspid valve

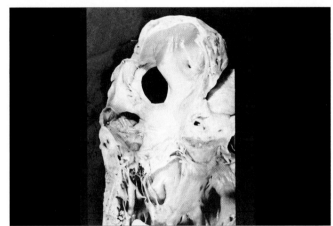

2   Secundum atrial septal defect. A single round defect occupies the site of the foramen ovale. The coronary sinus lies below and the tricuspid valve is separated from the defect by several centimeters of muscle tissue.

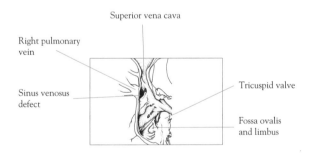

Right atrium

Defect in site of fossa ovalis

Limbus of foramen ovale

Coronary sinus

Tricuspid valve

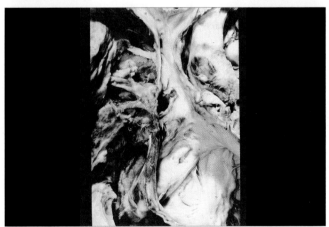

3   Sinus venosus defect. The defect is high in the wall of the superior vena cava and the right pulmonary veins drain to the right atrium via the defect.

Superior vena cava

Right pulmonary vein

Sinus venosus defect

Tricuspid valve

Fossa ovalis and limbus

4   The right atrium and ventricle in a heart with an ostium primum atrial septal defect. There is a deficiency in the base of the atrial septum, but separate annuli of the mitral and tricuspid valves.

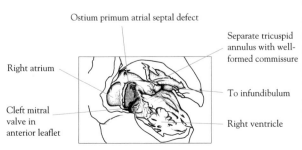

Ostium primum atrial septal defect

Separate tricuspid annulus with well-formed commissure

Right atrium

To infundibulum

Cleft mitral valve in anterior leaflet

Right ventricle

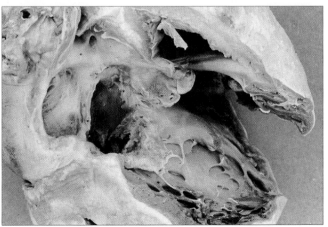

5 The left atrium and ventricle in a heart following operation, with an ostium primum atrial septal defect. There is a cleft in the mitral valve.

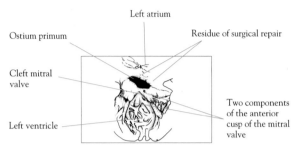

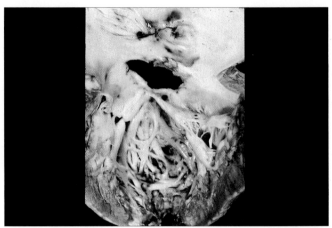

6 Auscultatory findings of atrial septal defect are characterized by relatively fixed splitting of the second heart sound during expiration and inspiration, and an ejection systolic murmur over the left second interspace due to increased pulmonary flow. Aortic and pulmonary components of the second heart sound are equally delayed during inspiration, explaining fixed split-ting. With a large shunt, a tricuspid flow murmur can be heard along the lower left sternal border. S_1=First heart sound; A_2=aortic component of the second heart sound; P_2=pulmonary component of the second heart sound; ESM=ejection systolic murmur; MDM=mid-diastolic murmur.

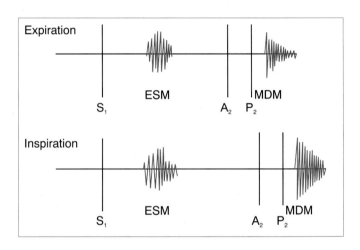

7 Chest X-ray in secundum atrial septal defect. There is pulmonary plethora, a large pulmonary trunk, and a small aortic knuckle.

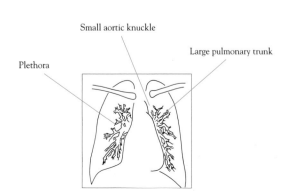

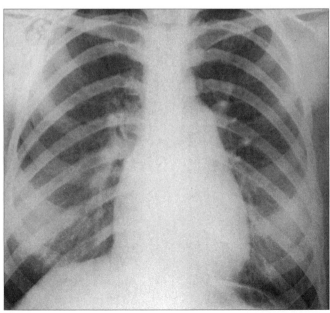

8   Chest X-ray in a secundum atrial septal defect showing cardiac enlargement.

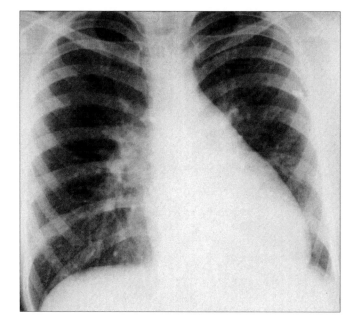

Cardiac enlargement

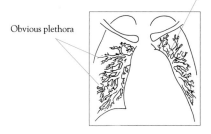

9   Chest X-ray in an atrial septal defect with pulmonary hypertension showing a large heart, a grossly dilated pulmonary trunk, and more obvious plethora.

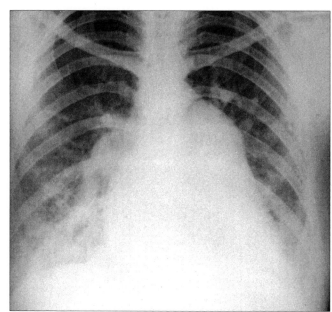

Grossly dilated pulmonary trunk

Obvious plethora

10   Chest X-ray in an atrial septal defect complicated by the Eisenmenger reaction. There is a grossly dilated pulmonary trunk.

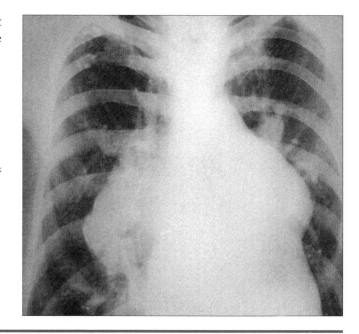

Very large central pulmonary arteries

Enormous pulmonary trunk

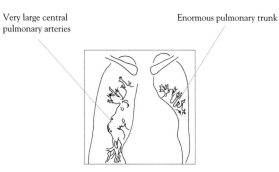

11   Chest X-ray showing a horizontal vessel above the right hilum representing an anomalous pulmonary vein.

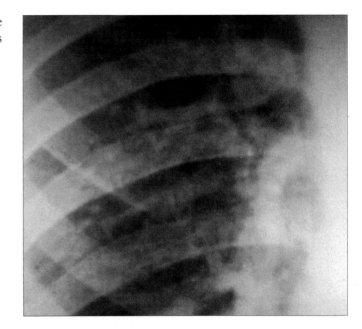

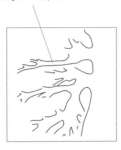

Anomalous pulmonary vein

12   Chest X-ray of a primum atrial septal defect with mitral regurgitation showing slight enlargement of the heart, a prominent pulmonary trunk, pulmonary plethora, and upper zone vessel dilatation.

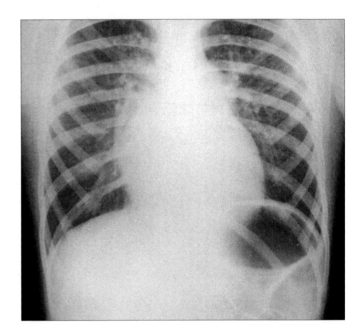

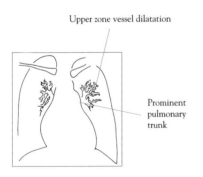

Upper zone vessel dilatation

Prominent pulmonary trunk

13

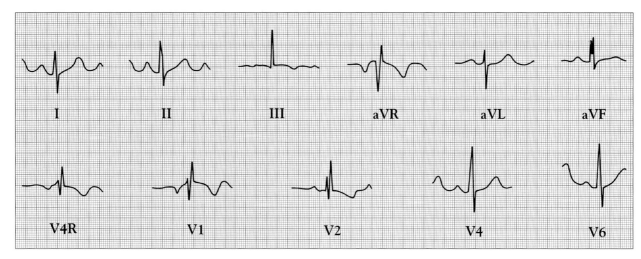

Electrocardiogram of a patient with a secundum atrial septal defect showing sinus rhythm, right axis deviation, and rsR complexes from V4R to V4 indicating incomplete right bundle branch block.

14

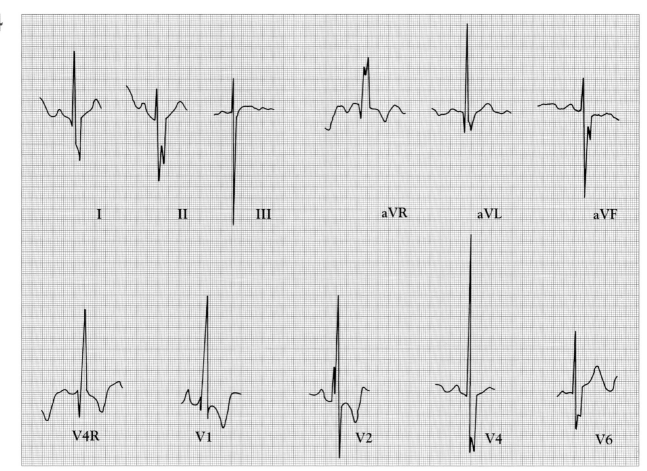

Electrocardiogram of a patient with ostium primum atrial septal defect showing left axis deviation and right bundle branch block.

15

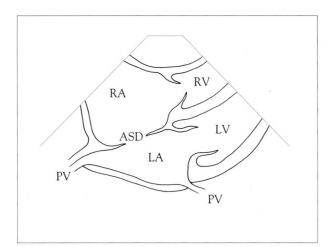 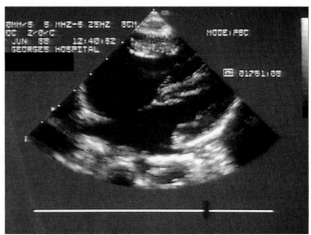

Two-dimensional subcostal view in a child with an ostium secundum atrial septal defect. There is consistent echo drop-out in the central region of the interatrial septum (fossa ovalis). The right heart chambers are enlarged and the pulmonary veins prominent.

16

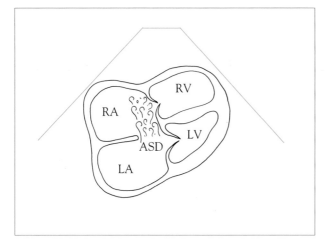 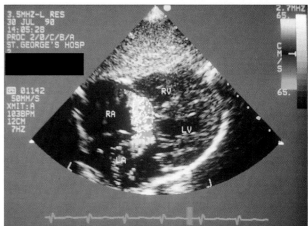

Two-dimensional subcostal view in a child with an ostium primum atrial septal defect. The defect extends right down to the atrioventricular valves and the normal 'step' between the insertion points of the tricuspid and mitral valves into the septum is absent. Color Doppler shows the left-to-right shunt.

17

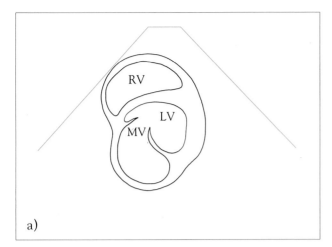

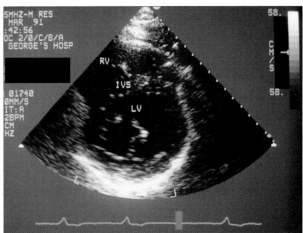

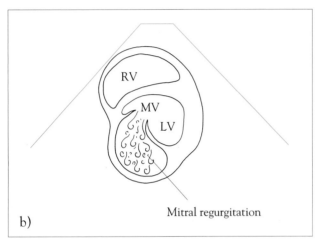

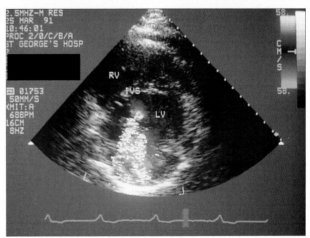

(a) Parasternal short-axis view showing the 'cleft' in the anterior mitral leaflet commonly present in patients with an ostium primum atrial septal defect. (b) Color Doppler shows the associated mitral regurgitation.

18

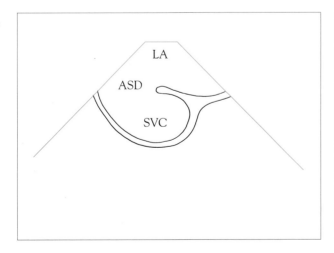

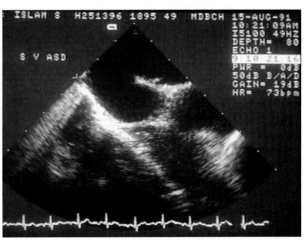

Transesophageal image showing a sinus venosus atrial septal defect right at the top of the atrial septum at the entry point of the superior vena cava. Since this region of the heart cannot normally be visualized by transthoracic echocardiography (except in infants), such defects can only be visualized by the transesophageal technique.

19

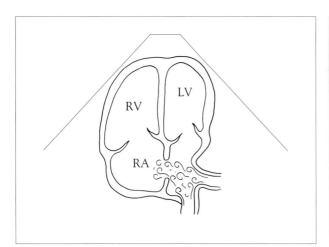
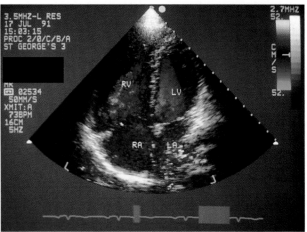

Two-dimensional apical four-chamber view with color Doppler of an ostium secundum atrial septal defect. Blood can be seen streaming from the enlarged pulmonary veins, across the defect into the right atrium.

20

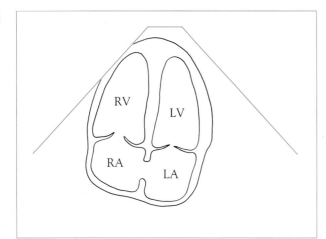
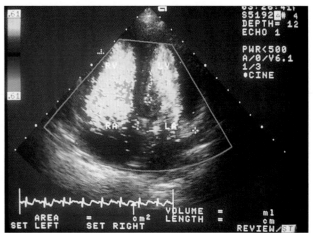

Two-dimensional apical four-chamber view of an ostium secundum atrial septal defect with color Doppler. The presence of a shunt is indicated by greater intensity of the color signal and increased color aliasing caused by higher flow velocities in the right heart chambers.

21   M-mode recording from a patient with an atrial septal defect showing the enlarged right ventricle and reversed ('paradoxical') septal motion signifying right ventricular volume overload.

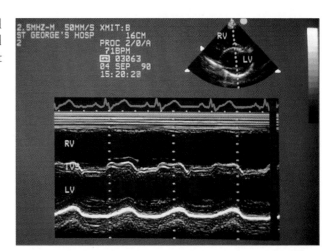

22

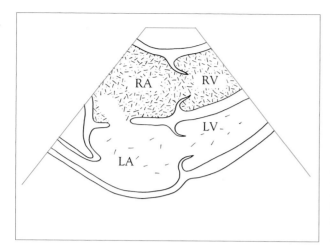

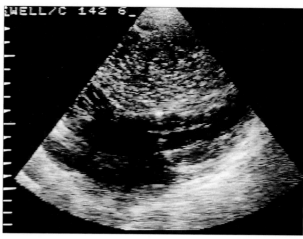

Two-dimensional subcostal view showing a bubble contrast study in a patient with an ostium secundum atrial septal defect. Agitated saline has been injected into an arm vein and a cloud of microbubbles is seen in the right heart chambers. There is a 'negative contrast' washout effect from non-opacified blood shunting from left to right across the defect. There is also a little right-to-left shunting, shown by the presence of a few bubbles in the left heart.

23 Magnetic resonance spin echo image in the transaxial plane showing atrial septal defect.

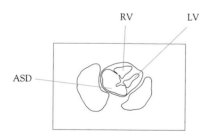

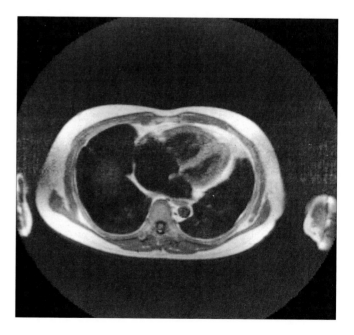

24 Magnetic resonance imaging of atrial septal defect. The left-hand panel shows a spin echo image in the transaxial plane demonstrating an atrial septal defect. The right-hand panel shows a velocity map in the same plane, and flow is clearly seen through the defect.

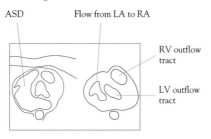

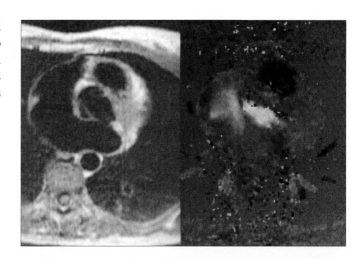

25 By measuring flow independently in the aorta and pulmonary artery, the pulmonary/systemic flow ratio can be calculated.

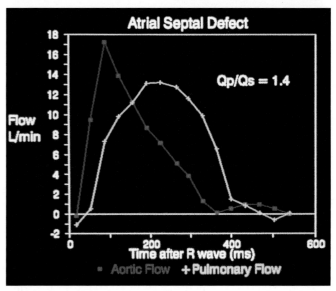

26 Left ventricular angiogram (antero-posterior projection) in an ostium primum atrial septal defect showing the 'goose-neck' deformity.

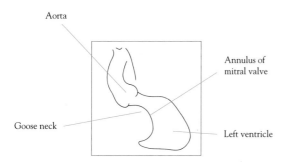

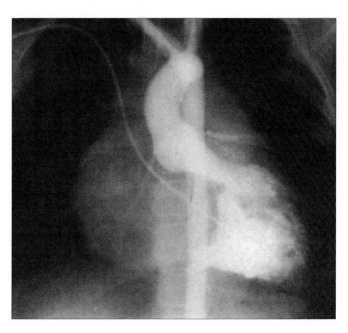

VENTRICULAR SEPTAL DEFECT

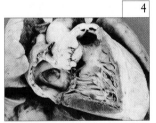

The incidence of ventricular septal defects is 2/1000 live births and constitutes about 20–30% of all congenital cardiac malformations. The prevalence of such defects in school age children is about 1/1000 and in adults approximately 0.5/1000. In the adult they may be part of a complex congenital cardiac malformation such as Fallot's tetralogy but in this section it will be considered as an isolated abnormality.

Pathophysiology

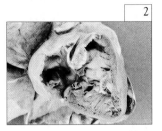

Ventricular septal defects can occur in the membranous septum [1] or in any part of the muscular septum. The defects may be single [2] or multiple [3]. Usually the defect permits communication between the two ventricles, but rarely when the defect is in the atrio-ventricular component of the membranous septum there will be a communication between the left ventricle and right atrium (Gerbode defect). The most common defects exist in and around the ventricular component of the membranous septum [4]. The size of the defect is variable and the hemodynamic consequences will therefore vary. Defects in the membranous septum are particularly likely to lead to aortic regurgitation due to aortic cusp prolapse [5]. Many of the ventricular septal defects which are present at birth close spontaneously. Later in life, if there has been long-standing left-to-right shunting, pulmonary vascular disease may develop [6]. When pulmonary vascular resistance is lower than systemic vascular resistance, a left-to-right shunt occurs. With increasing pulmonary vascular resistance, the magnitude of the left-to-right shunt decreases, and with equal pulmonary and systemic vascular resistance, reversal of shunt (right to left) occurs (Eisenmenger's complex).

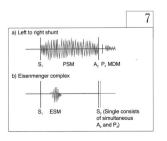

Infective endocarditis is an important complication even if the lesion is hemo-dynamically insignificant.

Presentation

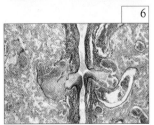

Symptoms
The patient with a small left-to-right shunting ventricular septal defect and a normal pulmonary artery pressure (maladie de Roger) is usually asymptomatic, the condition being diagnosed on routine clinical examination. The child or young adult with a large left-to-right shunt and elevation of the pulmonary artery pressure may complain of breathlessness and fatigue. If pulmonary vascular disease has developed (Eisenmenger ventricular septal defect) then patients may be asymptomatic or complain of breathlessness, fatigue or may even be noticed to be cyanosed.

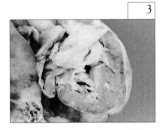

Signs
The patient with a 'Roger' ventricular septal defect has only a pansystolic murmur usually accompanied by a thrill at the left sternal edge. The second heart sound may be abnormally widely split in expiration but moves normally in inspiration.

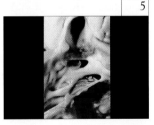

The patient with a large left-to-right shunt and pulmonary hypertension will have a hyperdynamic apical impulse reflecting the increased stroke volume of the left ventricle. On auscultation, in addition to the pansystolic murmur, the pulmonary valve closure sound is accentuated although the splitting is physiologic. There is often an additional mid-diastolic murmur over the apical area reflecting the increased flow through the normal mitral valve.

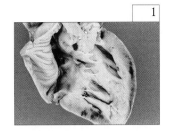

The patient with an Eisenmenger ventricular septal defect may be cyanosed and clubbed. The jugular venous pulse may show abnormal dominance of the 'a' wave while the arterial pulse is usually normal. On auscultation, the second heart sound is characteristically found to be single, although it incorporates both components (aortic closure and pulmonary closure), which have become fused. The second heart sound is accentuated due to the loud pulmonary closure sound. There may be no murmurs but a pulmonary ejection sound and a short ejection systolic murmur are common [7].

Investigations

Radiology
A small ventricular septal defect does not cause cardiac enlargement, but the central pulmonary arteries are usually slightly enlarged in the plain chest X-ray [8]. With a larger defect there is cardiac enlargement. The increased pulmonary flow and pressure are reflected in left atrial dilatation, a large pulmonary trunk, and obvious pulmonary plethora [9]. If pulmonary vascular disease has developed (Eisenmenger syndrome), there is enlargement of the pulmonary trunk and central pulmonary vessels [10], while the peripheral vessels are constricted.

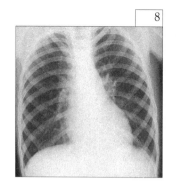

Electrocardiography
In a small left-to-right shunting defect the electrocardiogram may be normal. The adult with a moderately large left-to-right shunting defect may show voltage increases (tall R-waves in V5 and S-waves in V1) indicating left ventricular enlargement [11]. When a defect is complicated by the Eisenmenger reaction, the electrocardiogram shows right ventricular hypertrophy [12] although additional left ventricular hypertrophy is often also seen.

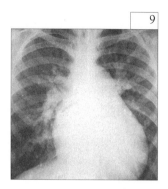

Echocardiography
Larger ventricular septal defects can be visualized directly, provided that care is taken to examine the whole of the interventricular septum using parasternal long- and short-axis, apical and subcostal views [13]. The majority of defects are, however, too small to be seen on imaging. Such lesions are said to be 'fully restrictive', i.e. a large pressure difference still exists between left and right ventricles and the resulting high jet velocity is readily detected by color Doppler. Thus, the presence of a ventricular septal defect is demonstrated even though the actual hole is invisible [14].

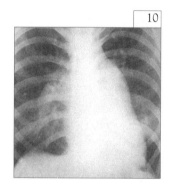

Provided that the ultrasound beam can be aligned with the color jet (not always easy in the case of muscular trabecular defects), continuous-wave Doppler can measure the pressure gradient between the left and right ventricles. In the absence of left ventricular outflow obstruction, left ventricular pressure can be determined using a cuff sphygmomanometer, hence the absolute value of right ventricular pressure can be calculated [15]. Alternatively, information on right ventricular pressure can be obtained from the velocity of tricuspid or pulmonary regurgitant jets.

The majority of perimembranous inlet defects, and many muscular trabecular defects, close spontaneously during the first decade of life. Perimembranous inlet defects close by

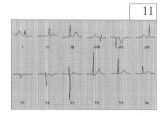
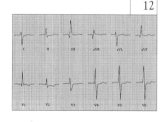
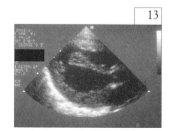
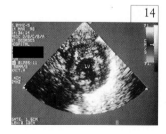

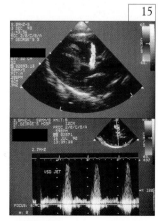

attaching tissue from the tricuspid valve septal leaflet across the hole [16]. Perimembranous outlet and doubly-committed subarterial defects cannot employ this mechanism and the former may be complicated by prolapse of the right coronary aortic cusp, leading to aortic regurgitation [17].

The degree of shunting can be assessed qualitatively from the appearance of the color jet, and semi-quantitatively from left ventricular dimensions. Doppler can be used to calculate the Qp/Qs ratio, as described in *Atrial Septal Defect.*

Large ventricular septal defects, or a multiplicity of small ones — so-called 'Swiss Cheese' lesion — offer essentially free communication between the two ventricles and are thus termed 'non-restrictive'. Jet velocities are low and shunts often bi-directional [18]. Additional signs of right ventricular hypertrophy and pulmonary hypertension may be present [19].

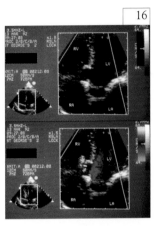

Magnetic Resonance Imaging (MRI)
MRI, like transesophageal echocardiography, delineates the anatomic location and size of the defect, as well as atrioventricular valve abnormalities and ventricular size [20,21]. The velocity map by MRI can quantify the left-to-right shunt through the ventricular septal defect [22].

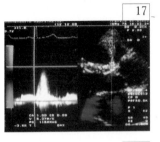

Cardiac Catheterization and Angiography
The left-to-right shunt or bi-directional shunt can be detected at cardiac catheterization and the pulmonary artery pressure measured. Pulmonary vascular resistance and pulmonary-to-systemic flow ratios may be calculated. A left ventricular angiogram shows the position of the ventricular septal defect and whether multiple defects are present [23–25].

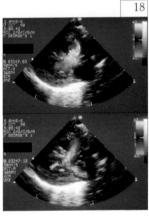

Principles of Management

Ventricular septal defects may close spontaneously. Defects with a large left-to-right shunt require catheter or surgical closure to prevent the development of pulmonary vascular disease. Cardiopulmonary transplant is the only effective treatment for the Eisenmenger syndrome. Antibiotic prophylaxis for infective endocarditis is recommended.

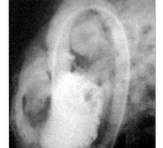
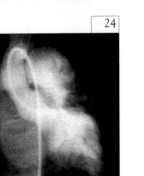
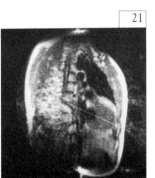
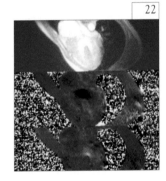

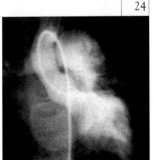
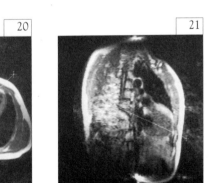
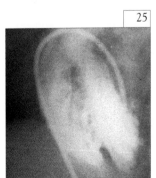

1 The parietal wall of the right ventricle has been removed, showing a slit-like defect at the site of the membranous septum.

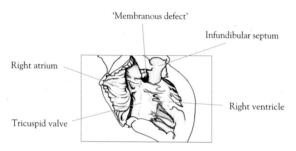

'Membranous defect'

Infundibular septum

Right atrium

Right ventricle

Tricuspid valve

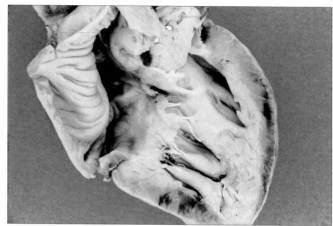

2 Posterior muscular septal defect.

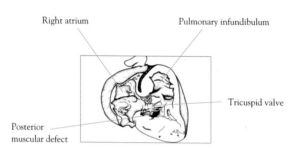

Right atrium

Pulmonary infundibulum

Tricuspid valve

Posterior muscular defect

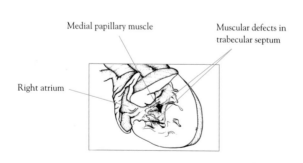

3 Multiple muscular defects in trabecular septum.

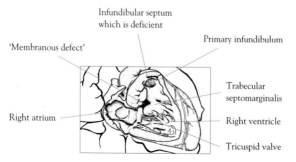

Medial papillary muscle

Muscular defects in trabecular septum

Right atrium

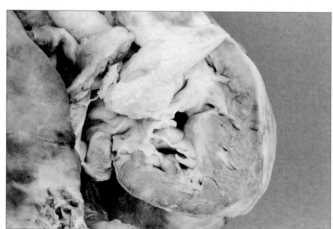

4 Heart opened in a similar fashion to [1], showing a large defect of the muscle surrounding the membranous septum.

Infundibular septum which is deficient

'Membranous defect'

Primary infundibulum

Right atrium

Trabecular septomarginalis

Right ventricle

Tricuspid valve

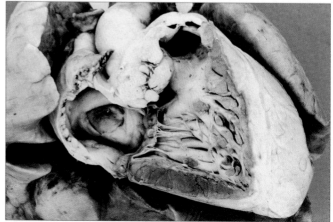

5 Infundibular septal defect with prolapsing aortic valve leaflet.

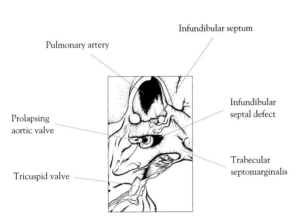

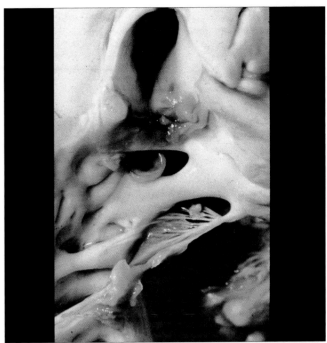

6 Pulmonary vascular disease secondary to a ventricular septal defect.

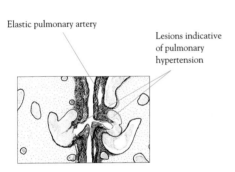

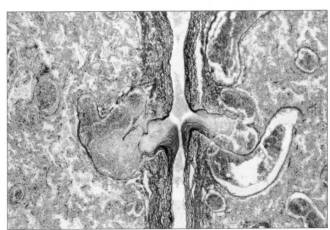

7 Auscultatory findings in ventricular septal defect. In the presence of left-to-right shunt (a), a pansystolic murmur, widely split second heart sound, and a flow murmur at the apex are usually present.

With Eisenmenger physiology (b), the second heart sound becomes single (a fusion of A_2 and P_2) due to identical right and left ventricular ejection times. Pansystolic murmur of VSD is usually absent. A short ejection systolic murmur associated with pulmonary hypertension can be present.

S_1=First heart sound; A_2=aortic component of the second heart sound; P_2=pulmonary component of the second heart sound; PSM=pansystolic mumur; ESM=ejection systolic murmur; MDM= mid-diastolic flow murmur.

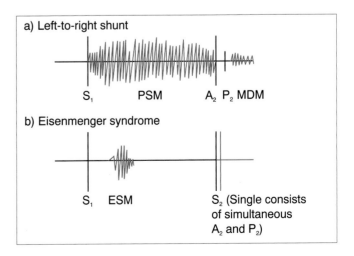

8   Chest X-ray showing normal sized heart with slight enlargement of the central pulmonary arteries in a small ventricular septal defect.

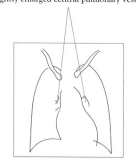

Slightly enlarged central pulmonary vessels

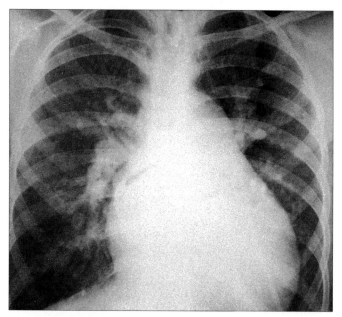

9   Chest X-ray showing increased cardiac size with dilatation of the left atrium, pulmonary trunk, and pulmonary plethora in a ventricular septal defect with pulmonary hypertension.

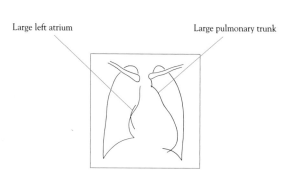

Large left atrium

Large pulmonary trunk

10   Chest X-ray in Eisenmenger ventricular septal defect showing slight enlargement of the heart and gross enlargement of the central pulmonary vessels.

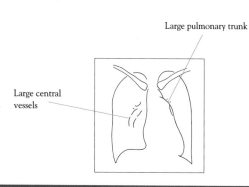

Large pulmonary trunk

Large central vessels

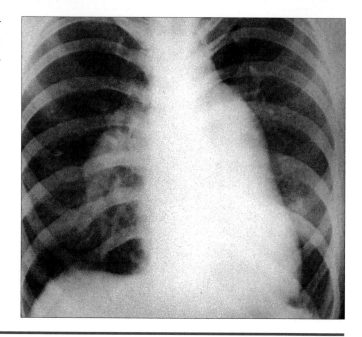

11

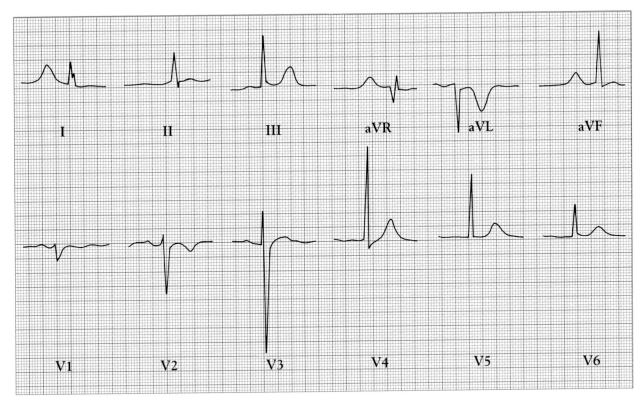

Electrocardiogram of a 10-year-old patient with ventricular septal defect. The pulmonary/systemic flow ratio was 2:1 and the pulmonary vascular resistance normal. There is evidence of slight left ventricular hypertrophy as shown by the increased voltage of R-waves in the left precordial leads. Note: V4 to V6, 1 mV=0.5 cm.

12

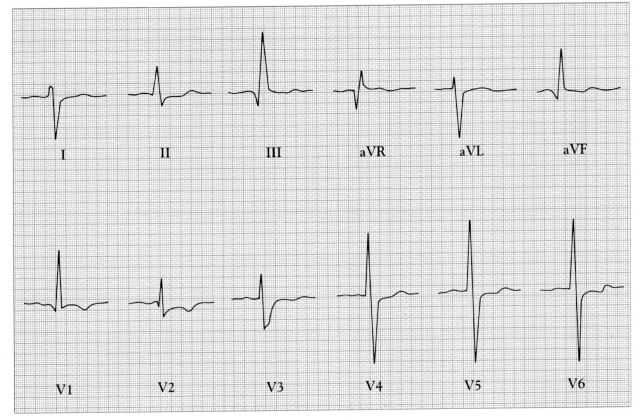

Electrocardiogram of a patient aged 21 with Eisenmenger ventricular septal defect, showing right axis deviation, with dominant R-waves, inverted T-waves in right chest leads, and deep S-waves in V5 and V6. Note: 1 mV=0.5 cm.

13

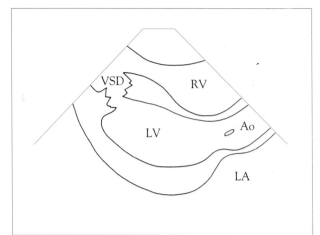 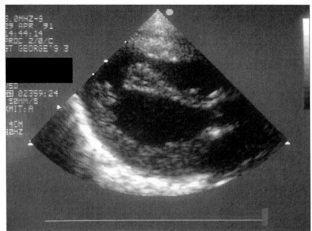

Two-dimensional parasternal long-axis view of an infant with a large ventricular septal defect in the apical part of the muscular septum.

14

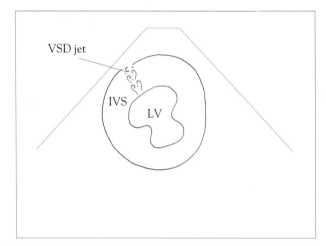 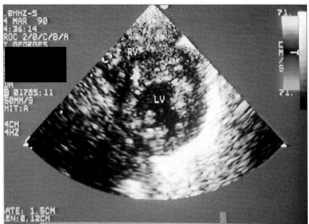

Two-dimensional parasternal short-axis view showing a tiny muscular trabecular ventricular septal defect. Presence of the defect is revealed only by the bright 'flame' seen by color Doppler.

15

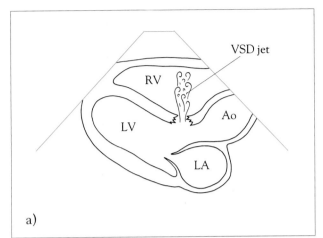

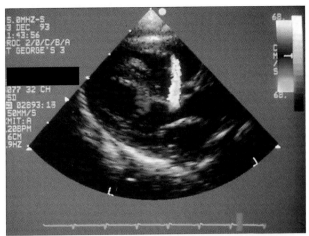

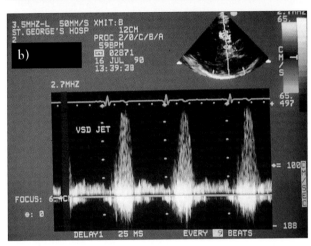

(a) Parasternal long-axis view showing a muscular outlet ventricular septal defect. The hole is large enough to be seen on the two-dimensional image, but the presence of the shunt is confirmed by color Doppler. (b) Continuous wave Doppler shows the high velocity (4.5 m/s) of the jet indicating a restrictive defect with a high pressure gradient (80 mmHg) between left and right ventricles.

16

(a) Magnified view of the atrioventricular septum in a 10-year-old child born with a perimembranous inlet ventricular septal defect. The extent of the original lesion can be seen. It has almost completely closed by growth of tissue at the base of the tricuspid valve forming an aneurysmal pouch over the hole. (b) Color Doppler shows the small residual shunt.

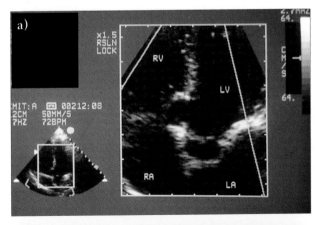

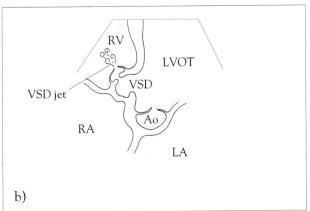

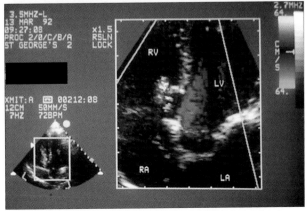

17

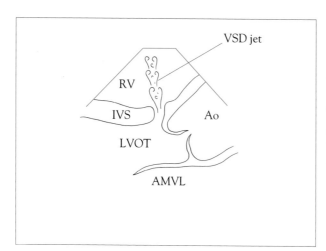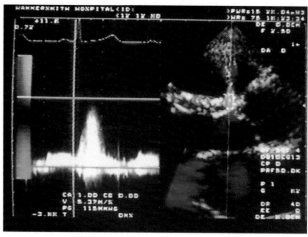

Magnified view of the left ventricular outflow tract in a parasternal long-axis view showing a small perimembranous outlet ventricular septal defect. Presence of a shunt is indicated by color Doppler and its restrictive nature is confirmed by continuous-wave Doppler.

18

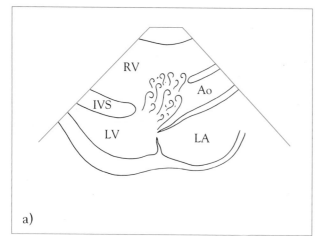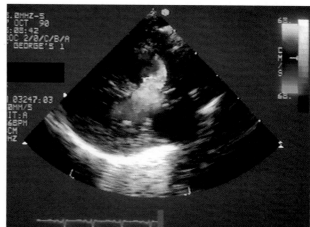

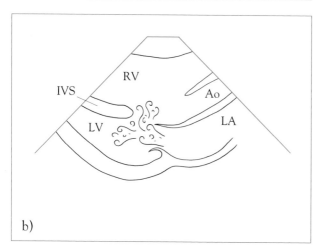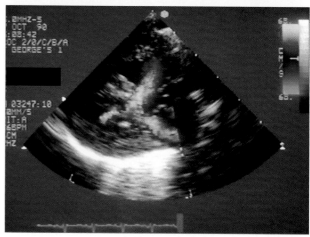

A very large, non-restrictive ventricular septal defect. (a) A systolic frame showing left-to-right shunting across the defect. Note that there is no color aliasing as the shunt velocity is low. (b) A diastolic frame showing blood flowing through the mitral valve into both ventricles. Hemodynamically, the heart is functioning as though it had only one ventricle.

19

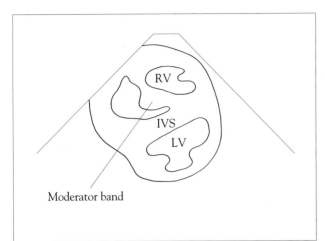

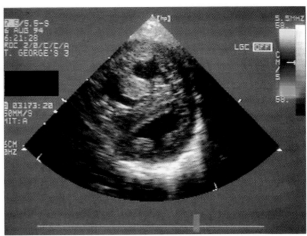

Two-dimensional parasternal short-axis view showing severe right ventricular hypertrophy associated with pulmonary hypertension secondary to a large ventricular septal defect. Note the thick moderator band and the flattened profile of the interventricular septum.

20   Magnetic resonance spin echo imaging of ventricular septal defect in the transaxial plane.

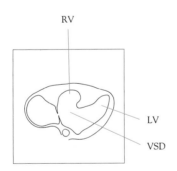

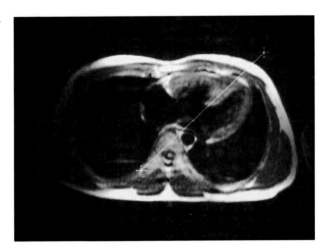

21   Magnetic resonance spin echo imaging of ventricular septal defect in the oblique plane. This
shows the septum *en face*, with a clear delineation
of the ventricular septal defect in the subaortic
position.

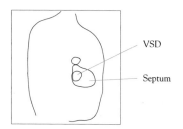

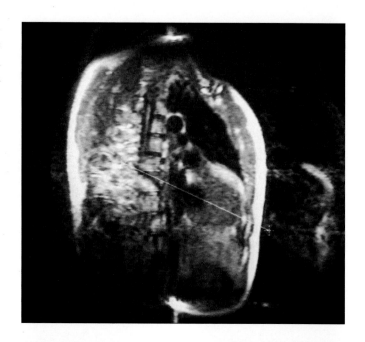

22   Magnetic resonance imaging in the horizontal
long-axis plane of ventricular septal defect. The
upper frame shows the gradient echo image, and
the septum is seen to be incomplete. The middle
image is a velocity map showing intense flow
from the left to the right ventricle during systole.
The bottom frame shows some reversed flow in
diastole.

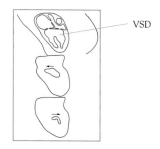

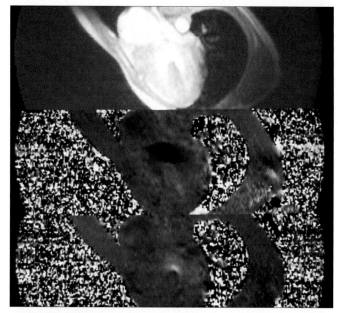

23   Left ventriculogram (lateral projection) showing
membranous ventricular septal defect.

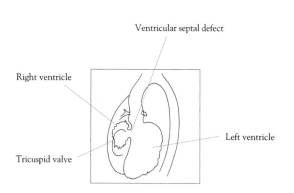

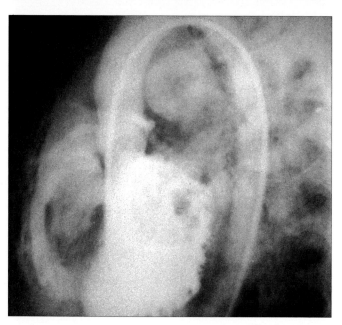

24   Left ventriculogram (antero-posterior projection) showing infundibular septal defect with shunt directly into the pulmonary trunk. The body of the right ventricle is not filled.

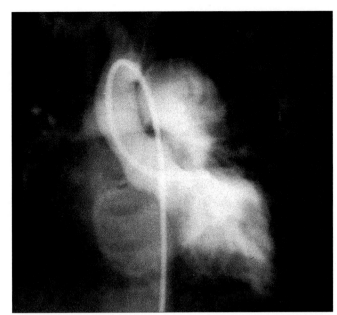

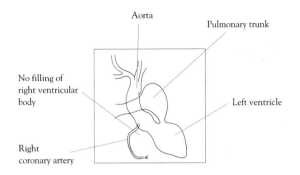

25   Left ventriculogram viewed in a projection which profiles the septum showing multiple defects in the trabecular septum.

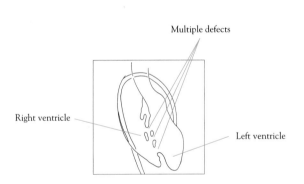

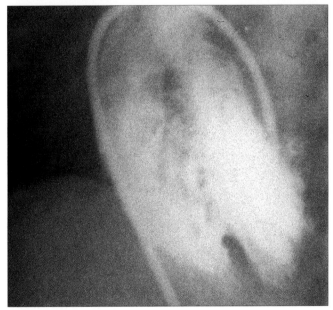

PERSISTENT DUCTUS ARTERIOSUS

Pathophysiology

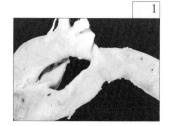

The ductus arteriosus connects the proximal left pulmonary artery to the arch of the aorta just distal to the origin of the left subclavian artery and forms a communication between the pulmonary and systemic circulation which persists throughout the whole of fetal life and into the neonatal period [1]. Normally, it closes shortly after birth but it may, for reasons which are not fully understood, remain patent throughout life. In children who have a persistent ductus arteriosus, a small proportion will have an additional cardiac abnormality. With normal pulmonary vascular resistance, the left-to-right shunt through the patent ductus causes volume overload of the left atrium and left ventricle, sparing the right atrium and ventricle. With increasing pulmonary vascular resistance, the magnitude of the left-to-right shunt decreases and when pulmonary vascular resistance exceeds systemic vascular resistance, a right-to-left shunt occurs preferentially to the descending aorta.

Presentation

Symptoms

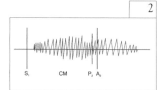

The lesion is rare in adults because it has usually been corrected by surgery in childhood. Adults presenting with an isolated persistent ductus arteriosus are usually asymptomatic and discovered by the chance finding of a murmur. Patients with a long-standing large left-to-right shunt may complain of breathlessness and even develop frank heart failure, particularly following the development of atrial fibrillation.

Signs

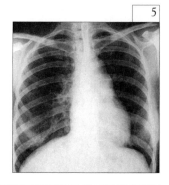

The physical signs of a left-to-right shunt through a persistent ductus arteriosus include a continuous murmur, best heard in the left infraclavicular area, which needs to be distinguished from a venous hum. If the shunt is small, there may be no other abnormal physical signs; if the shunt is large, there may be a sharp upstroke to the carotid pulse and a hyperdynamic left ventricle on palpation. Additionally, there may be a mid-diastolic flow murmur in the mitral area. In the presence of a large left-to-right shunt, the second heart sound can be paradoxically split due to selective prolongation of left ventricular ejection [2]. If pulmonary hypertension is present, the pulmonary valve closure sound will be accentuated.

The patient presenting with the Eisenmenger reaction and a persistent ductus arteriosus may be cyanosed, particularly in the lower limbs, with clubbing of the toes (differential cyanosis and clubbing). The remaining physical signs include physiologic splitting of the second heart sound but with an accentuated pulmonary valve closure sound, and right ventricular hypertrophy on palpation. There may be abnormal dominance of the 'a' wave in the jugular venous pulse. There may be either a short ejection systolic murmur or no murmur at all, but a pulmonary ejection sound may be present. An early diastolic murmur due to pulmonary regurgitation may be heard in those patients with the greatest dilatation of the central pulmonary arteries.

Investigations

Radiology

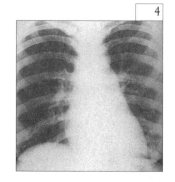

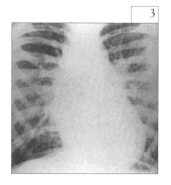

The patient with a large left-to-right shunt may show pulmonary plethora together with cardiac enlargement [3].

Characteristically, the aorta is dilated at the site of the ductus [4]. The older patient may show calcification in the region of the ductus [5].

The patient with an Eisenmenger persistent ductus arteriosus may have a normal sized heart but with dilated central pulmonary arteries and reduction in caliber of the peripheral pulmonary arteries [6].

Electrocardiography

If the ductus is small, the electrocardiogram will be normal. If the shunt is large, the left ventricle dilates and the electrocardiogram may show tall R-waves in V5 and deep S-waves in V1 (voltage changes of left ventricular hypertrophy) [7]. With the development of severe pulmonary vascular disease, the electrocardiogram reflects increasing right ventricular hypertrophy with tall R-waves and T-wave inversion in right ventricular leads and deep S-waves in the left ventricular leads [8]. Right axis deviation and right bundle branch block are also common features in persistent ductus arteriosus with severe pulmonary vascular disease.

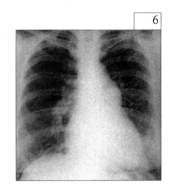

Echocardiography

Large persistent ducts can be imaged either in the parasternal short-axis or suprasternal views [9]. Smaller lesions cannot usually be seen, but as they are restrictive their presence is easily demonstrated by color Doppler [10]. Continuous-wave Doppler shows the undulating flow throughout the cardiac cycle [11].

If there is a large left-to-right shunt, the left ventricular end-diastolic dimension will be increased consistent with the increase in stroke volume. If the pulmonary vascular resistance is elevated, pressures in the aorta and pulmonary artery tend to equalize in diastole and this is shown by a deep 'sawtooth' pattern on the continuous-wave Doppler recording [12].

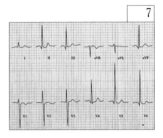

In the presence of a persistent fetal circulation, the duct is almost the same size as the aorta, and this gives rise to a characterisic 'three-finger' image, with bi-directional shunting [13]. Right-to-left ductal shunting can be hard to demonstrate with color Doppler; confirmation is provided by an echocardiographic contrast study showing passage of microbubbles from the pulmonary artery to the abdominal aorta.

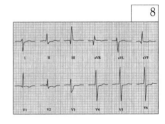

Magnetic Resonance Imaging (MRI)

MRI is a useful technique for determining the location and anatomic size of the patent ductus [14] and the pulmonary/systemic flow ratio (Qp/Qs).

Cardiac Catheterization and Angiography

Evidence of a left-to-right shunt can be detected by a step up in oxygen saturation in the pulmonary artery. The catheter can usually be passed directly from the left pulmonary artery into the descending aorta via the ductus arteriosus [15]. The presence of increased

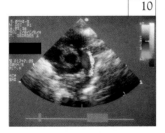
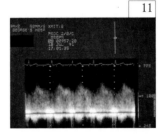
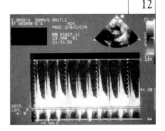

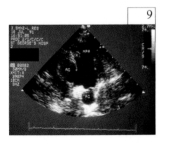

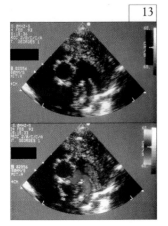
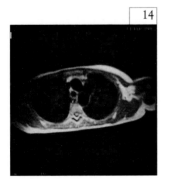
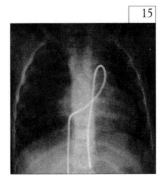

pulmonary artery pressure or increased pulmonary vascular resistance can be measured directly.

The aortogram is used to show the anatomy of the ductus [16,17].

Principles of Management

All patients with patent ductus arteriosus should be considered for catheter or surgical closure apart from those with the Eisenmenger reaction. Antibiotic prophylaxis for infective endocarditis is recommended. Cardiopulmonary transplantation is the only available treatment for the Eisenmenger situation.

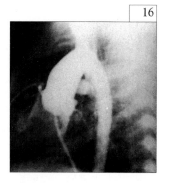

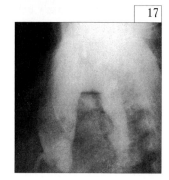

1 Pathologic specimen showing a persistent ductus arteriosus.

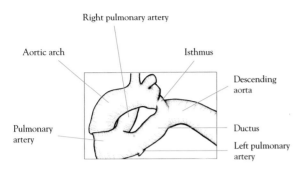

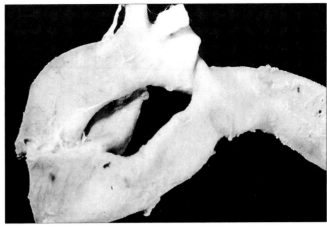

2 Continuous murmur throughout systole and diastole. The second heart sound can be paradoxically split.
S_1=First heart sound; P_2=pulmonary component of the second heart sound; A_2=aortic component of the second heart sound; CM=continuous murmur.

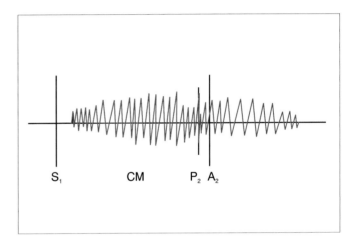

3 Chest X-ray in persistent ductus arteriosus with a large left-to-right shunt showing a large heart and pulmonary trunk, prominent aortic knuckle, and obvious pulmonary plethora.

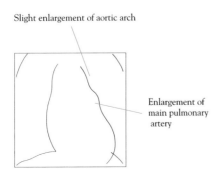

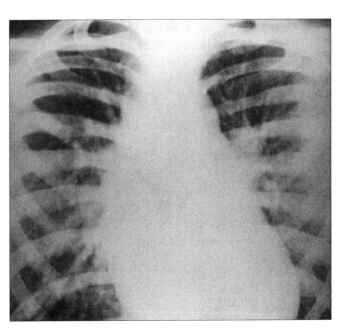

4   Chest X-ray showing a dilated aorta at the site of the persistent ductus.

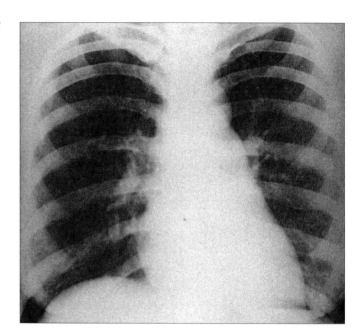

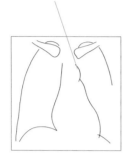

The aortic 'infundibulum' of persistent ductus

5   Chest X-ray showing calcification in a persistent ductus.

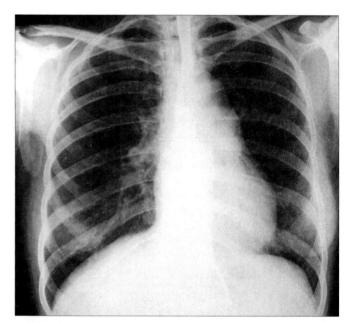

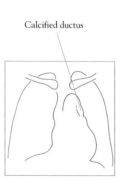

Calcified ductus

6   Chest X-ray in persistent ductus with the Eisenmenger situation showing a slightly enlarged heart, very large pulmonary trunk, and prominent aortic knuckle. The hilar vessels are large and the peripheral pulmonary vessels normal.

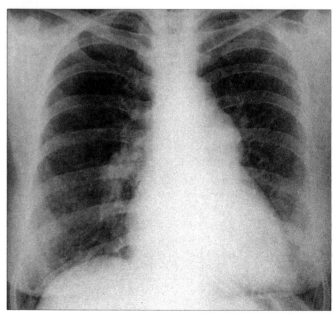

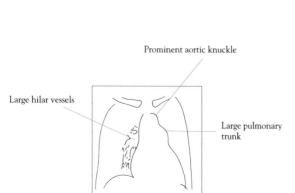

Prominent aortic knuckle

Large hilar vessels

Large pulmonary trunk

7

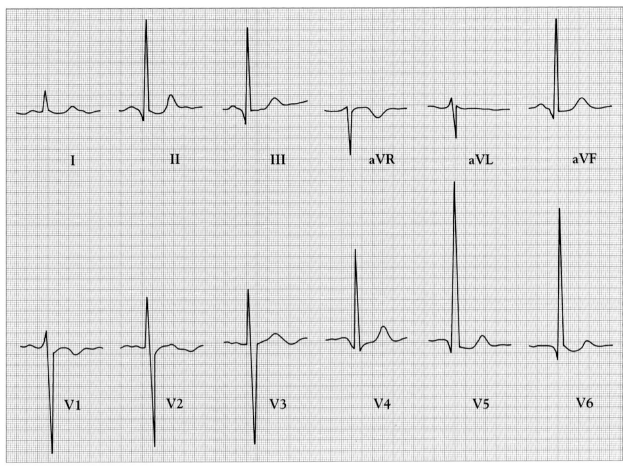

Electrocardiogram in persistent ductus arteriosus showing tall R-waves in left ventricular leads and deep S-waves in opposing leads — the pattern of diastolic overload.

8

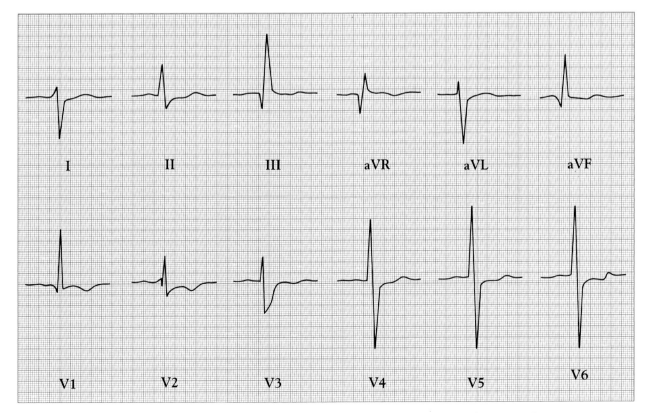

Electrocardiogram in Eisenmenger persistent ductus arteriosus, showing right axis deviation, dominant R-waves, inverted T-waves in right chest leads, and deep S-waves in V5 and V6. Note: 1 mV=0.5 cm.

9

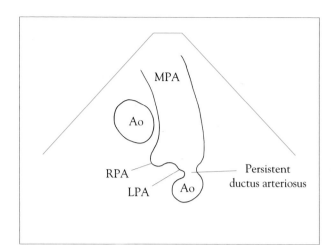
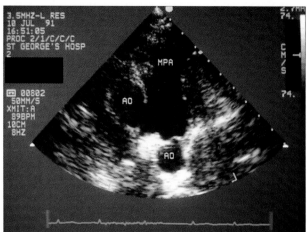

Two-dimensional parasternal short-axis view from a child with a persistent ductus arteriosus. The section cuts both the ascending and the descending limbs of the aortic arch. The duct is seen connecting the descending thoracic aorta with the pulmonary artery at the level of its bifurcation.

10

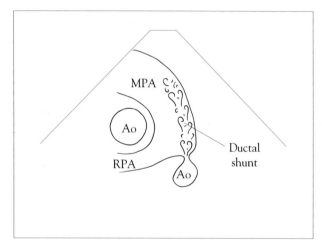
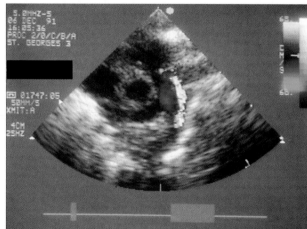

A small persistent ductus arteriosus visualized by color Doppler. A turbulent jet is seen flowing from the descending thoracic aorta into the pulmonary artery.

11   The restrictive character of a small PDA jet can be confirmed with continuous-wave spectral Doppler. A relatively high pressure gradient exists between the aorta and the pulmonary artery throughout the cardiac cycle, giving rise to undulating flow.

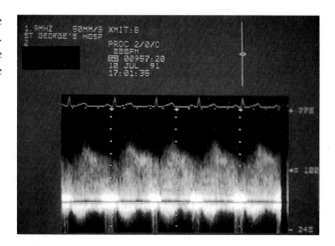

12   With a large PDA, high diastolic flow rapidly reduces the aorta–pulmonary artery pressure gradient, resulting in a deep 'sawtooth' flow pattern seen on continuous-wave spectral Doppler.

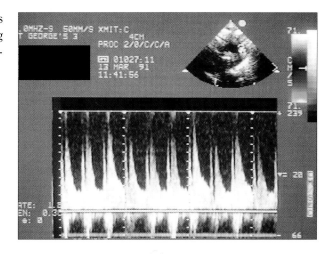

13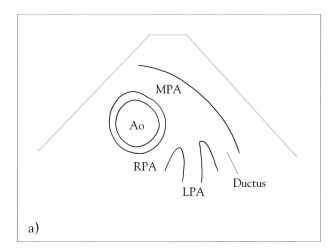

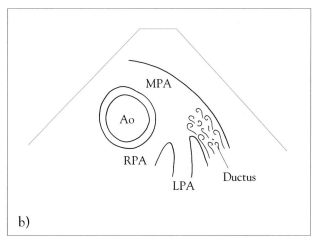
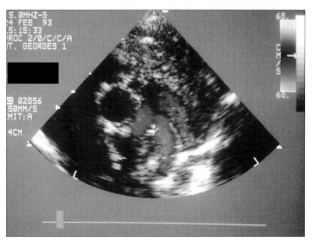

(a) When the fetal circulation persists, the ductus arteriosus is the same size as the aorta, shown by a characteristic 'three-finger' appearance to the main pulmonary artery in the parasternal short-axis view. (b) Color Doppler shows the normal pulmonary ejection (blue) with non-restrictive left-to-right shunting across the duct (red).

14 Magnetic resonance spin echo imaging in the transaxial plane of patent ductus arteriosus.

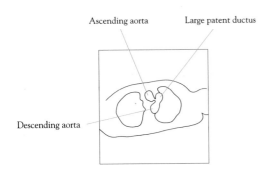

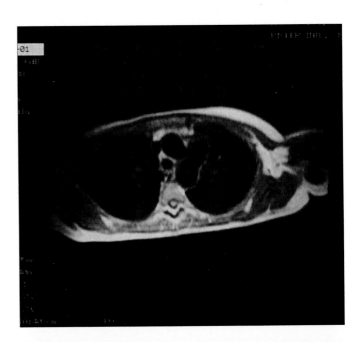

15 Chest X-ray showing typical position of a cardiac catheter passed across a persistent ductus from the pulmonary trunk to the descending aorta.

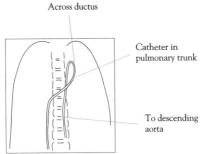

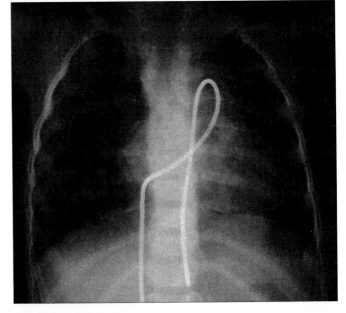

16 Aortogram (lateral projection) showing a small persistent ductus.

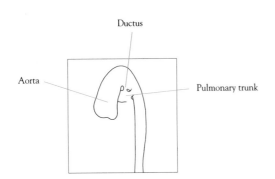

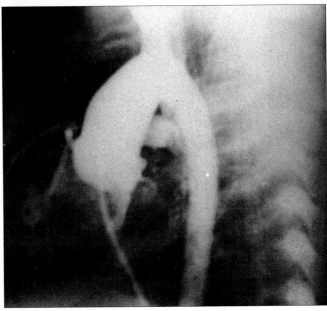

17   Aortogram (lateral projection) showing a large ductus.

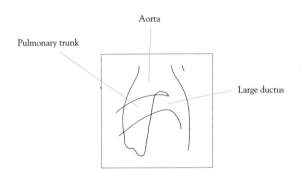

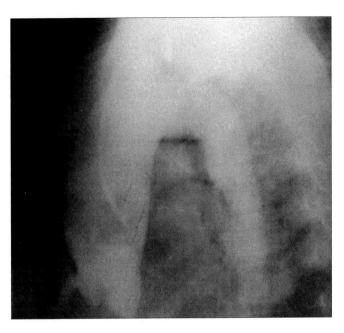

PULMONARY STENOSIS

Pathophysiology

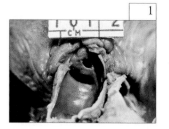

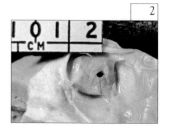

Right ventricular outflow tract obstruction can occur either at the pulmonary valve level or due to narrowing of the infundibular portion of the right ventricle, or both. In pulmonary valve stenosis, the valve is usually tricuspid and the valve cusps are fused along the margins to form an obstructing diaphragm [1]. The valve orifice may vary from 2–10mm in diameter [2] and the valve may tend to become thickened and calcified. Right ventricular hypertrophy will develop with time [3] even if the orifice is mildly narrowed. Dilatation of the pulmonary arteries beyond the valve occurs gradually. Rarely, pulmonary valve stenosis may be due to the carcinoid syndrome.

Infundibular stenosis may be due to hypertrophy of the outflow tract [3]. Obstruction may rarely occur if there is a compression externally from a tumor or an aberrant muscle bundle within the right ventricle. Infundibular stenosis may develop in patients with a large left-to-right shunt due to ventricular septal defect, or may be present in hypertrophic cardiomyopathy. With right ventricular outflow obstruction, a pressure gradient across the outflow tract develops. The more severe the outflow obstruction, the higher will be the pressure gradient. Secondary hypertrophy of the right ventricle invariably occurs in the presence of hemodynamically significant outflow obstruction. Secondary right ventricular failure is the end result of the uncorrected severe right ventricular outflow obstruction.

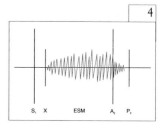

Presentation

Symptoms

The majority of adults with pulmonary valve stenosis, even with significant obstruction, deny symptoms. Occasionally, patients may complain of fatigue or dyspnea. The presence of angina or syncope would indicate severe obstruction, as would the development of right heart failure.

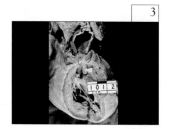

Signs

Most patients with right ventricular outflow obstruction presenting in adult life are detected because of the chance finding of a murmur. The murmur is ejection in type and finishes before pulmonary valve closure. In mild or moderate pulmonary valve stenosis, the second heart sound is abnormally widely split in expiration, although the split widens further on inspiration, as would occur in normal patients. The severity of the stenosis determines the width of splitting: the wider the expiratory split, the more severe the stenosis [4]. Pulmonary valve closure becomes inaudible when the stenosis is very severe. The abrupt halting of the abnormal pulmonary valve at the onset of systole gives rise to a pulmonary ejection sound. In infundibular stenosis, the ejection sound will be absent. Associated right ventricular hypertrophy may be detected by palpation and would give rise to abnormal dominance of the 'a' wave in the venous pulse.

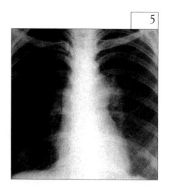

Investigations

Radiology

Pulmonary valve stenosis is characterized on the chest X-ray by a normal sized heart with post-stenotic dilatation of the pulmonary trunk, characteristically extending into the left branch [5]. Pulmonary artery dilatation in some cases may be gross [6]. Pulmonary oligemia may sometimes be visible.

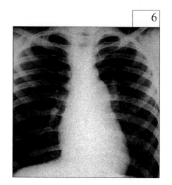

Electrocardiography

The electrocardiogram in mild or moderate pulmonary stenosis may be normal. In severe pulmonary stenosis, right ventricular hypertrophy is usually present [7]. In severe cases with right heart dilatation, right atrial enlargement may be present in addition to right ventricular hypertrophy.

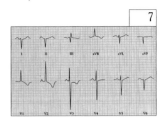

Echocardiography

The two-dimensional echocardiographic appearances of mild pulmonary valve stenosis are usually normal. In more severe cases, thickening and 'doming' of the valve in systole may be seen, together with enlargement of the proximal pulmonary arteries and right ventricular hypertrophy [8]. Color Doppler may show turbulent flow in the pulmonary artery [9], while continuous-wave Doppler can be used to measure the velocity. It can, however, be difficult to differentiate valve pathology from normal high stroke output in healthy children.

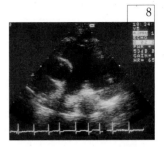

The transvalvular gradient in more severe cases is measured by continuous-wave Doppler. With the development of secondary infundibular outflow obstruction, an additional velocity component is shown either by placing a pulse-wave Doppler sample in the right ventricular outflow tract or as a double density on the continuous-wave recording [10,11].

In mild pulmonary valve stenosis, the M-mode echocardiogram is normal. With moderate or severe obstruction, the pulmonary valve echo shows marked exaggeration of its 'a' dip [12] and in extreme cases the valve may appear to open completely after atrial contraction and before the R-wave of the electrocardiogram. In most cases of pulmonary valve stenosis, even when severe, there is no M-mode echocardiographic evidence of right ventricular hypertrophy but occasionally the septum is thickened and echoes from the anterior wall of the right ventricle are unusually prominent. The septal motion is normal in direction unless the right ventricle fails with secondary tricuspid regurgitation.

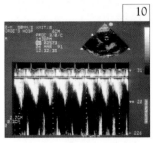

Magnetic Resonance Imaging (MRI)

MRI also delineates pulmonary valve and pulmonary artery anatomy [13].

Cardiac Catheterization and Angiography

The right ventricular outflow tract obstruction is detected at cardiac catheterization by a systolic pressure difference. The site of obstruction will also be determined.

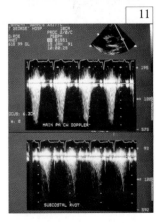

On right ventricular angiography, the site of the outflow obstruction can be seen when it is at valve level [14], infundibular level, or in the right ventricular cavity. In pulmonary valve stenosis, the cusps will be thickened, domed in systole, with a central jet and post-stenotic dilatation of the pulmonary artery [15].

Principles of Management

Most young patients can be treated by catheter valvuloplasty. If the pulmonary valve stenosis is severe, surgical pulmonary valvulotomy is required.

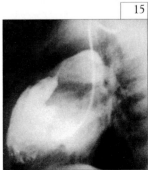

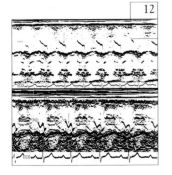

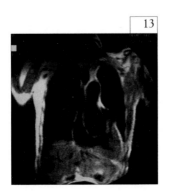

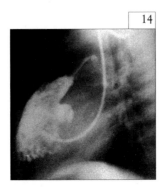

1 Moderate pulmonary valve stenosis viewed from above, through the opened pulmonary artery.

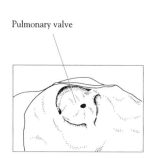

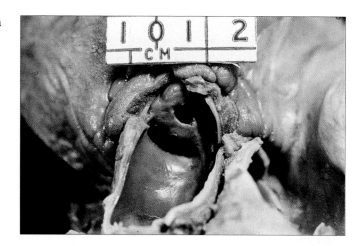

2 Severe pulmonary valve stenosis viewed from above, through the opened pulmonary artery.

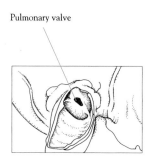

3 Critical pulmonary valve stenosis (red arrow) and secondary infundibular stenosis (white arrow) due to gross right ventricular hypertrophy, the wall being over 1 cm in thickness.

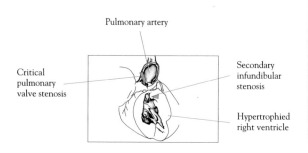

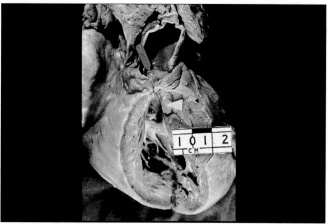

4   Auscultatory findings in pulmonary valve
stenosis. Characteristically, there is a long
ejection systolic murmur (ESM), often drowning
the aortic component of the second heart sound
(A_2) but ending before the pulmonary component
of the second heart sound, (P_2). Pulmonary
ejection sound (X), which characteristically
decreases in intensity during inspiration, is
frequently heard.
S_1=First heart sound.

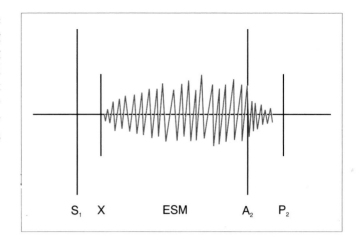

5   Chest X-ray in mild pulmonary stenosis showing
post-stenotic dilatation of the pulmonary trunk
and a prominent left pulmonary artery.

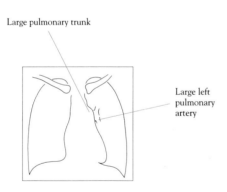

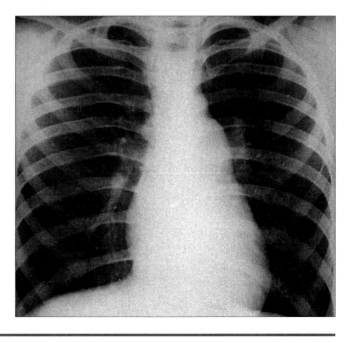

6   Chest X-ray showing obvious post-stenotic
dilatation of the left pulmonary artery in
pulmonary valve stenosis.

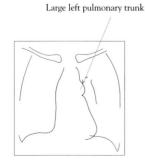

7

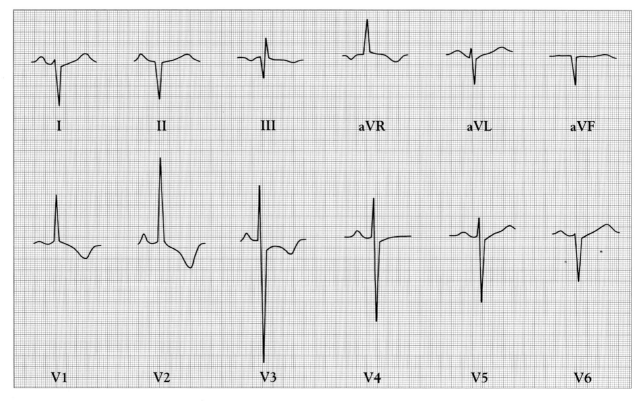

Electrocardiogram in severe pulmonary valve stenosis, showing deep S-wave in lead 1, a dominant R-wave in V1, and T-wave inversion in right chest leads.

8

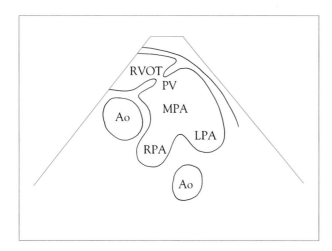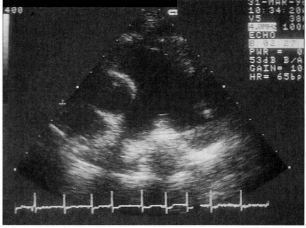

Two-dimensional parasternal short-axis image showing a mildly thickened pulmonary valve and enlarged proximal pulmonary arteries (post-stenotic dilatation) in a child with moderately severe pulmonary valve stenosis.

9

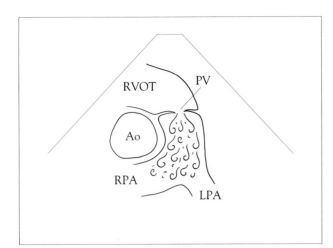

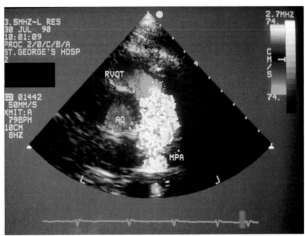

Two-dimensional parasternal short-axis image with color Doppler showing turbulent flow distal to the pulmonary valve in a child with mild pulmonary stenosis.

10 With increasing severity of pulmonary stenosis, the patient develops some infundibular hypertrophy and this can generate an additional outflow gradient, which increases as the muscle contracts during systole. This is best demonstrated with pulsed Doppler and gives rise to a characteristic pattern of the spectral display.

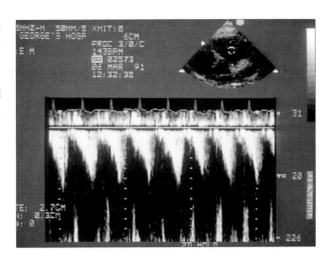

11

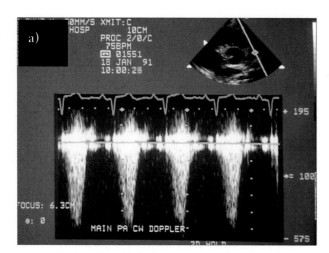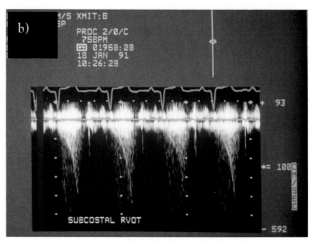

Severe pulmonary stenosis discovered by chance in a young adult. (a) Continuous-wave spectral Doppler shows an outflow velocity of 5 m/s, corresponding to a peak systolic gradient of 100 mmHg. (b) By directing the ultrasound beam along the right ventricular outflow tract, the dynamic infundibular gradient is shown. This has a peak end-systolic value of about 65 mmHg.

12

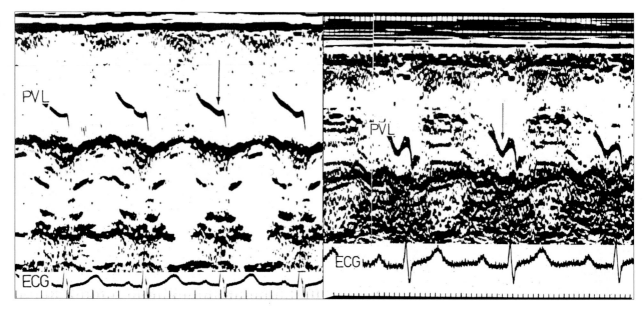

M-mode echocardiogram of the pulmonary valve showing the normal small downward dip (left-hand panel, arrowed) associated with atrial systole. In the right-hand panel, this dip (arrowed) is greatly exaggerated, indicating the presence of a large right ventricular 'a' wave in a patient with severe pulmonary stenosis.

13   Coronal spin-echo image of a 70-year-old patient with pulmonary stenosis (as part of Fallot's tetralogy which was uncorrected). The right ventricle is hypertrophied, and the infundibulum is narrowed and thickened with post-stenotic dilatation of the pulmonary trunk. A dilated aortic root is also visible.

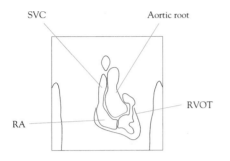

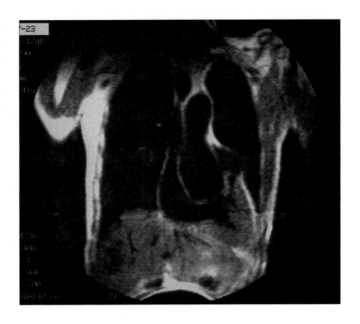

14   Right ventricular angiogram (lateral projection) in pulmonary valve stenosis showing a thickened and domed valve with a central systolic jet.

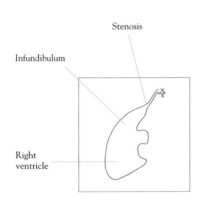

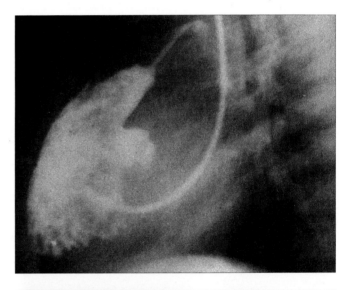

15   Another frame from the same patient as above, showing post-stenotic dilatation of the pulmonary artery.

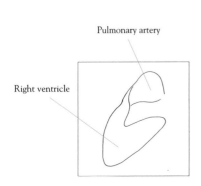

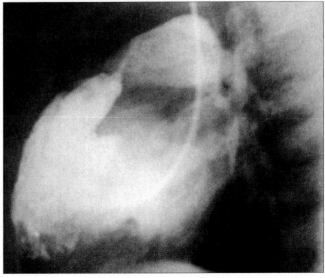

FALLOT'S TETRALOGY

Pathophysiology

Fallot's tetralogy consists of four discrete anatomic lesions: pulmonary infundibular stenosis with or without valvular stenosis, a ventricular septal defect, an aorta which overrides the ventricular septum, and right ventricular hypertrophy [1–3]. The foramen ovale frequently remains patent, although contributing little to the main right-to-left shunt which occurs at ventricular level. A right-sided aortic arch persists in 25% of patients. Hypertrophy of the right ventricle occurs as a result of right ventricular outflow obstruction. Right ventricular ejection predominantly occurs into the overriding aorta (right-to-left shunt) and there is decreased pulmonary flow.

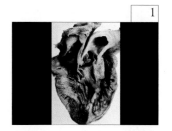

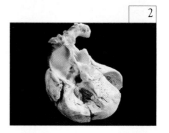

Presentation

Symptoms

Fallot's tetralogy will invariably present and be diagnosed in childhood. In adult life, the major complications include cerebral thrombosis (associated with polycythemia), cerebral abscess, infective endocarditis, and, rarely, cyanotic spells. Paradoxical embolism may occur in Fallot's tetralogy.

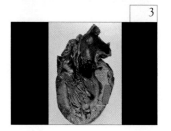

Signs

In Fallot's tetralogy, the 'a' wave in the venous pulse is not exaggerated (as it is in isolated pulmonary valve stenosis) because of the associated ventricular septal defect. Usually, there is an ejection systolic murmur, which may become abbreviated with severe obstruction. The pulmonary ejection sound and the pulmonary valve closure sound are often not heard as the valve is immobile. Central cyanosis and clubbing are an integral part of the condition.

Investigations

Radiology

The radiologic features of Fallot's tetralogy are a cardiac silhouette of normal size and lung fields which are either normally vascularized or under-vascularized [4]. The cardiac silhouette will not be enlarged in this condition, since chamber dilatation is negligible. The shape of the cardiac silhouette is normal in about 50% of cases and the remainder show a 'boot shape' [5]. This is produced by the hypertrophy of the right ventricle in the absence of left ventricular enlargement, leading to a lifting of the apex away from the left dome of the diaphragm, combined with an absence of shadow normally produced by the pulmonary artery (the pulmonary artery in Fallot's tetralogy being small). The absence of shadows in this area may be even more striking when a right-sided aortic arch is present [6].

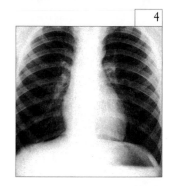

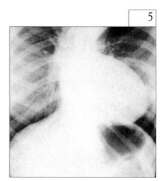

Electrocardiography

In Fallot's tetralogy the electrocardiogram will show moderate right ventricular hypertrophy, usually less striking than in severe pulmonary valve stenosis without ventricular septal defect. Right atrial hypertrophy is also less common in Fallot's tetralogy than in pulmonary valve stenosis [7].

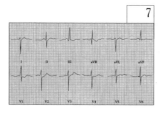

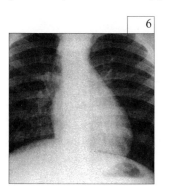

Echocardiography
The characteristic echocardiographic feature of Fallot's tetralogy is overriding of the interventricular septum by a displaced aortic root, resulting in a large, non-restrictive ventricular septal defect [8]. Color Doppler shows the systolic outflow from both ventricles into the aorta [9]. The associated right ventricular hypertrophy and outflow obstruction are evaluated as for pulmonary stenosis.

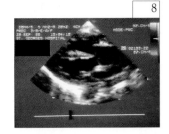

Magnetic Resonance Imaging (MRI)
MRI has been used to reveal the anatomic features of tetralogy [10].

Cardiac Catheterization and Angiography
Evidence of a right-to-left shunt at ventricular level will be seen from the desaturation of the left ventricular and aortic blood. A systolic pressure difference is seen between the right ventricular outflow tract and the pulmonary artery.

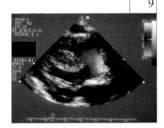

On right ventricular angiography, the outflow tract obstruction can be seen, as can the right-to-left shunt across the ventricular septal defect, by the passage of contrast from right ventricle to left ventricle [11]. The aortic override and the infundibular stenosis will also be seen [12].

Principles of Management

Total correction is preferable, if feasible, in young patients. A shunt procedure may be required initially to increase pulmonary flow before total correction can be undertaken in very young, severe cases.

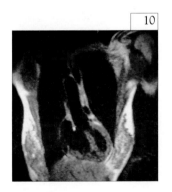
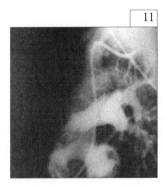
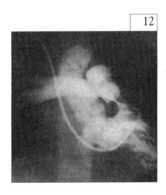

1   Right ventricular view in Fallot's tetralogy. The aorta is seen overriding the ventricular septal defect and the infundibular septum is deviated anteriorly to produce infundibular pulmonary stenosis.

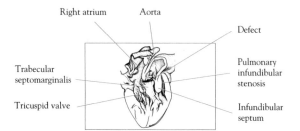

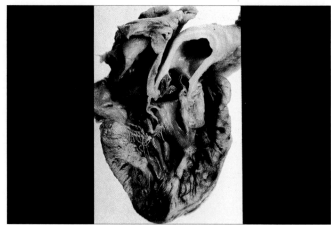

2   Fallot's tetralogy viewed from the anterior aspect with the anterior wall of the right ventricle cut away. Due to extreme aortic override, the great arteries have a side-by-side relationship.

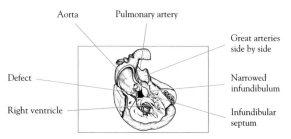

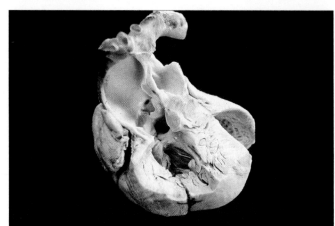

3   Fallot's tetralogy viewed from the right aspect showing extreme anterior deviation of the infundibular septum. The right ventricular outflow tract is a slit (arrowed).

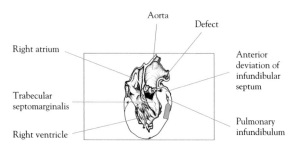

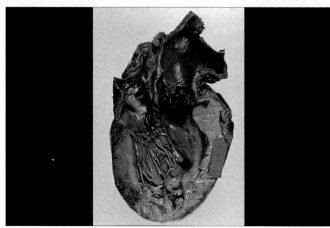

4 Chest X-ray in Fallot's tetralogy showing normal appearance apart from a slightly prominent aorta.

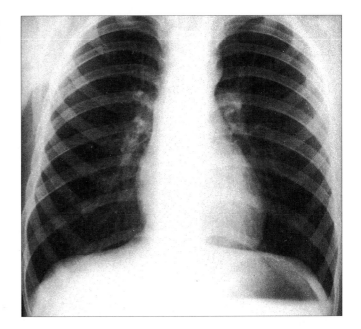

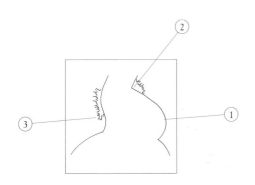

Slightly prominent aorta

5 Chest X-ray of Fallot's tetralogy showing a typical cardiac silhouette produced by 1) the tipped-up apex, 2) prominent pulmonary bay due to a small pulmonary artery, and 3) underfilling of the pulmonary vasculature.

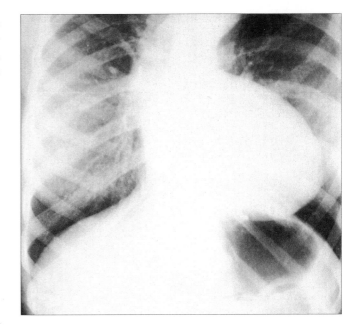

6 Chest X-ray showing right-sided aortic arch.

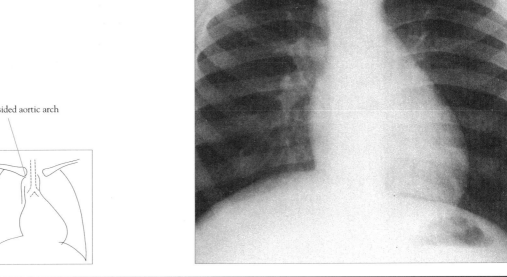

Right-sided aortic arch

7

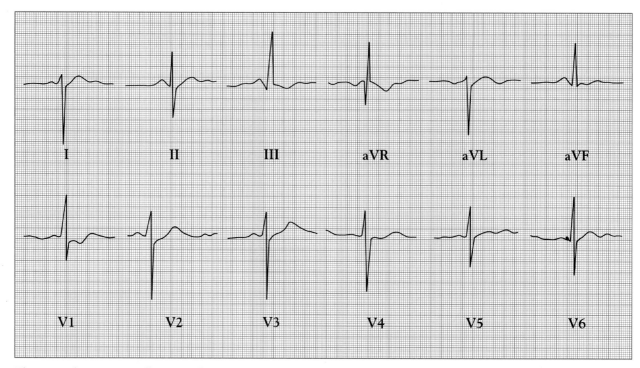

Electrocardiogram in Fallot's tetralogy showing moderate right ventricular hypertrophy.

8

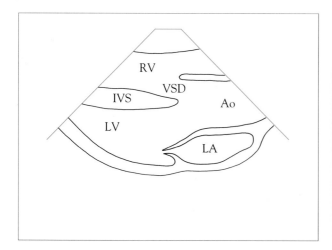 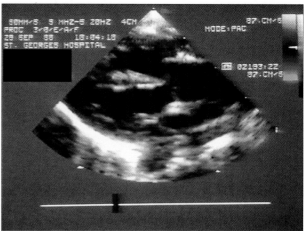

Parasternal long-axis view of a child with Fallot's tetralogy, showing the large aorta straddling the interventricular septum and creating a ventricular septal defect.

9   Parasternal long-axis view with color Doppler, showing systolic outflow from both ventricles into the large aorta, which straddles the hypertrophied interventricular septum.

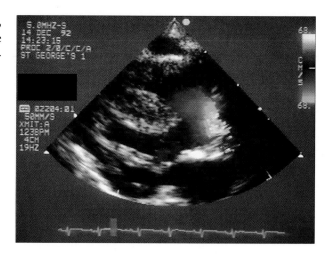

10   Magnetic resonance spin echo imaging in the coronal plane of Fallot's tetralogy. The ventricular septal defect and overriding aorta are clearly shown.

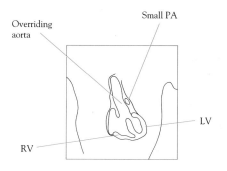

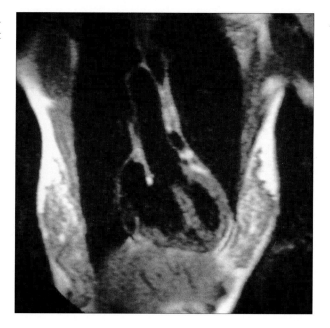

11   Right ventriculogram (lateral projection) showing right-to-left shunt across the ventricular septal defect.

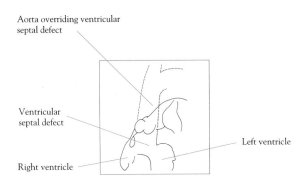

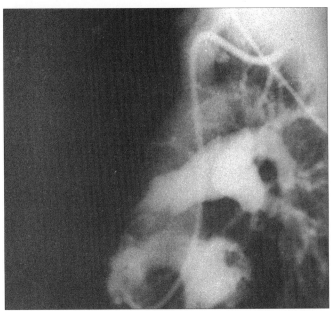

12   Right ventricular angiogram (antero-posterior projection) showing infundibular stenosis with aortic override.

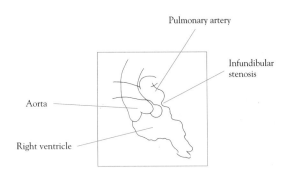

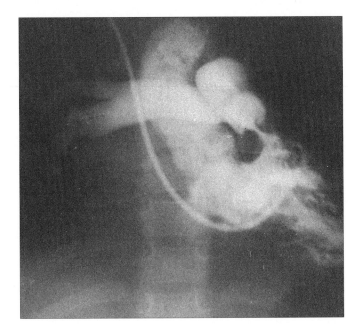

COARCTATION OF THE AORTA

Pathophysiology

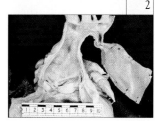

Coarctation of the aorta is a congenital constriction or narrowing of the aortic arch or descending aorta. It is of variable position, extent, and severity and may be associated with other congenital abnormalities such as a bicuspid aortic valve. Acquired coarctation of the aorta occurs at variable and multiple sites (Takayasu disease).

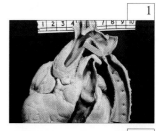

When coarctation of the aorta presents in adult life, the lesion is usually a sharply localized constriction just beyond the origin of the left subclavian artery and proximal to the insertion of the ligamentum arteriosum (postsubclavian) [1]. In less than 10% of cases the coarctation extends over several centimeters. An associated bicuspid aortic valve is present in about 85% of cases [2]. In the presence of isolated coarctation, a collateral circulation usually develops between the upper and lower parts of the body [3].

Coarctation of the aorta increases resistance to left ventricular ejection, which induces left ventricular hypertrophy. As the coarctation in adults is beyond the origin of the left subclavian artery, hypertension in the upper extremities only is observed. However, hypertension due to stimulation of the renin-angiotensin system, resulting from renal hypoperfusion, may also occur. A bicuspid aortic valve and coarctation may predispose to the development of bacterial endocarditis.

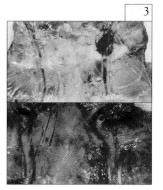

Presentation

Symptoms
Adults presenting with coarctation usually have no symptoms. The lesion is discovered at routine examination when hypertension is found or a murmur is heard. Occasionally, patients present with complications, e.g. angina, endocarditis, myocardial infarction, or dissection of the aorta. Cerebrovascular complications are not infrequent and are usually due to cerebral hemorrhage, often with rupture of a berry aneurysm. Leg claudication is infrequent.

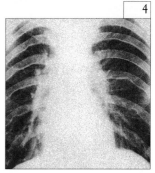

Signs
Blood pressure is usually elevated. The pulses in the legs are often weak and the femoral pulse delayed by comparison with the right brachial pulse. Prominent arterial pulsation in the suprasternal notch may be present. The development of the collateral circulation between the upper and lower parts of the body may be revealed by palpating arterial pulsation around the scapulae. The left ventricle becomes hypertrophied in response to hypertension and this may be clinically obvious on palpation with a double apical impulse. A classic auscultatory finding is an ejection systolic murmur arising at the site of the coarctation, which may be best heard high up on the back over the spine. This murmur is delayed relative to an aortic valve ejection murmur and consequently appears to spill through the aortic valve closure sound. Additional auscultatory findings may be due to a coexistent bicuspid aortic valve with an ejection sound and an ejection systolic murmur. Other murmurs may be produced by turbulent blood flow in the dilated and anastomotic arteries around the scapulae. These also sound like delayed ejection or sometimes continuous murmurs.

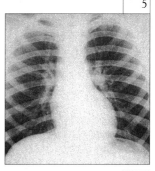

Investigations

Radiology
The characteristic features in the chest X-ray of a discrete coarctation are rib notching [4], abnormalities of the aortic knuckle [5], and cardiac enlargement [6]. Rib notching is usually seen after puberty. The aortic knuckle may be flat, high or low

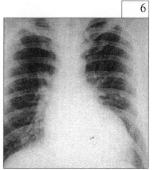

or, more rarely, double [7]. Post-stenotic dilatation of the descending aorta is a common feature.

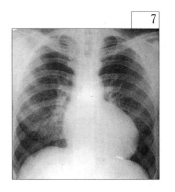

Electrocardiography
The electrocardiogram in coarctation may be normal or show features of left ventricular hypertrophy with ST-T abnormalities in the left ventricular leads [8].

Echocardiography
In the young child, the presence of aortic coarctation can usually be demonstrated by seeing a 'kink' in the upper thoracic aorta close to the origin of the left subclavian artery. The appearance is often as though an echo-dense wedge has been driven into the aortic wall [9a]. Color Doppler shows flow acceleration at this point [9b].

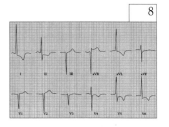

In the older child, or adult, it is usually not possible to image a coarctation directly, or to obtain a good color Doppler signal. Transesophageal imaging is sometimes helpful, but it can be difficult to image the aortic arch in the region of the left subclavian artery. Clues to the presence of coarctation include enlargement of the aortic arch and right brachiocephalic (innominate) artery, left ventricular hypertrophy, often with a non-stenotic bicuspid aortic valve, and lack of pulsatile flow in the abdominal aorta.

While continuous-wave Doppler may show some increase in flow velocity at the site of a coarctation, the presence of collateral vessels can minimize, or even completely mask, the severity of the lesion. The cardinal Doppler feature is not a *high* velocity, but rather a *prolongation* of flow into diastole [10].

Magnetic Resonance Imaging (MRI)
MRI has been used to determine the anatomic severity of coarctation and the anatomy of the aorta [11], as well as the pressure gradient and amount of collateral flow.

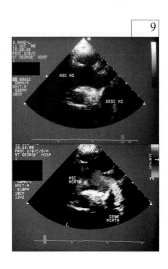

Cardiac Catheterization and Angiography
There will be a systolic pressure difference between the region above the site of coarctation and the region below. The aortogram of a typical discrete coarctation shows a shelf-like narrowing at the junction between the isthmus and descending aorta [12]. With long-standing severe coarctation there is visible dilatation of the internal mammary and other collateral arteries.

Principles of Management

Hemodynamically significant coarctation requires surgical correction. Catheter dilatation of the coarctation is less effective. Antibiotic prophylaxis for bacterial endocarditis is recommended.

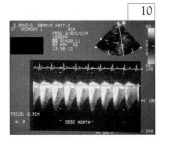

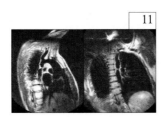

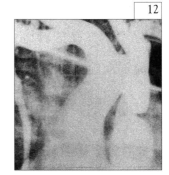

1   Arch arteries showing coarctation of the aorta (arrow) just beyond the left subclavian artery. The orifices of the intercostal arteries in the descending aorta are greatly enlarged.

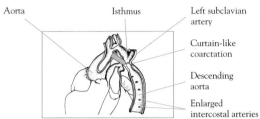

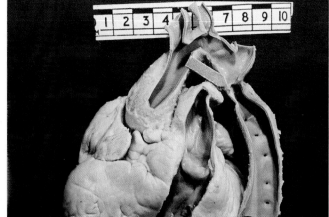

2   Arch arteries showing coarctation of the aorta with dilatation of the ascending aorta and bicuspid aortic valve.

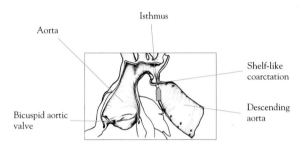

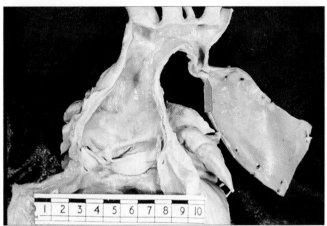

3   Panels showing the internal mammary arteries from a normal patient and a patient with coarctation. The patient with coarctation has gross dilatation of the arteries due to collateral flow.

NORMAL

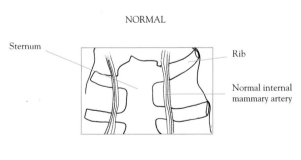

COARCTATION

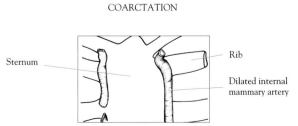

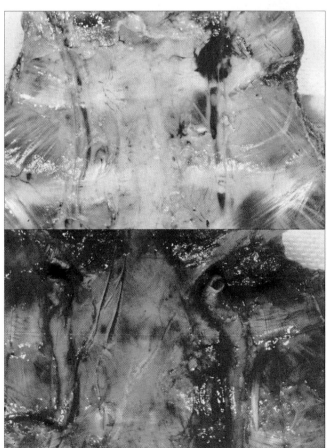

4   Chest X-ray in coarctation showing marked rib notching.

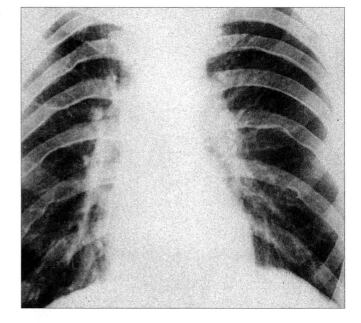

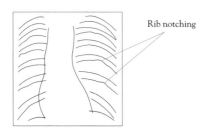

5   Chest X-ray in coarctation showing a flat aortic knuckle and rib notching.

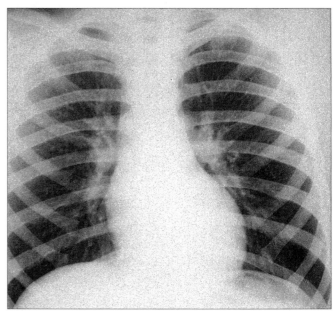

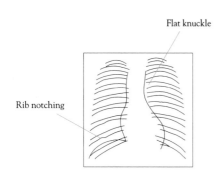

6   Chest X-ray in coarctation showing a large heart with left atrial and upper lobe vessel dilatation, which indicates pulmonary venous hypertension.

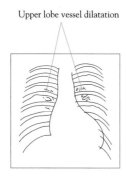

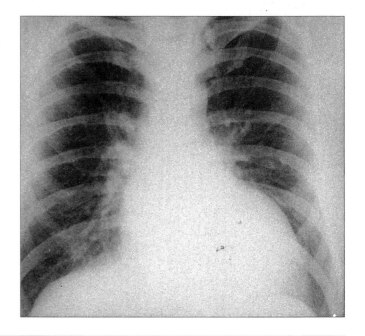

7 Chest X-ray in coarctation. The '3' sign is present. The upper bulge, in the position of a rather high aortic knuckle, is formed by a large left subclavian artery, coming off the aortic arch before the coarctation. The lower bulge is formed by post-stenotic dilatation of the descending aorta below the coarctation.

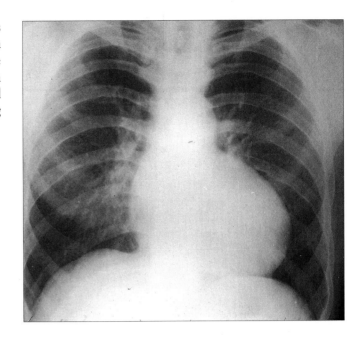

Enlarged left subclavian artery, the '3' sign

Post-stenotic dilatation

8

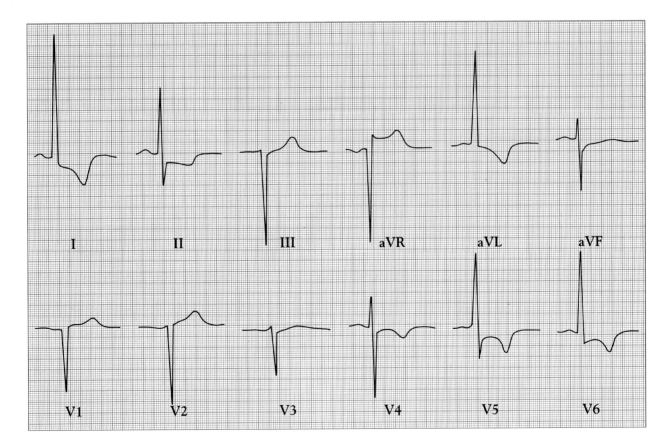

Electrocardiogram of a patient with coarctation of the aorta. Note high-voltage QRS complexes and ST-T changes in leads I, II, aVL and V4-V6 indicating left ventricular hypertrophy. For V1 to V6, 1 mV=0.5 cm.

9

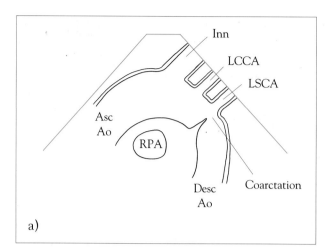

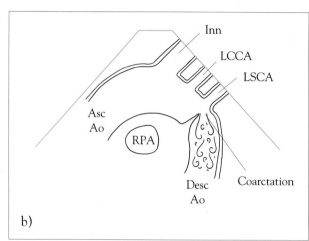

(a) Two-dimensional suprasternal view showing the aortic arch and upper-body vessels. There is a bright 'wedge' of tissue restricting the aortic lumen just distal to the left subclavian artery. (b) Color Doppler shows an increase in velocity and turbulence at this point.

10   Continuous-wave spectral Doppler from a child with aortic coarctation. There is a double density caused by superimposition of flows proximal and distal to the lesion. Note that there is not a great increase in peak flow velocity, but flow beyond the restriction is continuous throughout the cardiac cycle.

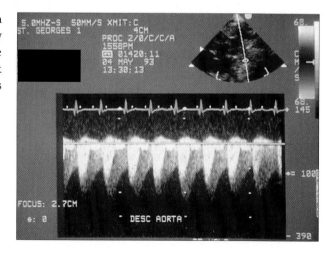

11

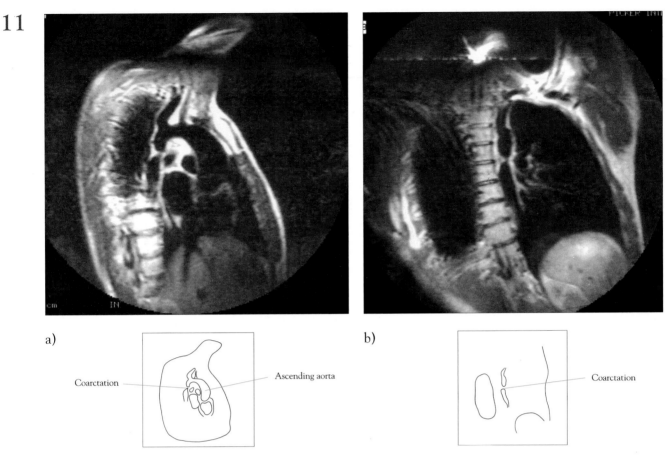

a)

b)

Coarctation of the descending thoracic aorta. Spin-echo images in the sagittal plane (a) and oblique coronal plane (b). The site of the coarctation is clearly shown, originating after the head and upper arm vessels.

12 Aortogram (antero-posterior projection) showing a shelf-like narrowing at the junction of the isthmus with the descending aorta. Note the dilated internal mammary artery.

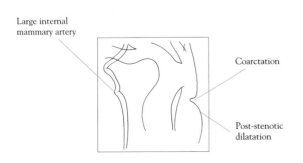

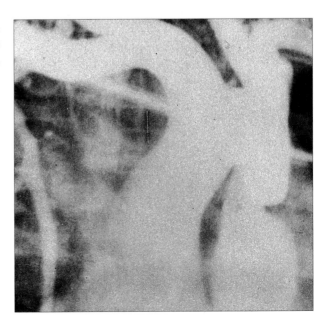

CHAPTER 6
The Cardiomyopathies

DILATED CARDIOMYOPATHY

HYPERTROPHIC CARDIOMYOPATHY

RESTRICTIVE CARDIOMYOPATHY

Abbreviations

AF	Atrial filling		LV	Left ventricle
Ao	Aorta		LVEDP	Left ventricular end-diastolic pressure
AVL	Aortic valve leaflet		MV	Mitral valve
ED	End-diastole		PVW	Posterior ventricular wall
ES	End-systole		RA	Right atrium
HCM	Hypertrophic cardiomyopathy		RF	Rapid filling
IAS	Interatrial septum		RV	Right ventricle
IVS	Interventricular septum		RVEDP	Right ventricular end-diastolic pressure
LA	Left atrium		RVO	Right ventricular outflow
LAA	Left atrial appendage		S	Septum

DILATED CARDIOMYOPATHY

Definition and Pathophysiology

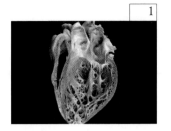

The term cardiomyopathy is used to describe pathophysiologic abnormalities of cardiac muscle. The essential morphologic and functional abnormalities of dilated cardiomyopathy comprise a dilated left ventricular cavity and impaired systolic function due to myocardial disease without an obvious cause. The cavity/mass ratio is increased, even though left ventricular mass is increased. Due to ventricular cavity dilatation, left ventricular wall stress is also increased. The pathologic features comprise a dilated, globular, thin-walled left ventricle with a large cavity [1]. The histology of virtually all forms of dilated cardiomyopathy shows interstitial fibrosis and vacuolated muscle fibers [2]. Etiologic factors include alcohol or a previous viral infection, but usually an obvious etiology cannot be established. Chronic left ventricular damage from coronary artery disease, with or without prior myocardial infarction (known as ischemic cardiomyopathy) may result in morphologic, functional, hemodynamic, and neuroendocrine abnormalities similar to those of idiopathic dilated cardiomyopathy. Acute myocarditis from any cause may also lead to pathologic and functional changes indistinguishable from those of idiopathic dilated cardiomyopathy.

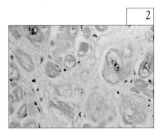

Irrespective of the etiology of dilated cardiomyopathy, left ventricular contractile function, ejection fraction, and 'Starling' function are depressed [3].

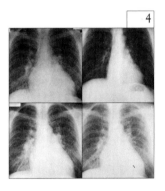

Presentation

Symptoms

Although patients with dilated cardiomyopathy may occasionally be asymptomatic and present with cardiomegaly on routine chest X-ray, the presentation usually includes breathlessness and fatigue, or even frank fluid retention due to heart failure. Rarely, a patient will present as a result of a systemic embolus (e.g. with a stroke) or the consequences of arrhythmias (such as dizziness or syncope).

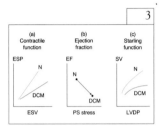

Signs

The signs are those of left ventricular dysfunction with a double apical impulse and gallop rhythm on auscultation. Sinus tachycardia is common with a small, sharp upstroke arterial pulse, reflecting reduced stroke volume. Pulsus alternans may be present. A pansystolic murmur due to secondary mitral or tricuspid regurgitation may be present. The jugular venous pressure may show an increased 'v' or systolic wave if there is additional tricuspid regurgitation. Signs of pulmonary hypertension, including a loud pulmonary valve closure sound (P_2), may also be present. Patients with fluid retention usually have pulmonary hypertension and an elevated systemic (jugular) venous pressure.

Investigations

Radiology

In dilated cardiomyopathy, the chest X-ray shows non-specific cardiac enlargement and signs of elevated pulmonary venous pressure, which include upper lobe blood diversion, Kerley B-lines, or even frank pulmonary edema [4]. In long-standing left ventricular failure, the radiologic features of pulmonary venous hypertension may be absent even when pulmonary venous pressure is significantly elevated.

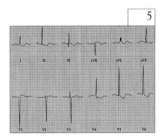

Electrocardiography

Dilated cardiomyopathy (when not ischemic in etiology) is not associated with specific diagnostic electrocardiographic abnormalities. Usually, the electrocardiogram shows non-specific ST-T abnormalities [5] or left bundle branch block [6]. Some patients may show Q-waves in the precordial leads simulating myocardial infarction [7]. Intraventricular conduction defects and varying degrees of atrioventricular block and sinus node dysfunction may also be present. Supraventricular or ventricular arrhythmias may occur.

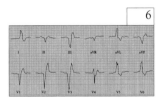

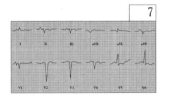

Echocardiography
Dilated cardiomyopathy is characterized by an enlarged, thin-walled, globular heart showing generalized hypokinesis [8,9], although segmental wall motion abnormalities are also seen occasionally. Left ventricular systolic shortening fraction is reduced below the normal 30% minimum and can be so low as almost to be unmeasurable. Generally, all four chambers are enlarged but the presence of functional tricuspid and mitral regurgitation due to dilatation of the valve annuli can greatly influence the degree of enlargement of individual chambers. Such appearances in idiopathic dilated cardiomyopathy can also result from extensive ischemic heart disease, although it tends to be more segmental in its presentation. The frequent presence of left bundle branch block in association with dilated cardiomyopathy causes some left ventricular dyskinesis, which further complicates the distinction between idiopathic and ischemic dilated cardiomyopathy.

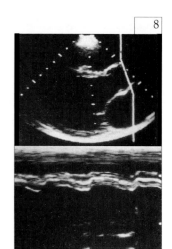

Many patients with dilated cardiomyopathy have thrombus in the left atrium (especially the appendage), best detected by transesophageal echocardiography [10]. Frank mural thrombus in the ventricles is usually associated with localized endocardial damage (e.g. myocardial infarction).

Color Doppler detects the presence of functional mitral and/or tricuspid valve regurgitation and provides a semi-quantitative assessment of severity [11]. Measurement of tricuspid regurgitation jet velocity with continuous-wave Doppler allows pulmonary artery pressures to be measured. Stroke output and systolic acceleration can be determined and serial measurements used to evaluate the efficacy of therapy.

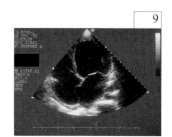

Nuclear Techniques
Increased end-systolic and end-diastolic volumes with a reduced ejection fraction can be demonstrated either by first-pass or by gated blood pool scintigraphy [12]. Such global abnormalities of left ventricular wall motion are more frequent in idiopathic dilated cardiomyopathy than in patients with coronary artery disease, who commonly demonstrate regional wall motion abnormalities including left ventricular aneurysm.

Magnetic Resonance Imaging (MRI) and Computed Tomography (CT)
MRI demonstrates a dilated left ventricle with little or no increase in left ventricular wall thickness and a reduced ejection fraction [13]. CT demonstrates similar findings [14].

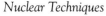
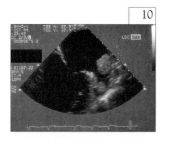
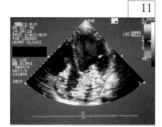
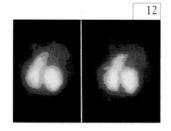
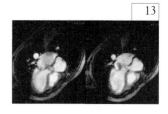

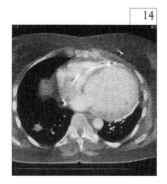
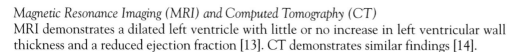

Cardiac Catheterization and Angiography
Echocardiography is so characteristic in dilated cardiomyopathy that cardiac catheterization is usually unnecessary unless there is a need to exclude coronary artery disease as the etiologic factor. Left ventricular angiography will show a large volume left ventricle with reduced ejection fraction [15].

The hemodynamics in symptomatic patients with overt heart failure include an elevated pulmonary capillary wedge pressure and decreased cardiac output [16]. These hemodynamic abnormalities are more pronounced during exercise. In some patients, cardiac output may remain normal at rest and during exercise.

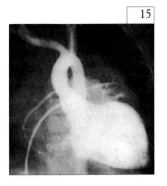

Principles of Management

The treatment of non-ischemic and ischemic cardiomyopathy is similar. The natural history of the condition is very variable. Severe heart failure with fluid retention and the presence of arrhythmias are associated with a worse prognosis. Mortality is reduced, particularly for patients in heart failure, and symptoms are improved by ACE inhibitors and to a lesser extent by certain vasodilators such as hydralazine and isosorbide dinitrate [17]. Diuretics are necessary to control fluid retention (pulmonary or systemic edema), as well as restriction of salt and water intake. Controlled, submaximal, regular exercise may be useful. Digitalis may be beneficial in patients with atrial arrhythmias, particularly atrial fibrillation, and sometimes in severe cases in sinus rhythm. Patients with refractory symptoms on vasodilators and ACE inhibitors should be considered for cardiac transplantation if appropriate. If cardiac transplantation is not feasible, positive inotropic agents, such as intermittent dobutamine or phosphodiesterase inhibitors or combinations of vasodilators and ACE inhibitors, or, in occasional patients, beta-adrenergic blocking agents should be considered. Low-dose amiodarone may also improve symptoms, left ventricular function, and prognosis in patients with heart failure due to dilated cardiomyopathy.

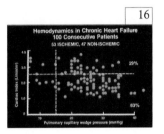

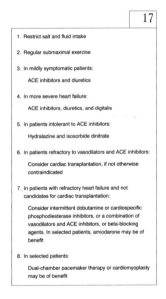

1. Restrict salt and fluid intake

2. Regular submaximal exercise

3. In mildly symptomatic patients:
   ACE inhibitors and diuretics

4. In more severe heart failure:
   ACE inhibitors, diuretics, and digitalis

5. In patients intolerant to ACE inhibitors:
   Hydralazine and isosorbide dinitrate

6. In patients refractory to vasodilators and ACE inhibitors:
   Consider cardiac transplantation, if not otherwise contraindicated

7. In patients with refractory heart failure and not candidates for cardiac transplantation:
   Consider intermittent dobutamine or cardiospecific phosphodiesterase inhibitors, or a combination of vasodilators and ACE inhibitors, or beta-blocking agents. In selected patients, amiodarone may be of benefit

8. In selected patients:
   Dual-chamber pacemaker therapy or cardiomyoplasty may be of benefit

1   Long-axis view in dilated cardiomyopathy showing markedly dilated ventricular cavities and thinning of the ventricular walls.

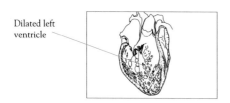

Dilated left ventricle

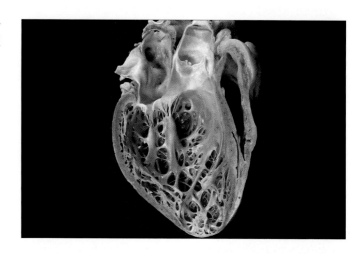

2   Histologic appearance of non-specific dilated cardiomyopathy. The muscle fibers vary in size and are vacuolated. Fibrosis is increased between the muscle fibers.

Fibrosis

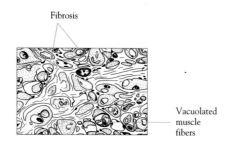

Vacuolated muscle fibers

3   Schematic representation of changes in ventricular function in dilated cardiomyopathy (DCM). (a) A rightward and downward shift of the relation of end-systolic pressure (ESP) to end-systolic volume (ESV) compared with normal (N) indicates depressed contractile function in DCM. (b) Ejection fraction (EF) in DCM is decreased compared with normal. EF reduction is due not only to decreased contractility but also to increased left ventricular peak systolic (PS) stress. (c) Left ventricular function curve relating stroke volume (SV) to left ventricular diastolic pressure (LVDP) shows a shift downwards and to the right in DCM compared with normal.

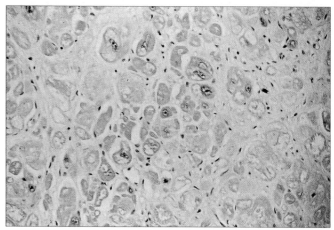

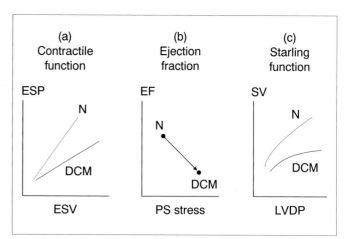

4

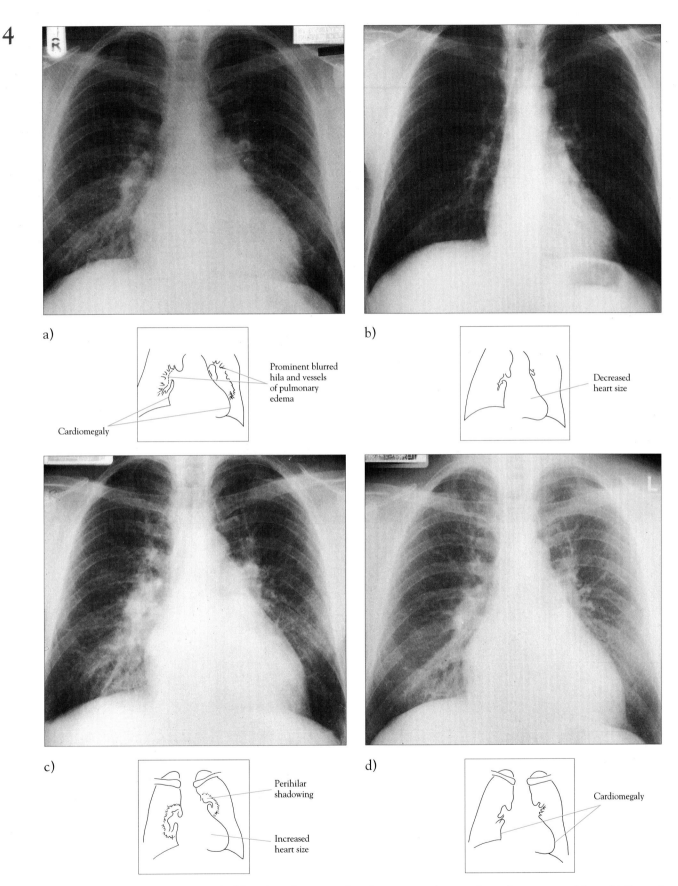

(a) Chest X-ray of a patient with dilated cardiomyopathy, showing cardiomegaly and prominent blurred hila and vessels, and pulmonary edema. (b) Following treatment, there was a decrease in heart size and resolution of pulmonary edema. (c) With recurrence of heart failure, heart size increased again and there was blurring of vessel outlines and perihilar shadowing suggesting pulmonary edema. (d) With treatment, although pulmonary edema cleared, cardiomegaly persisted.

5

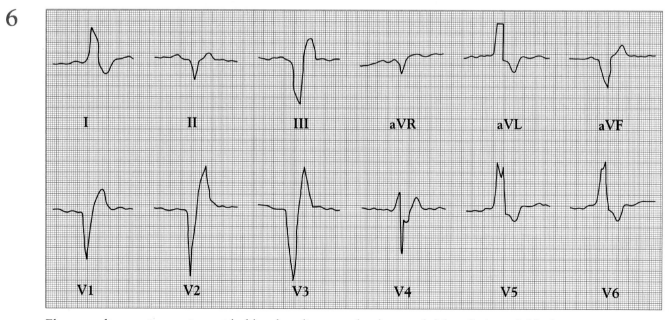

Electrocardiogram in a patient with dilated cardiomyopathy showing non-specific ST-T abnormalities.

6

Electrocardiogram in a patient with dilated cardiomyopathy showing left bundle branch block.

7

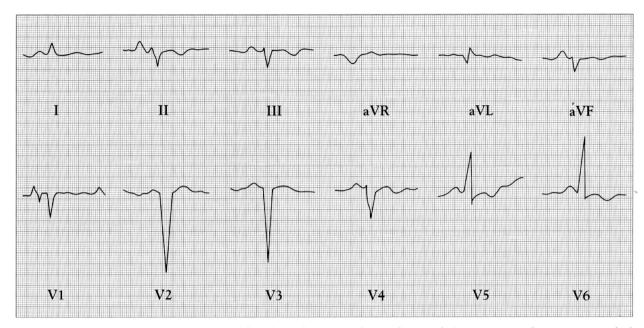

Electrocardiogram in a patient with dilated cardiomyopathy with septal Q-waves simulating myocardial infarction.

8

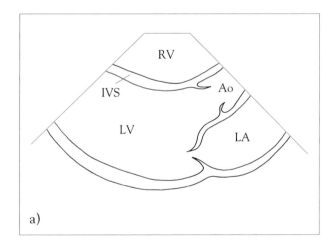

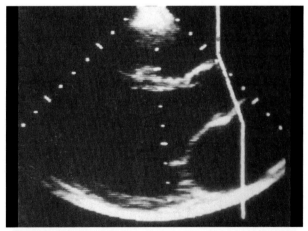

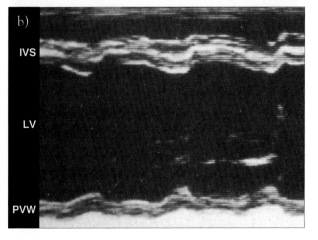

(a) Parasternal long-axis view of dilated cardio-myopathy. The left atrium is enlarged and the mitral valve annulus dilated leading to functional regurgitation. The left ventricle is large, thin-walled, and globular in shape. (b) The M-mode recording shows the enlarged left ventricle with severely impaired systolic function.

9

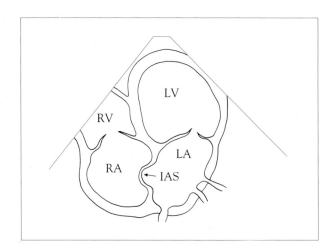 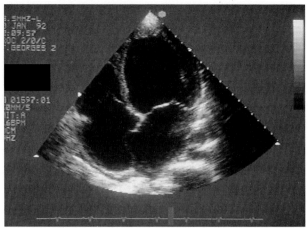

Apical four-chamber view showing enlargement of all four cardiac chambers. As a consequence of elevated left atrial pressure, the fossa ovale is stretched and the pulmonary veins are prominent.

10

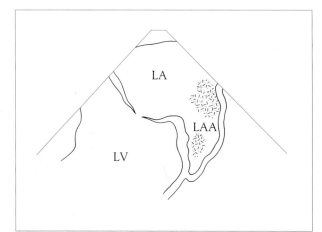 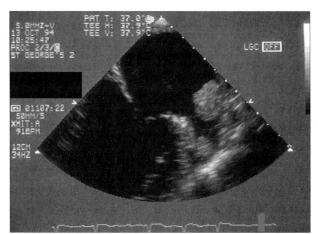

Transesophageal study showing a close-up view of thrombus in the left atrial appendage.

11

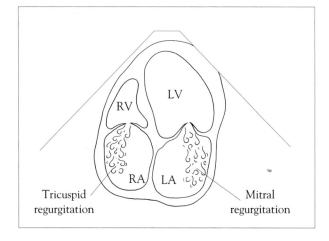 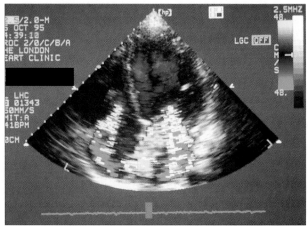

Apical four-chamber view with color-flow Doppler showing moderately severe functional mitral and tricuspid regurgitation in a patient with dilated cardiomyopathy.

12　Gated blood pool scan showing little difference in the size of the ventricular cavities between end-diastole (left) and end-systole (right).

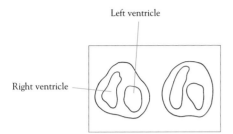

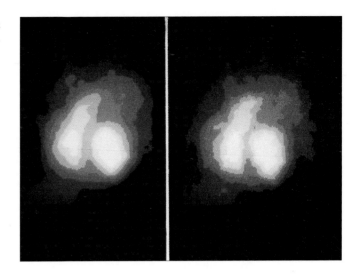

13

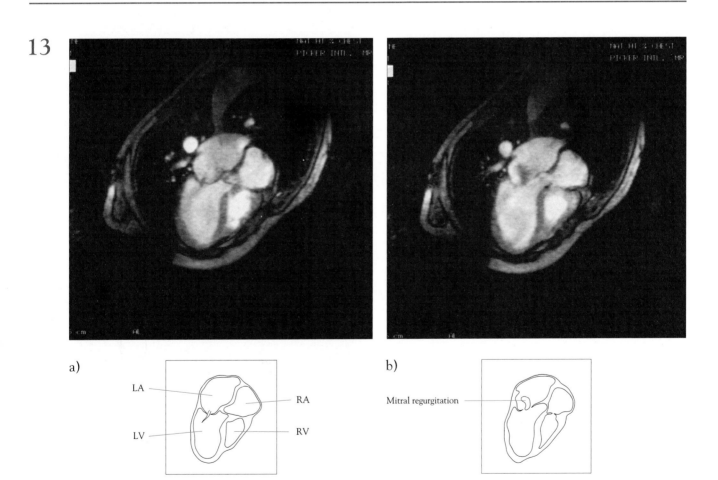

a)

b)

Magnetic resonance gradient echo imaging in the horizontal long-axis plane of a patient with dilated cardiomyopathy. The left ventricle is dilated and there is marked impairment of wall motion from end-diastole (a) to end-systole (b), demonstrating reduced ejection fraction.

14 Contrast computed tomography of a patient with dilated cardiomyopathy showing left ventricular enlargement and normal wall thickness. It also shows automated implantable cardioverter defibrillator patches.

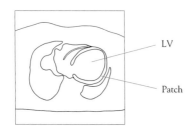

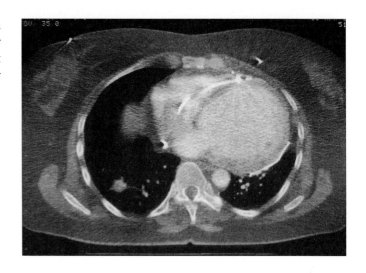

15 Left ventricular angiogram (antero-posterior projection) showing a dilated left ventricle in systole.

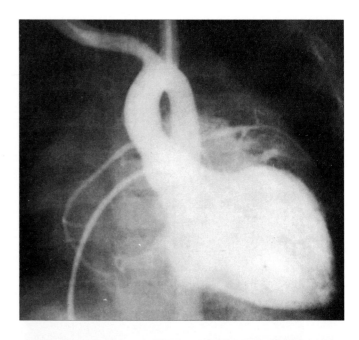

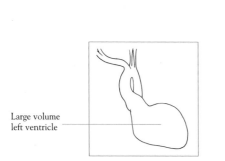

16 Hemodynamics at rest in patients with ischemic and non-ischemic dilated cardiomyopathy. In the majority of patients cardiac output is lower and pulmonary capillary wedge pressure higher than normal.

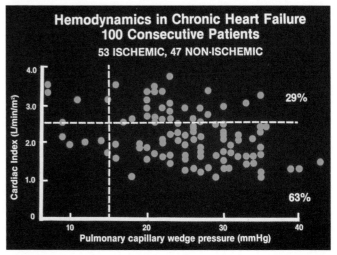

17   Principles of management of dilated cardio-
          myopathy.

1. Restrict salt and fluid intake

2. Regular submaximal exercise

3. In mildly symptomatic patients:

   ACE inhibitors and diuretics

4. In more severe heart failure:

   ACE inhibitors, diuretics, and digitalis

5. In patients intolerant to ACE inhibitors:

   Hydralazine and isosorbide dinitrate

6. In patients refractory to vasodilators and ACE
   inhibitors:

   Consider cardiac transplantation, if not otherwise
   contraindicated

7. In patients with refractory heart failure and not
   candidates for cardiac transplantation:

   Consider intermittent dobutamine or cardiospecific
   phosphodiesterase inhibitors, or a combination of
   vasodilators and ACE inhibitors, or beta-blocking
   agents. In selected patients, amiodarone may be of
   benefit

8. In selected patients:

   Dual-chamber pacemaker therapy or cardiomyoplasty may be of benefit

HYPERTROPHIC CARDIOMYOPATHY

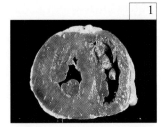

Definition and Pathophysiology

Hypertrophic cardiomyopathy (HCM) is a condition in which there is hypertrophy of the left ventricle, and occasionally of the right ventricle, without obvious cause. The distribution of hypertrophy is variable: it may be concentric [1]; or the hypertrophy of the septum may be disproportionately greater than that of the free walls, particularly that of the posterior wall [2]; there may be localized hypertrophy of the apex (apical HCM), or of the mid-ventricle (mid-ventricular HCM). When there is asymmetric septal hypertrophy, the septum may project into the left or right ventricle, or both [3]. In those cases where hypertrophy results in obstruction to outflow, a patch of endocardial thickening develops over the septum due to contact with the anterior cusp of the mitral valve [4]. The mitral leaflets are frequently longer than normal, but myxomatous degeneration with mitral valve prolapse is uncommon. Mitral annular calcification is frequently associated with HCM.

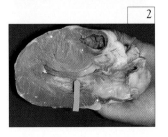

Histologic examination reveals hypertrophied muscle bundles with misalignment of myocytes (disarray). Muscle fibers may be arranged in circular whorls or in clusters with fibers radiating from a central point [5]. Examination at ultrastructural level shows myofibrillar disorganization within individual cells. Decreased lumen size with increased wall thickening of the intramyocardial coronary arteries is also frequently observed.

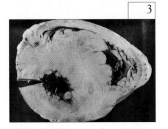

The left ventricular cavity is small or normal, with a marked increase in wall thickness [6]. The cavity/mass ratio is decreased. Contractile function, fiber shortening, and ejection fraction are normal. End-diastolic volume is normal or decreased, but the end-systolic volume is consistently smaller than normal. Left ventricular distensibility is decreased due to increased muscle and chamber stiffness. Left ventricular compliance and myocardial relaxation are decreased, resulting in impairment of ventricular filling.

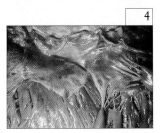

Presentation

Symptoms
Many patients are asymptomatic and the diagnosis of HCM is made either from the chance finding of a cardiac murmur, or by screening members of the family of a patient with HCM. Approximately 50% of cases of HCM are familial, the remainder occurring in sporadic form. The inherited familial type appears to be autosomal dominant with a high degree of penetration. Mutations in the beta-cardiac myosin heavy chain gene have been identified as the genetic abnormality in the familial form. Symptomatic patients may complain of typical angina, atypical chest pain, dyspnea, palpitation, presyncope, or frank exertional or spontaneous syncope. Increased myocardial oxygen requirements and impaired myocardial perfusion due to reduced coronary flow reserve may induce myocardial ischemia and angina. Ischemia-induced or spontaneous ventricular arrhythmias (rarely bradyarrhythmia) produce syncope. Abnormalities of ventricular filling can lead to a reduction in stroke volume and symptoms of low cardiac output such as fatigue and poor exercise tolerance. Syncope may be the result of a reduction in stroke volume or arrhythmias.

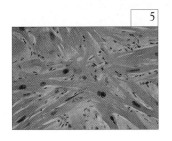

End-diastolic volume:	Normal or decreased
End-systolic volume:	Decreased
Left ventricular thickness:	Increased
Cavity/mass ratio:	Decreased
Ejection fraction:	Normal or increased
Fiber shortening:	Normal or increased
Peak systolic stress:	Normal or increased
Muscle stiffness:	Increased
Chamber stiffness:	Increased

Signs
In non-obstructive HCM the only abnormal physical finding may be a double apical impulse due to a palpable augmented left atrial contraction and a sustained left ventricular systolic outward movement. The upstroke of the carotid pulse is sharp or jerky, reflecting an increase in early systolic ejection from the left ventricle, sometimes with a 'bisferiens' quality as obstruction reduces emptying from the left ventricle later in systole. A prominent 'a' wave in the jugular venous pulse may be due to a non-compliant right ventricle as a result of generalized right ventricular hypertrophy or the hypertrophied

septum encroaching on the right ventricular cavity. The second heart sound may be split physiologically or may be reversed due to prolongation of left ventricular ejection. The clinical diagnosis of obstructive HCM depends on the presence of an ejection systolic murmur with its characteristic changes in intensity with various maneuvers [7]. A murmur due to additional mitral regurgitation is also present in many patients.

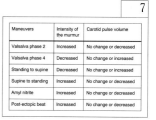

Maneuvers	Intensity of the murmur	Carotid pulse volume
Valsalva phase 2	Increased	No change or decreased
Valsalva phase 4	Decreased	No change or increased
Standing to supine	Decreased	No change or increased
Supine to standing	Increased	No change or decreased
Amyl nitrite	Increased	No change or decreased
Post-ectopic beat	Increased	No change or decreased

Investigations

Radiology
The heart size may be normal or enlarged with or without the findings of pulmonary venous hypertension [8]. A bulge on the high left border of the heart due to septal hypertrophy may be recognized in some patients [9], and left atrial enlargement is common.

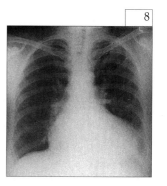

Electrocardiography
The electrocardiogram (ECG) is rarely normal in symptomatic patients but may be normal in 20–30% of asymptomatic patients. Increased left ventricular voltage with ST-T abnormalities [10], QS patterns in the precordial leads, or non-specific ST-T abnormalities are common electrocardiographic findings. Deep Q-waves in leads II, III, aVF, or the lateral precordial leads [11] due to abnormal localized septal depolarization are present in 20–50% of patients. Rarely, the ECG may resemble the Wolff–Parkinson–White syndrome with a short PR interval and slurring of the QRS complex [12]. Giant T-wave inversion in the lateral precordial leads with voltage criteria of left ventricular hypertrophy suggests apical HCM [13]. Intraventricular conduction defects and left bundle branch block are more common than right bundle branch block.

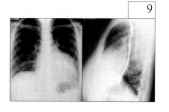

Ambulatory ECG, Electrophysiologic Studies and Signal-Averaged ECG
Ambulatory ECG recordings reveal non-sustained ventricular tachycardia in approximately 25–30% of patients [14], established atrial fibrillation in about 10%, and paroxysmal atrial fibrillation or supraventricular tachycardia in approximately 30% of patients. As ventricular tachycardia and syncope are important risk factors for sudden death (other risk factors are young age, history of sudden death in the family, and history of aborted sudden death), electrophysiologic studies are increasingly being performed in patients with a history of syncope or aborted sudden death. Electrophysiologic studies in such patients may reveal inducible sustained ventricular tachycardia (approximately 40% of patients), sino-atrial and His-Purkinje dysfunction, and accessory pathways. Abnormal, signal-averaged ECGs (low amplitude–high frequency) may identify up to 50% of patients with ventricular tachycardia.

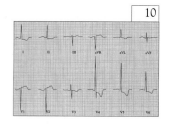

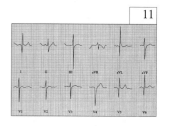

Echocardiography
M-mode echocardiography demonstrates increased septal thickness, exceeding that of the posterior wall, a small left ventricular cavity, and systolic anterior movement (SAM) of the mitral valve [15]. Fractional shortening is normal or increased despite septal hypokinesis. Aortic valve closure to mitral valve opening time, i.e. isovolumic relaxation time,

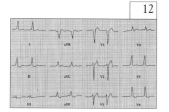

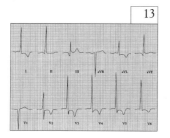

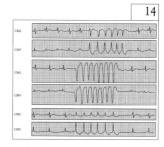

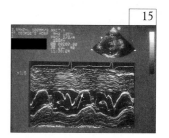

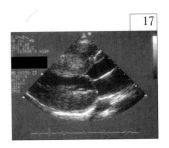

is prolonged. Early systolic closure of the aortic valve, which indicates the presence of left ventricular outflow gradient, can also be recognized by M-mode echocardiography [16]. Transthoracic and transesophageal two-dimensional echocardiography is helpful to delineate anatomic and functional abnormalities of the mitral valve as well as the distribution of left ventricular hypertrophy [17–19]. Since the hypertrophy is regional, and not always primarily in the septum, it is important to make a number of measurements of wall thickness. This is usually done from the short-axis views, with measurements made at the cardinal compass points at the level of the mitral leaflet tips, top of papillary muscles, and possibly papillary muscle bases as well [20]. The mitral valve leaflets may be longer than normal and thickened. Following initial rapid ejection with increased velocity, angulation of the mitral leaflets proximal to their edges and drawing in of the leaflets towards the left ventricular outflow tract (SAM) due to the Venturi effect causes outflow obstruction which is followed by mitral regurgitation (ejection, obstruction, regurgitation sequence) [21].

Doppler echocardiography reveals mitral regurgitation in the majority of patients [22], and is also useful in estimating the left ventricular outflow gradient [23].

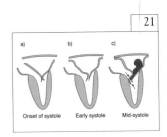

Nuclear Techniques
Gated blood pool scintigraphy shows a normal or increased left ventricular ejection fraction. The time–activity curve demonstrates rapid early ejection but, more importantly, reduced peak filling rate and increased time to peak filling rate [24].

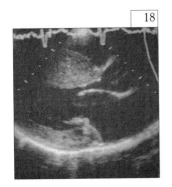

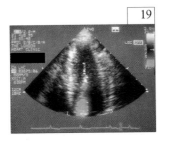

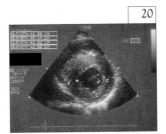

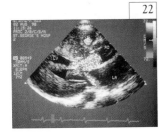

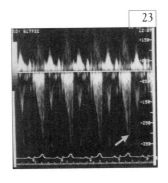

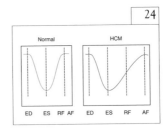

Magnetic Resonance Imaging (MRI) and Computed Tomography (CT)
MRI and CT demonstrate a normal or increased left ventricular ejection fraction and a normal or small left ventricular cavity. The distribution of hypertrophy can also be recognized [25,26], as well as the outflow gradient.

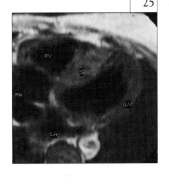

Cardiac Catheterization and Angiography
The consistent hemodynamic abnormality is an elevated left ventricular end-diastolic pressure due to increased left ventricular stiffness. A pressure difference between the left ventricular cavity and the outflow tract indicates obstruction, which can be present at rest or can be induced by various maneuvers (Valsalva, amyl nitrite inhalation, isoprenaline infusion). The pressure gradient may be decreased by vasopressors [27]. In contrast to aortic valve stenosis, following a premature ventricular beat, the aortic pressure may fall while the left ventricular pressure increases. Left ventricular angiography shows a small cavity, apical obliteration, and prominent papillary muscles [28,29]. The ventricle often has an irregular outline and there may be mitral regurgitation. Right ventricular angiography may show infundibular obstruction due to septal hypertrophy [30].

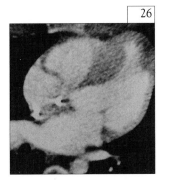

Principles of Management

In asymptomatic patients, no specific therapy is indicated, except determination of adverse risk factors [31]. Very strenuous physical activity should be avoided. Antibiotic prophylaxis for bacterial endocarditis is recommended. In mildly symptomatic patients without a significant resting left ventricular outflow gradient, calcium entry blocking agents may be effective. In patients intolerant to calcium entry blocking agents, beta-adrenergic blocking agents should be considered. In patients with arrhythmias, amiodarone may be of benefit. Disopyramide may be helpful in controlling arrhythmias and decreasing left ventricular outflow obstruction by its negative inotropic effect in selected patients. Dual-chamber pacing with a short atrioventricular interval decreases outflow gradient and improves symptoms. In symptomatic patients refractory to pharmacotherapy, myotomy and myomectomy should be considered. In some patients, cardiac transplantation becomes necessary.

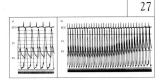

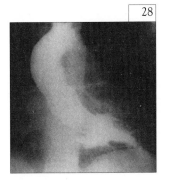

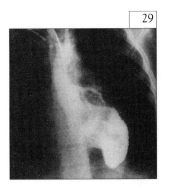

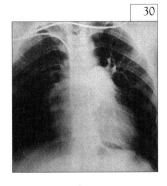

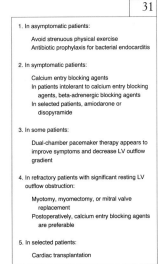

1. In asymptomatic patients:

   Avoid strenuous physical exercise
   Antibiotic prophylaxis for bacterial endocarditis

2. In symptomatic patients:

   Calcium entry blocking agents
   In patients intolerant to calcium entry blocking agents, beta-adrenergic blocking agents
   In selected patients, amiodarone or disopyramide

3. In some patients:

   Dual-chamber pacemaker therapy appears to improve symptoms and decrease LV outflow gradient

4. In refractory patients with significant resting LV outflow obstruction:

   Myotomy, myomectomy, or mitral valve replacement
   Postoperatively, calcium entry blocking agents are preferable

5. In selected patients:

   Cardiac transplantation

1   Transverse section through the heart in hypertrophic cardiomyopathy showing concentric left ventricular hypertrophy.

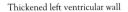

Thickened left ventricular wall

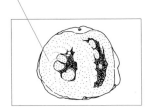

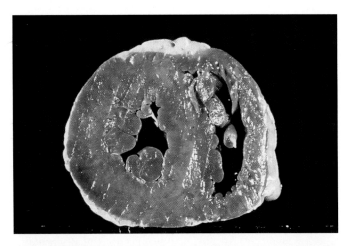

2   The left ventricle from a patient with hypertrophic cardiomyopathy showing a small cavity with a very thick wall. The septal region is asymmetrically thickened, being at least twice as thick as the parietal wall. The septum bulges into the outflow tract of the left ventricle and impinges onto the anterior cusp of the mitral valve (arrow).

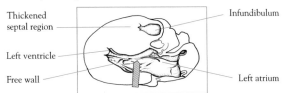

Thickened septal region   Infundibulum

Left ventricle

Free wall   Left atrium

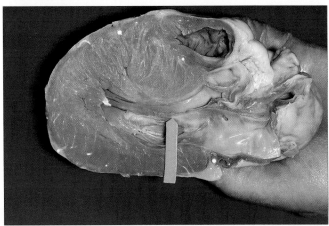

3   Transverse section across the left and right ventricles in hypertrophic cardiomyopathy. The septum is approximately two and a half times the thickness of the left ventricular free wall and bulges into the right ventricular outflow tract.

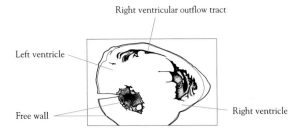

Right ventricular outflow tract

Left ventricle

Free wall   Right ventricle

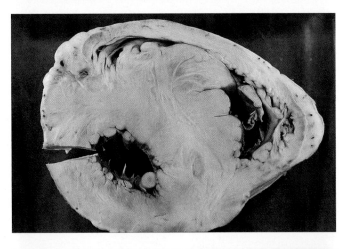

4   Pathologic specimen showing thickening of the anterior leaflet of the mitral valve with a corresponding thickening on the ventricular septum opposite, indicating contact in life with an obstruction to ventricular flow.

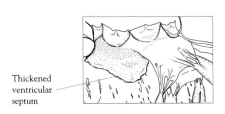

Thickened ventricular septum

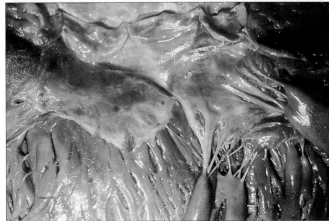

5   Histologic section of the myocardium in hypertrophic cardiomyopathy. The muscle fibers are arranged in a characteristic cross-over pattern radiating out in all directions rather than being arranged in parallel fashion.

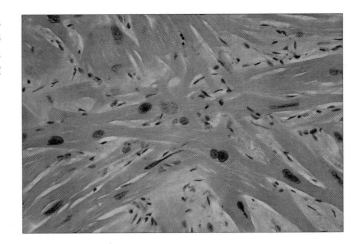

Muscle fibers

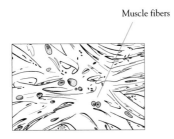

6   Functional and morphologic changes in hypertrophic cardiomyopathy.

End-diastolic volume:	Normal or decreased
End-systolic volume:	Decreased
Left ventricular thickness:	Increased
Cavity/mass ratio:	Decreased
Ejection fraction:	Normal or increased
Fiber shortening:	Normal or increased
Peak systolic stress:	Normal or increased
Muscle stiffness:	Increased
Chamber stiffness:	Increased

7   Changes in the intensity of the ejection systolic murmur and the carotid pulse volume during various maneuvers.

Maneuvers	Intensity of the murmur	Carotid pulse volume
Valsalva phase 2	Increased	No change or decreased
Valsalva phase 4	Decreased	No change or increased
Standing to supine	Decreased	No change or increased
Supine to standing	Increased	No change or decreased
Amyl nitrite	Increased	No change or decreased
Post-ectopic beat	Increased	No change or decreased

8   Chest X-ray showing large heart and left atrium with pulmonary venous hypertension.

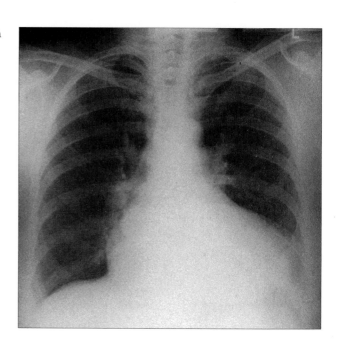

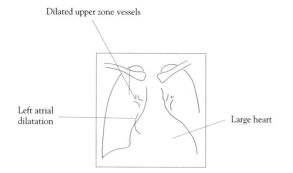

9

a)

b)

a) The frontal chest X-ray shows an obvious bulge on the high border of the cardiac silhouette due to septal hypertrophy. b) The lateral view shows a slight bulge of the myocardial mass behind the barium-filled esophagus.

10

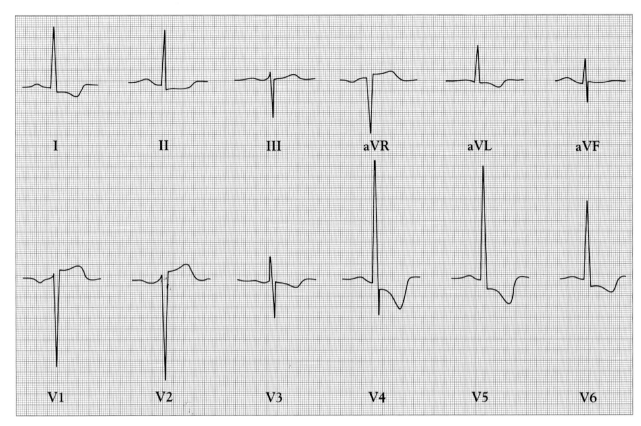

Electrocardiogram of a patient with hypertrophic cardiomyopathy. Note high voltage in chest leads and T-wave inversion in left ventricular leads. All chest leads, 1 mV=0.5 cm.

11

Electrocardiogram of a patient with hypertrophic cardiomyopathy, showing well developed Q-waves in leads I, aVL, and V4 to V6, simulating myocardial infarction.

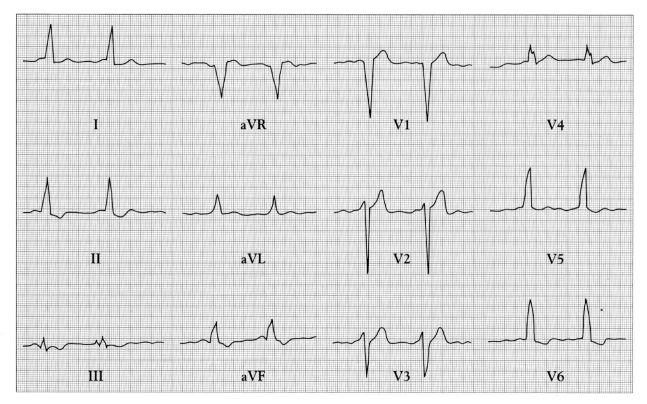

Electrocardiogram showing shortening of the PR interval, widening of the QRS complex, and a delta wave indicative of pre-excitation. This is an occasional feature of hypertrophic cardiomyopathy.

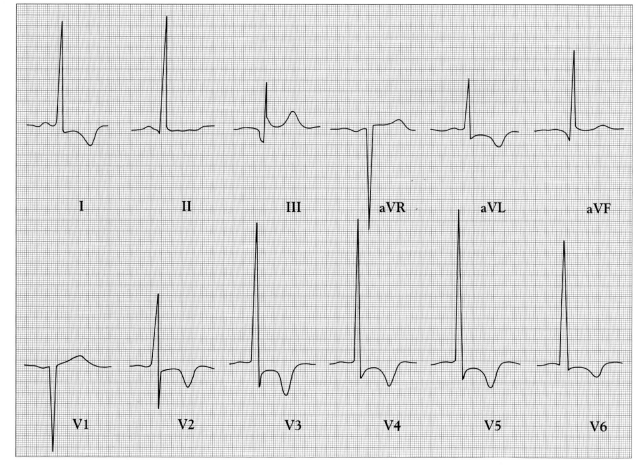

Giant T-wave inversions with tall QRS complexes in lateral precordial leads suggest apical hypertrophic cardiomyopathy.

14

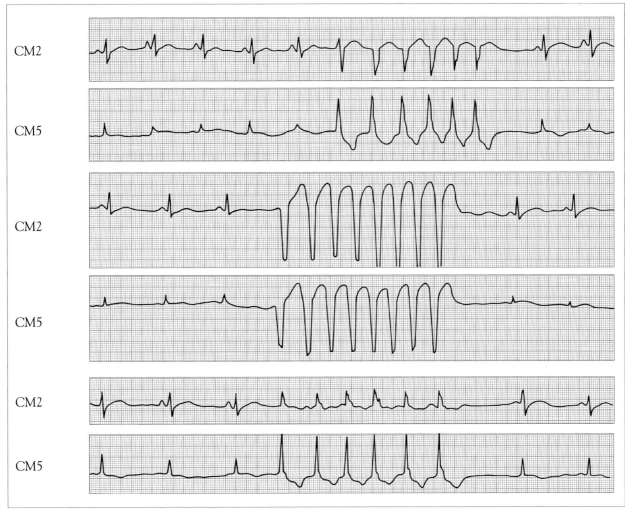

Ambulatory electrocardiogram of a patient with hypertrophic cardiomyopathy showing three episodes of non-sustained ventricular tachycardia.

15 M-mode recording showing massive septal thickening in a patient with hypertrophic cardiomyopathy. The motion pattern of the anterior mitral valve leaflet is very abnormal: the septal thickening and small left ventricle restrict its opening in early diastole and there is striking systolic anterior motion ('SAM') (arrow).

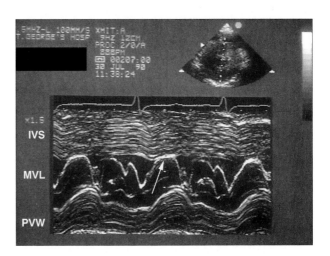

16 High-speed M-mode recording of the aortic valve in hypertrophic cardiomyopathy. As systole commences, the valve cusps initially separate normally. However, after a short period, almost all blood in the small ventricle has been ejected and the cusps start to close again with an irregular 'shattering' motion.

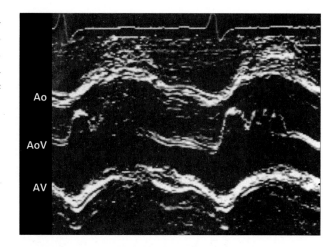

17

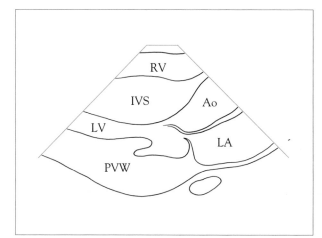

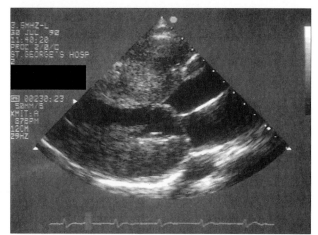

Parasternal long-axis view taken in mid-systole showing the abnormal 'SAM' of the mitral valve. Note the massive hypertrophy and very small left ventricular cavity.

18

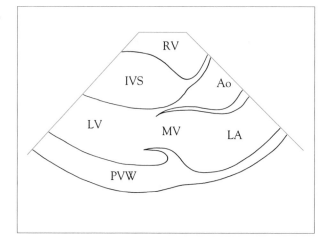

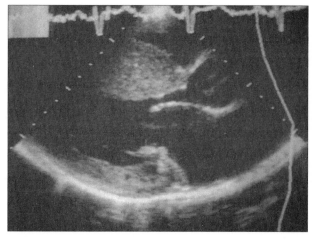

Parasternal long-axis view showing severe hypertrophy of the upper septum below the left ventricular outflow tract. This is the most commonly affected region of the myocardium.

19

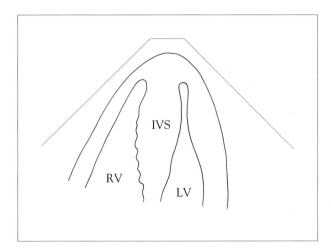
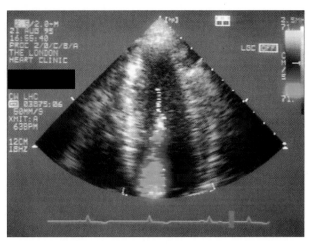

Apical four-chamber view showing hypertrophy restricted to the apical region. Color-flow Doppler shows virtual obliteration of the ventricular cavity in this region. Such patients do not show mitral valve motion abnormalities.

20

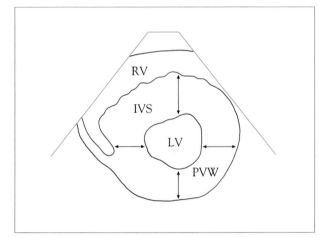
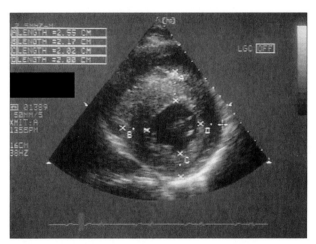

Parasternal short-axis view showing the technique of measuring myocardial wall thickness at quadrantal points. These measurements are made at the level of the mitral valve leaflets, at the top of the papillary muscles, and the papillary muscle bases.

21 Diagram showing the sequence of mitral valve motion associated with hypertrophic cardiomyopathy. (a) At the onset of systole, the high ejection velocity around the thickened upper septum lowers pressure in the outflow tract (Venturi effect) and draws the mitral leaflets towards the septum. (b) The 'SAM' exacerbates the degree of outflow obstruction. (c) Distortion of the valve apparatus results in secondary mitral regurgitation.

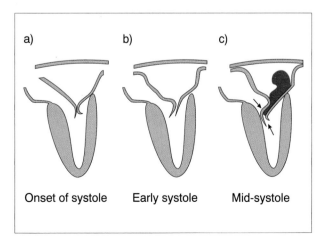

22

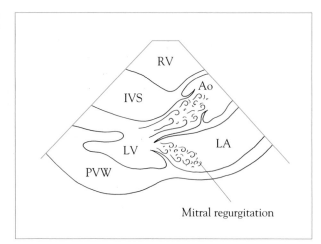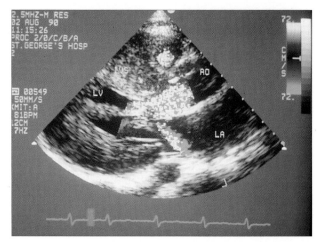

Parasternal long-axis view with color-flow Doppler in late systole showing the hemodynamics described in [21c].

23 Continuous-wave spectral Doppler showing the characteristic increasing velocity associated with a dynamic outflow gradient in hypertrophic cardiomyopathy. In this patient, the maximum velocity is 3.3 m/s, corresponding to a peak gradient of 44 mmHg.

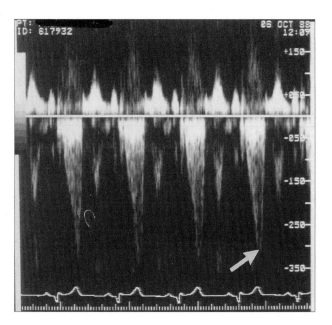

24 Schematic illustration of the time–activity curve in hypertrophic cardiomyopathy (HCM). Compared with normal, peak filling rate is reduced and time to peak filling rate is prolonged, indicating abnormal diastolic function. Ejection fraction and ejection rate remain normal.

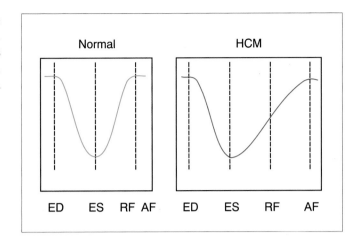

25 Magnetic resonance image showing localized septal hypertrophy.

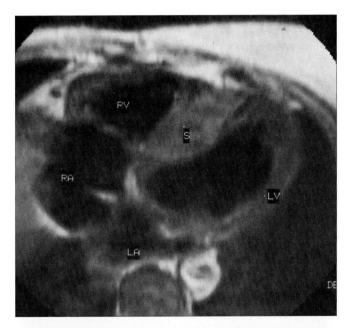

26 Ultrafast cine CT image of hypertrophic cardiomyopathy showing the grossly thickened interventricular septum.

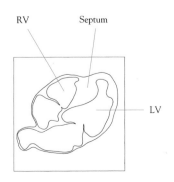

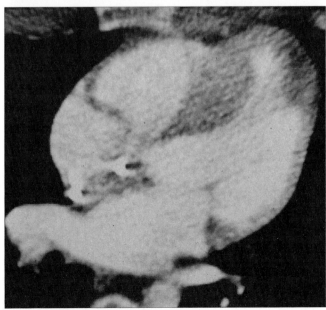

27

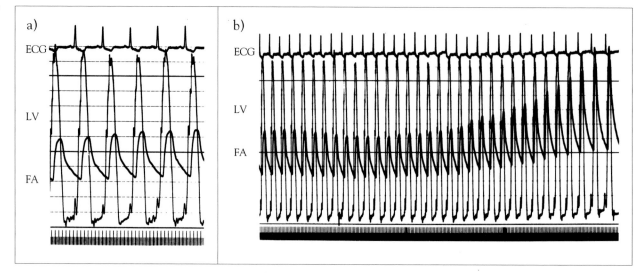

Simultaneous aortic and left ventricular pressures in a patient with hypertrophic cardiomyopathy. (a) Resting ventricular gradient between femoral arterial (FA) pressure and left ventricular (LV) systolic pressure. (b) During infusion of phenylephrine, which increases FA pressure, the outflow gradient is obliterated.

28 Left ventricular angiogram in systole (antero-posterior projection) showing a small irregular cavity.

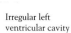

Irregular left
ventricular cavity

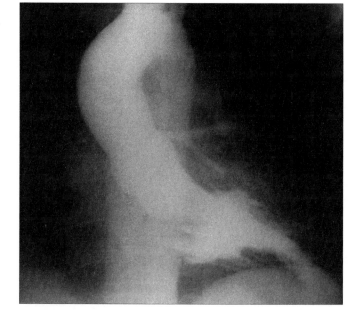

29 Left ventricular angiogram in diastole (antero-posterior projection) showing an irregular outline and inferior indentation from asymmetric septal hypertrophy.

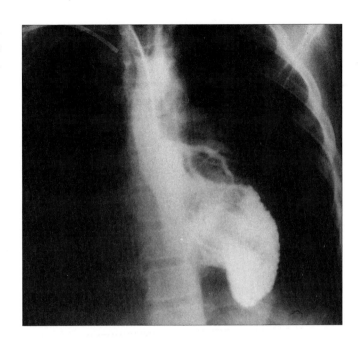

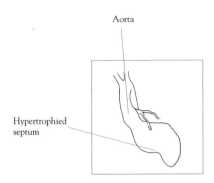

30 Right ventricular angiogram (antero-posterior projection) showing infundibular obstruction due to septal hypertrophy.

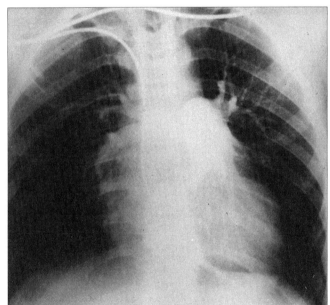

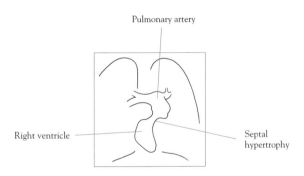

31 Principles of management of hypertrophic cardiomyopathy.

1. In asymptomatic patients:

   Avoid strenuous physical exercise
   Antibiotic prophylaxis for bacterial endocarditis

2. In symptomatic patients:

   Calcium entry blocking agents
   In patients intolerant to calcium entry blocking
     agents, beta-adrenergic blocking agents
   In selected patients, amiodarone or disopyramide

3. In some patients:

   Dual-chamber pacemaker therapy appears to
   improve symptoms and decrease LV outflow
   gradient

4. In refractory patients with significant resting LV outflow
   obstruction:

   Myotomy, myomectomy, or mitral valve
     replacement
   Postoperatively, calcium entry blocking agents
     are preferable

5. In selected patients:

   Cardiac transplantation

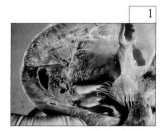

RESTRICTIVE CARDIOMYOPATHY

Definition and Pathophysiology

Impaired ventricular distensibility with abnormal, restrictive diastolic filling and relatively preserved systolic function are the characteristic functional derangements of restrictive cardiomyopathy. While the purest and rarest form is due to idiopathic myocardial fibrosis (idiopathic restrictive cardiomyopathy), the most common cause worldwide is endomyocardial fibrosis with or without eosinophilia [1,2]. Involvement of the atrioventricular valves is common, causing mitral and/or tricuspid regurgitation. Mural thrombi near the apex may cause cavity obliteration in advanced cases. Amyloid infiltration of the myocardium is another common cause of restrictive cardiomyopathy [3,4]. Other conditions, including hemochromatosis, sarcoidosis, autoimmune disease, glycogen storage disease, mucopolysaccharoidosis, and neoplastic disease may infiltrate the myocardium, resulting in hemodynamic abnormalities characteristic of restrictive cardiomyopathy. Both ventricles are usually involved, although one ventricle may be more involved than the other. The ventricular cavity size is substantially reduced in endomyocardial fibrosis. Ventricular wall thickness is normal or slightly increased except in amyloid infiltration, when a marked increase in wall thickness occurs, but without further increase in systolic thickening. The pericardium is normal except when a pericardial effusion coexists.

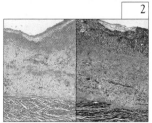

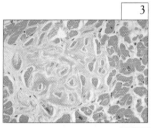

Presentation

Symptoms

Patients usually present with dyspnea, and ankle and abdominal swelling — signs and symptoms resulting from pulmonary and systemic venous hypertension. The stiff indistensible ventricles cause the pressure–volume relation to be shifted to the left compared with normal. Normal ventricular filling, required to maintain an adequate stroke volume, is achieved only by a marked increase in ventricular filling pressures with a passive increase in systemic and pulmonary venous pressures [5]. Post-capillary pulmonary hypertension also contributes to right heart failure and a further increase in systemic venous pressure. In advanced cases, cardiac output may decrease due to marked impairment of ventricular filling.

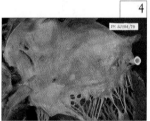

There may be gross peripheral edema and ascites, but paroxysmal nocturnal dyspnea, orthopnea, and frank pulmonary edema are uncommon. Ascites may be more marked than peripheral edema. Syncope may be a presenting symptom resulting from ventricular arrhythmias or conduction disturbances. Orthostatic hypotension due to impaired autonomic function may be a presenting symptom in amyloid heart disease.

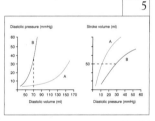

Signs

Physical examination reveals evidence of restrictive filling of the right ventricle with an elevated jugular venous pressure, a prominent 'y' descent, and Kussmaul's sign (increase or lack of fall of jugular venous pressure during inspiration). Mitral and/or tricuspid regurgitation murmurs are usually present in endomyocardial fibrosis. The signs of restrictive cardiomyopathy may be very similar to those of constrictive pericarditis with myocardial involvement.

Investigations

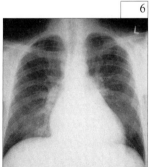

Radiology

Cardiac size is usually normal but may be enlarged due to bi-atrial dilatation [6].

Radiologic findings of pulmonary venous hypertension are more common in restrictive cardiomyopathy than in constrictive pericarditis. Pericardial calcification is absent in restrictive cardiomyopathy and, when present, the diagnosis of constrictive pericarditis is virtually confirmed [7], although additional involvement of the myocardium may be present.

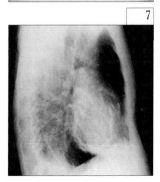

Electrocardiography

The electrocardiogram may show sinus rhythm, supraventricular arrhythmias (usually atrial fibrillation), intraventricular conduction defects including right and left bundle branch block, and evidence of sino-atrial and atrioventricular nodal dysfunction. Low-voltage QRS complexes are common in amyloid heart disease [8]. Q-waves, simulating myocardial infarction, are present in approximately one-third of patients with amyloid heart disease. Non-specific ST-T changes probably indicate myocardial fibrosis.

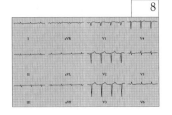

Echocardiography

The primary echocardiographic features shown by two-dimensional imaging are enlargement of both atria in the presence of normal ventricular size and the absence of organic mitral valve disease. Systolic function may be normal or only mildly impaired [9]. Amyloid infiltration causes a marked increase in wall thickness, but with minimal systolic thickening, and an increase in the echogenicity of the myocardium [10,11]. In endo-myocardial disease and eosinophilic heart disease, obliteration of one or both ventricular apices and global subendocardium by a thrombotic fibro-calcific process can be recognized [12]. Raised right-sided filling pressure may be evident from dilatation of the caval and hepatic veins.

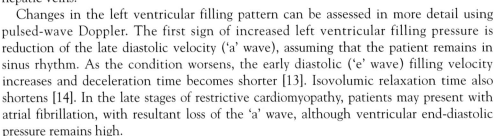

   Changes in the left ventricular filling pattern can be assessed in more detail using pulsed-wave Doppler. The first sign of increased left ventricular filling pressure is reduction of the late diastolic velocity ('a' wave), assuming that the patient remains in sinus rhythm. As the condition worsens, the early diastolic ('e' wave) filling velocity increases and deceleration time becomes shorter [13]. Isovolumic relaxation time also shortens [14]. In the late stages of restrictive cardiomyopathy, patients may present with atrial fibrillation, with resultant loss of the 'a' wave, although ventricular end-diastolic pressure remains high.

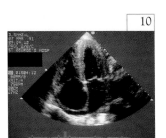

   The significance of diastolic filling measurements is age related. In a young person with a compliant ventricle, the majority of filling takes place in early diastole and the 'a' wave is usually small (typically less than 50% of the 'e' wave amplitude. With increasing age, and particularly in the presence of hypertension, the 'e' wave becomes smaller, deceleration time lengthens, and the 'a' wave amplitude increases.

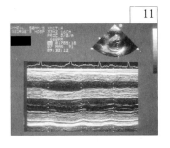

Nuclear Techniques

Gated blood pool scintigraphy may show reduced end-systolic and end-diastolic volumes with normal or slightly impaired ejection fraction. Time–activity curves may demonstrate impaired ventricular filling.

Magnetic Resonance Imaging (MRI) and Computed Tomography (CT)

MRI and CT are most useful in the differential diagnosis between restrictive cardio-myopathy and constrictive pericarditis. Both techniques can reveal the presence, severity, and distribution of pericardial thickening in constrictive pericarditis [15]. Pericardial calcification can also be detected. Pericardial abnormalities are absent in restrictive cardiomyopathy. Ventricular function, cavity size, and wall thickness can be assessed. Although these imaging techniques can reveal anatomic abnormalities, it is the func-tional abnormalities which best permit a distinction between restrictive cardiomyopathy and constrictive pericarditis to be made.

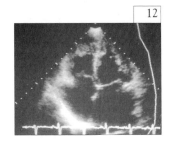

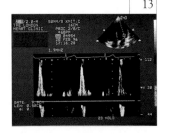

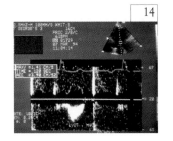

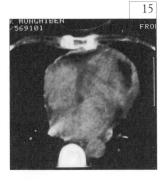

Cardiac Catheterization and Angiography
Catheterization reveals elevated filling pressures in both right and left ventricles. The filling pressures in the two ventricles usually differ, with left ventricular end-diastolic pressure being greater than that of the right ventricle by 5 mmHg or more [16]. In constrictive pericarditis, the end-diastolic pressures of both ventricles are equal. A prominent early diastolic dip followed by mid- to late-diastolic plateau ($\sqrt{}$) is seen in both restrictive cardiomyopathy and constrictive pericarditis. In restrictive cardio-myopathy, however, right ventricular end-diastolic pressure is usually less than one-third of the right ventricular peak systolic pressure, which exceeds 40–45 mmHg.

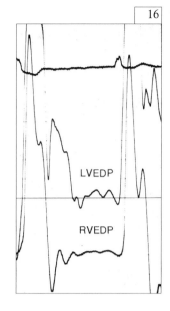

In endomyocardial fibrosis, left ventricular angiography frequently demonstrates cavity obliteration and mitral regurgitation [17]. Left ventricular ejection is usually normal. Right ventricular angiography shows cavity obliteration and tricuspid regurgitation [18]. Endomyocardial biopsy is often required to establish the etiology of restrictive cardio-myopathy.

Principles of Management

Diuretics are required to control fluid retention [19]. No specific therapy is available for amyloid heart disease. Atrioventricular sequential pacing may be considered if heart block is present. In severe endomyocardial fibrosis, surgical removal of the endocardium and replacement of the atrioventricular valves may be considered. Cardiac transplantation is indicated in selected patients.

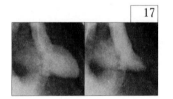

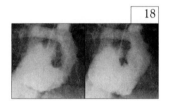

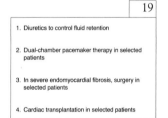

19
1. Diuretics to control fluid retention

2. Dual-chamber pacemaker therapy in selected patients

3. In severe endomyocardial fibrosis, surgery in selected patients

4. Cardiac transplantation in selected patients

1   Restrictive cardiomyopathy due to endomyocardial fibrosis (section through the left ventricle).
There is marked left ventricular apical obliteration with endocardial thickening and super-added
thrombus.

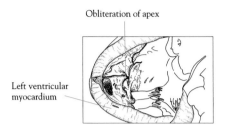

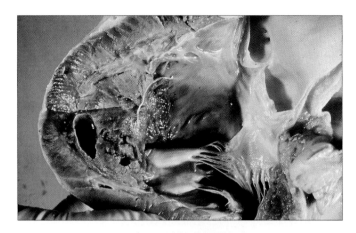

2   Histology of endomyocardial fibrosis. The
endocardium is markedly thickened and, using
hematoxylin and eosin (left panel), it is not easy
to distinguish the cause of this thickening.
However, staining by a trichrome method (right
panel) reveals that the endocardial thickening is
due to a deep layer of collagen, staining blue, and
a more superficial layer of fibrin.

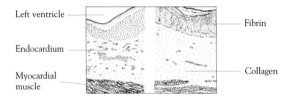

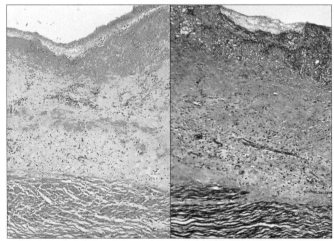

3   Restrictive cardiomyopathy due to amyloid
deposition in the myocardium. In hematoxylin
and eosin stained histologic sections, amyloid is a
pale pink homogeneous material. Amyloid is laid
down between myocardial cells and ultimately
completely surrounds them, leaving a lattice
of amyloid within which are embedded a few
residual muscle cells staining a deeper pink color.

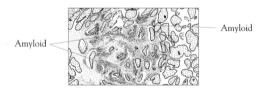

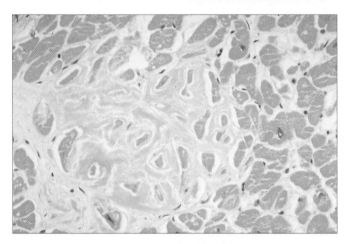

4   Macroscopic view of the heart with cardiac
amyloid showing amyloid deposits in the left
atrium. After fixation in formalin, inspection of
the surface of the left atrium shows deposits of
amyloid as brown translucent nodules, 1–2 mm in
diameter, just beneath the endocardium. Similar
deposits are present in this specimen within the
posterior cusp of the mitral valve but not in the
anterior cusp.

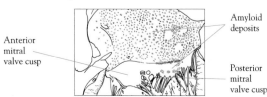

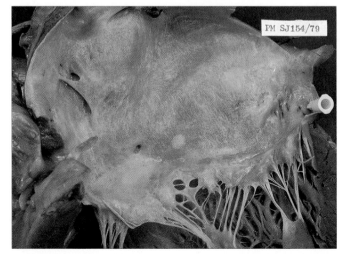

5 Schematic illustrations of changes in the pressure–volume curves (left) and left ventricular function curves (right) in restrictive cardiomyopathy. The diastolic pressure–volume curve is shifted to the left; to maintain adequate stroke volume, left ventricular pressure has to be elevated. (A) Normal pressure–volume and ventricular function curves. (B) Pressure–volume and ventricular function curves in restrictive cardiomyopathy. To maintain a stroke volume of 50 ml, if a diastolic volume of 70 ml is required, diastolic pressure is elevated to 30 mmHg. Note that despite the normal ejection fraction (71%), the ventricular function curve is shifted downwards and to the right.

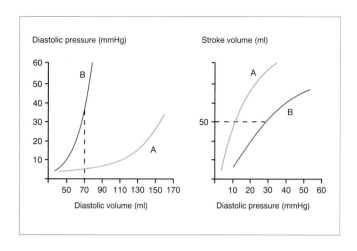

6 Chest X-ray showing cardiomegaly due to bi-atrial enlargement.

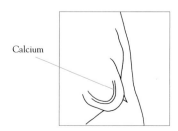

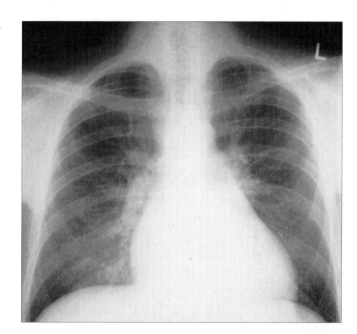

7 Lateral chest X-ray showing marked pericardial calcification.

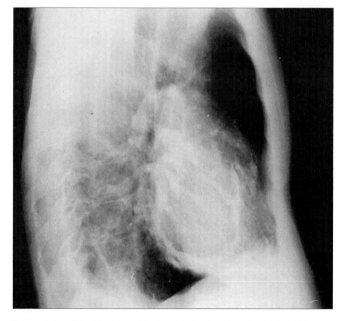

8

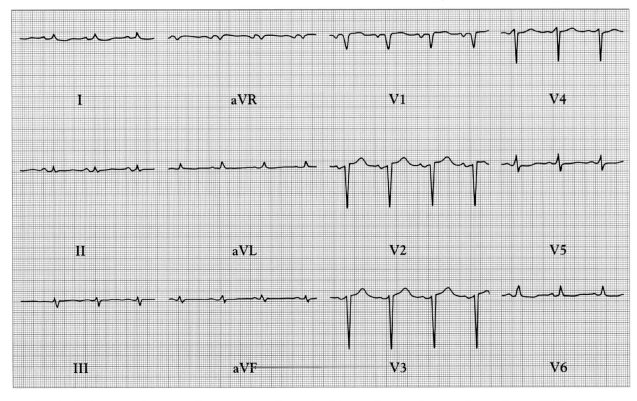

Twelve-lead electrocardiogram of a patient with amyloid heart disease showing low-voltage QRS complexes, particularly in the limb leads.

9

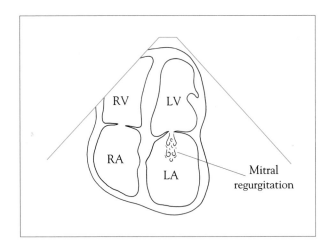 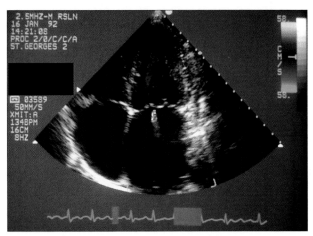

Apical four-chamber view of a case of restrictive cardiomyopathy. The left ventricle is not enlarged or hypertrophied, but the left atrium is dilated due to the high filling pressures and color-flow Doppler shows a little functional mitral regurgitation.

10

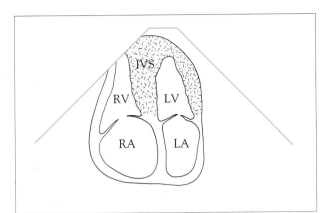 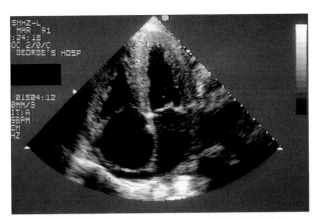

Apical four-chamber view of amyloid heart disease showing marked increase in left ventricular wall thickness with increased echogenicity of the myocardium.

11 M-mode recording from the same patient as in [10], showing severely impaired left ventricular systolic function.

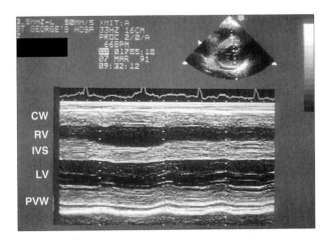

12

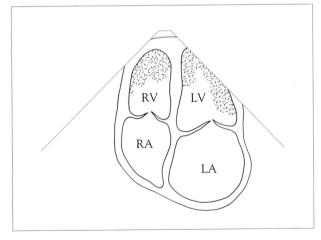 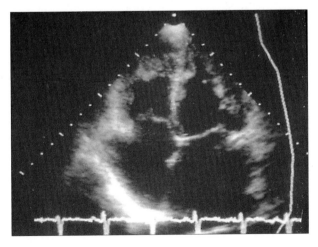

Apical four-chamber views of a patient with eosinophilic heart disease showing thrombus deposits in the apices of both ventricles. This both reduces static diastolic volume and 'splints' the ventricles, preventing adequate contraction and relaxation.

13 Pulsed Doppler recording of transmitral diastolic flow in a patient with restrictive cardiomyopathy. Early diastolic filling causes the brief, high velocity 'spike' with rapid deceleration and there is virtually no filling during atrial systole.

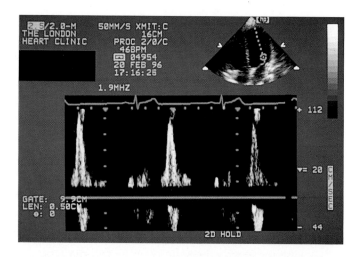

14 High-speed pulsed Doppler recording of aortic and mitral flow. In restrictive cardiomyopathy, the isovolumic relaxation time is very short (typically <60 ms).

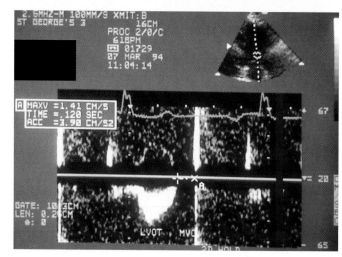

15 Computed tomography illustrating thickened pericardium in a patient with constrictive pericarditis. Pericardial effusion was also present.

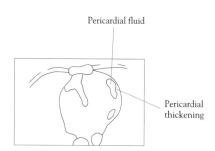

Pericardial fluid

Pericardial thickening

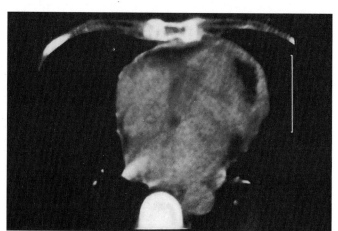

16 Pressure recordings taken from the right and left ventricles simultaneously in endomyocardial fibrosis showing the typical 'dip and plateau' and the elevated and different end-diastolic pressure measurements.

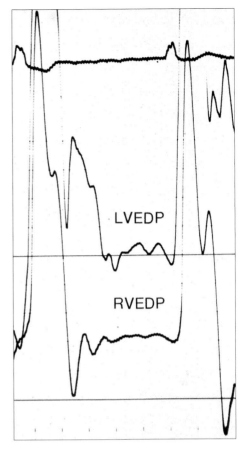

17

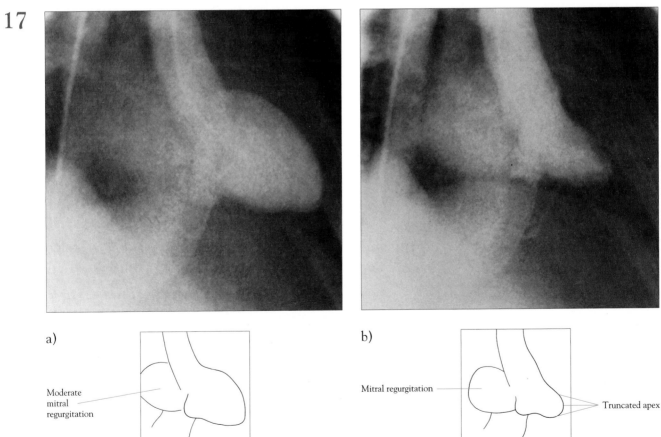

a)

Moderate mitral regurgitation

b)

Mitral regurgitation

Truncated apex

Restrictive cardiomyopathy in (a) diastole and (b) systole. The left ventricle is normal in size, smooth in outline, and contracts well from diastole to systole. There is moderate mitral regurgitation. The smooth outline of the ventricle and the degree of truncation of the apex are typical of restrictive cardiomyopathy.

18

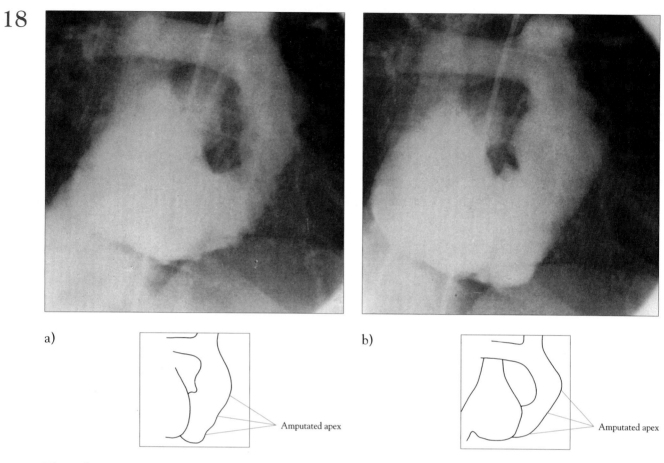

a)

b)

Amputated apex

Amputated apex

The right ventriculogram in systole (a) and diastole (b) shows that the ventricle, although contracting well, has its entire apex amputated. There is also gross tricuspid regurgitation. These appearances are typical of the type of restrictive cardiomyopathy associated with eosinophilic heart disease.

19 Principles of management of restrictive cardio-
    myopathy.

1. Diuretics to control fluid retention

2. Dual-chamber pacemaker therapy in selected patients

3. In severe endomyocardial fibrosis, surgery in selected patients

4. Cardiac transplantation in selected patients

CHAPTER 7
Miscellaneous Cardiac Conditions

CARDIAC TUMORS

PULMONARY EMBOLIC AND PULMONARY VASCULAR DISEASE

PERICARDIAL DISEASE

Abbreviations

a	Anterior	MV	Mitral valve
Ao	Aorta	MVL	Mitral valve leaflet
AP	Antero-posterior	p	Posterior
CW	Chest wall	PA	Postero-anterior
Eff	Effusion	PE	Pericardial effusion
En	Endocardium	Per	Pericardium
Ep	Epicardium	PVW	Posterior ventricular wall
IVC	Inferior vena cava	RA	Right atrium
IVS	Interventricular septum	RL	Right lateral
LA	Left atrium	RPA	Right pulmonary artery
LL	Left lateral	RV	Right ventricle
LV	Left ventricle	SVC	Superior vena cava
LVOT	Left ventricular outflow tract		

CARDIAC TUMORS

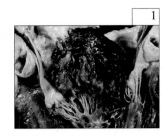

The incidence of primary cardiac tumors in unselected autopsy series is between 0.001% and 0.05%; 80% of all primary neoplasms are benign.

Pathology

The most common primary cardiac tumor is the atrial myxoma; all others are very rare. Atrial myxomata arise on the interatrial septum around the site of the foramen ovale; 80% project into the left atrium [1] and 20% into the right atrium [2]. The myxoma is a shining gelatinous multicolored mass, often with an irregular surface [3]. Some myxomata extend into the mitral or tricuspid valve orifice producing obstruction, and with time the valve may be destroyed by direct mechanical trauma. Thrombus forms over the tumor, and embolization of thrombus or actual tumor fragments is common. The tumors often contain areas of hemorrhage along with myxoid areas [4]. Histologically, the tumor consists of nests of epithelial ('lipidic') cells in a myxomatous stroma. The tumor is not malignant but recurrence following partial removal occurs. Other primary benign tumors are rare, but include rhabdomyoma (hamartoma) and fibroma. The primary malignant cardiac tumors are also rare but include rhabdomyosarcoma [5] and hemangiosarcoma.

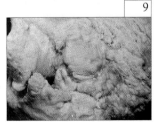

Children with tuberose sclerosis develop multiple rhabdomyomata consisting of large clear cells often interpreted as being masses of Purkinje cells. Occasionally, isolated masses of fibrous tissue (fibromata or rhabdomyomata) are found in otherwise normal children [6].

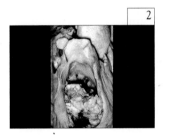

Secondary cardiac tumors are more common than primary neoplasms. Multiple small nodules may occur throughout the myocardium in carcinoma of the breast, malignant melanoma [7], or bronchial tumors. More rarely, a single large tumor deposit occurs [8]. Occasionally, renal carcinoma or hepatoma spreads to the right atrium via the vena cava, or bronchial carcinoma may spread to the left atrium via the pulmonary veins.

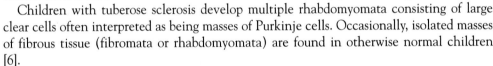

Primary pericardial tumors are very rare. The most common are the hemangiosarcoma and the mesothelioma. Secondary pericardial tumors are not uncommon. Tumors may occur as isolated nodules or plaques [9] or as florid fibrinous pericarditis, in which occasional tumor cells can be found. Spread of the tumor into the pericardium may occur via the lymphatics (e.g. in carcinoma of the breast) or by direct invasion (e.g. in carcinoma of the bronchus).

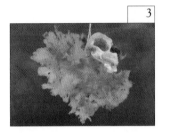

Presentation

Symptoms

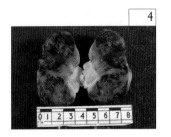

Cardiac tumors may be clinically silent. Myxomata may present with constitutional symptoms such as weight loss, fatigue, fever, arthralgias, and, less frequently, rashes, clubbing of the fingers, and Raynaud's phenomenon. Tumors on the left side of the heart may present with single or multiple systemic emboli. Positional dyspnea, orthopnea, paroxysmal nocturnal dyspnea, and syncope can be presenting symptoms. Right atrial myxomata may present with embolism into the pulmonary circulation. In some cases, a myxoma will present by the chance finding of abnormal auscultatory signs.

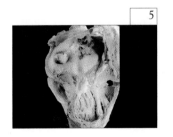

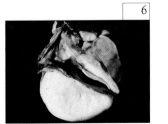

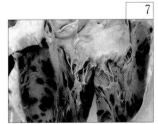

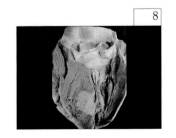

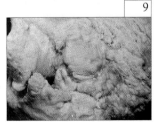

Signs

The physical signs of a left atrial myxoma may be indistinguishable from those of rheumatic mitral valve disease in sinus rhythm, including the same auscultatory features and the signs of pulmonary hypertension. Occasionally, a characteristic tumor 'plop' and a tumor ejection sound may be recognized [10]. Similarly, right atrial myxoma will closely mimic the physical signs of tricuspid valve disease. An elevated jugular venous pressure, either with a sharp (tricuspid regurgitation) or slow (tricuspid stenosis) 'y' descent, is recognized.

Tumors involving the pericardium may present as a pericardial effusion or as cardiac tamponade. In cases where tumors extensively involve cardiac muscle, the clinical features will be those of a restrictive cardiomyopathy.

Investigations

Radiology

In left atrial myxoma, the chest X-ray may be normal or the appearance may reflect mitral valve obstruction with pulmonary venous hypertension [11]. Massive left atrial enlargement is rare. With a right atrial myxoma, the chest X-ray may show evidence of pulmonary infarcts — the result of tumor emboli [12]. An increased cardiac silhouette may be seen if there is a pericardial effusion. Calcification of the myxoma can occasionally be recognized by plain chest X-ray or by fluoroscopy.

Electrocardiography

When left atrial myxoma obstructs the mitral valve, the electrocardiogram usually shows left atrial enlargement and may additionally show right ventricular hypertrophy [13] reflecting severe pulmonary hypertension. When right atrial myxoma obstructs the tricuspid valve, the electrocardiogram may show right atrial enlargement [14]. When a pericardial effusion is present, non-specific ST-T changes and low-voltage QRS complexes may be seen. Primary cardiac tumors or secondary metastases can be associated with deep T-wave inversions, non-specific ST-T changes, or findings of myocardial infarction. Sinus rhythm is most common, but atrial and ventricular tachyarrhythmias, atrioventricular block, and intraventricular conduction defects may occur.

Echocardiography

The typical left atrial myxoma, attached by a narrow pedicle to the interatrial septum at the fossa ovalis, moving into the mitral valve orifice in diastole, and not associated with any pericardial effusion or clinical signs of malignancy, presents a classical picture sufficiently diagnostic to preclude the need for further investigations [15]. M-mode echocardiography typically shows an amorphous cloud of echoes behind the mitral valve [16]. Transesophageal echocardiography provides excellent visualization of masses associated with the atria [17], and more readily aids differentiation of a myxoma from thrombus, which usually originates within the atrial appendage, although it can be trapped in a partially patent foramen ovale and present an impossible differential diagnosis. The echoes appear just after the upward opening movement of the anterior mitral

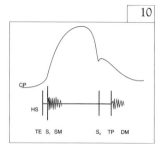

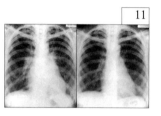

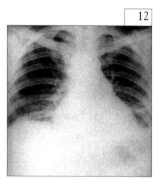

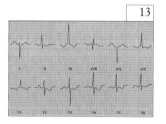

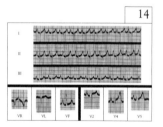

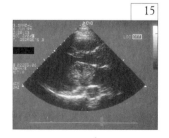

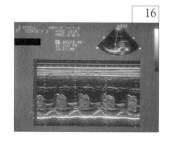

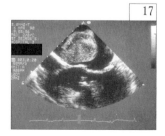

valve leaflet, and arise from well behind the valve, i.e. in the left atrium. If the tumor is very mobile, it descends through the mitral orifice into the left ventricle during diastole and returns to the left atrium during systole.

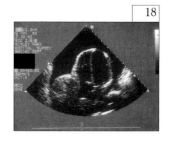

Malignant neoplasms, either primary or secondary, normally have a broad base and are seen to be intimately involved with the myocardium, but may manifest only as localized thickening of the myocardium. They are almost always accompanied by pericardial effusion; indeed, this is the most common clinical presentation [18].

Tumors can also enter the heart via the systemic or pulmonary veins. Examples include metastases from bronchial carcinoma and renal tumors such as hypernephroma [19].

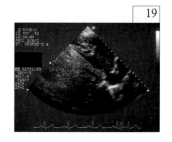

Although some types of tumor have characteristic locations and attachments, it is never possible to identify with certainty the nature of a mass, or to distinguish benign tumors from neoplasms, thrombus, or vegetations.

Laboratory Findings
In patients with myxomata, elevated sedimentation rate, leukocytosis, hemolytic anemia, thrombocytopenia, polycythemia, and hypergammaglobulinemia may be detected. The elevated immunoglobulins are usually of the IgG fraction. The embolic material, when available, should be examined histologically to confirm the diagnosis of the type of tumor.

Radionuclide Ventriculography
This technique may show a filling defect with different locations or size during systole and diastole corresponding to tumor movement.

Magnetic Resonance Imaging (MRI), Computed Tomography (CT), and Cardiac Catheterization and Angiography
Both cine MRI and CT can detect intracardiac masses and tumors. The location and size of the tumor and involvement of the pericardium can also be detected [20]. MRI can also delineate benign or malignant primary or secondary ventricular tumors [21,22].

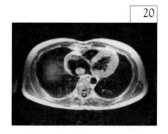

In patients with atrial myxomata, the hemodynamics may reflect obstruction of the atrioventricular valves. Although rarely necessary for diagnostic purposes (particularly with the development of two-dimensional echocardiography), when angiography is performed it may show filling defects in the atria [23]. Ventricular tumors also produce ventricular filling defects [24]. Selective coronary angiography sometimes reveals tumor neovascularization [25].

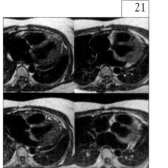
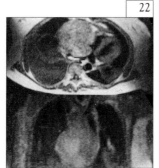
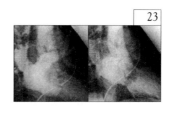
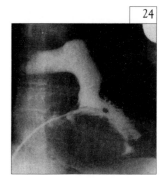

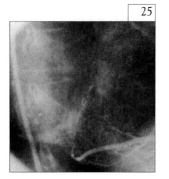

When tumors involve the myocardium, the hemodynamics may mimic restrictive cardiomyopathy, while angiography may reveal encroachment on normal cardiac chambers [26].

Principles of Management

All myxomata should be surgically removed as soon as the diagnosis is made [27]. The recurrence rate is lower than 5% and the results of surgery are excellent. Rhabdomyomata and fibromata should also be partially or completely removed if they produce hemodynamic abnormalities. No effective therapy is available for primary or secondary malignant tumors.

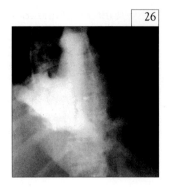

26

27

1. Echocardiographic evaluation as soon as the diagnosis is suspected

2. Surgical removal of atrial myxomata as soon as the diagnosis is established

3. Recurrence of myxomata is less than 5%

4. Partial or complete resection of fibromata and rhabdomyomata in symptomatic patients

1 Left atrial myxoma. The tumor extends down into the mitral valve. Fibrous thickening is seen on the anterior cusp of the valve due to mechanical trauma from the tumor mass.

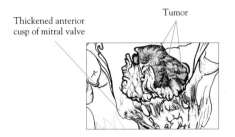

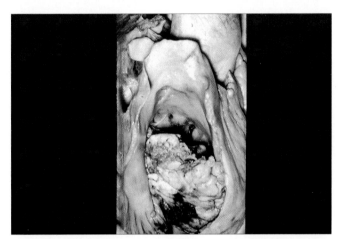

2 Right atrial myxoma. The tumor is a lobulated mass filling the cavity of the right atrium.

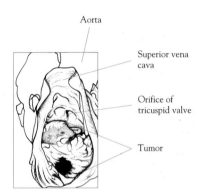

3 Excised left atrial myxoma, attached to the stalk, showing a markedly irregular external surface.

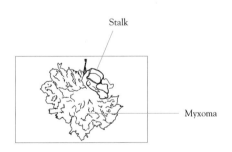

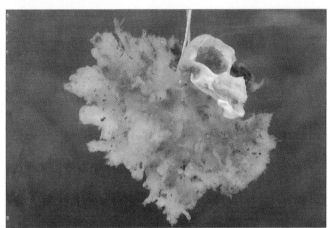

4 Section through an excised left atrial myxoma showing a heterogeneous surface, with hemorrhagic and myxoid areas.

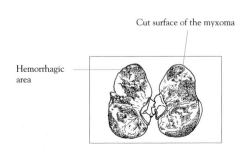

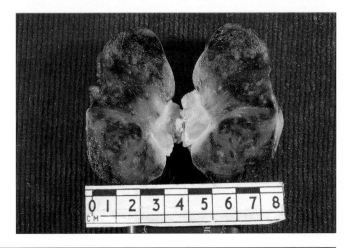

5   Rhabdomyosarcoma in the atrial septum. The right atrium is opened to show the bulging tumor mass which occupies the septum.

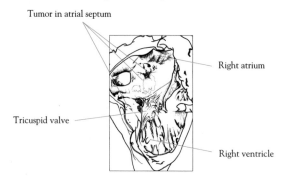

Tumor in atrial septum

Right atrium

Tricuspid valve

Right ventricle

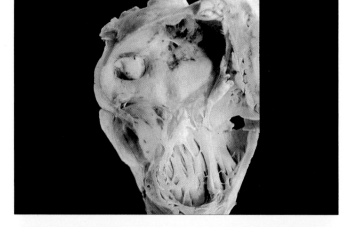

6   Right ventricular rhabdomyoma. A large solid white mass of tumor replaces most of the normal ventricular muscle.

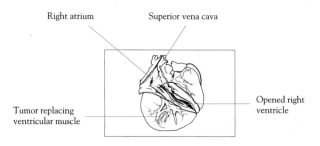

Right atrium   Superior vena cava

Tumor replacing ventricular muscle

Opened right ventricle

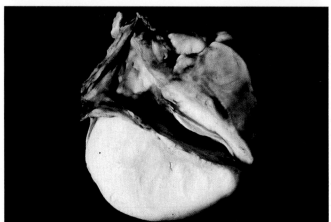

7   Secondary deposits of tumor in the heart. Multiple black deposits are seen in the myocardium secondary to malignant melanoma of the skin.

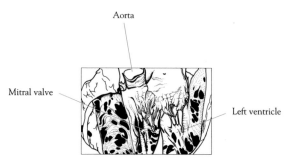

Aorta

Mitral valve

Left ventricle

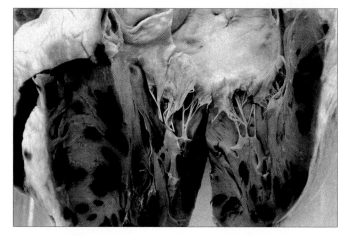

8   Single deposit of secondary carcinoma in the heart. The large tumor mass lies in the interventricular septum. The primary tumor site was in the kidney.

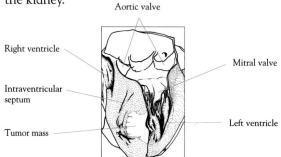

Aortic valve

Right ventricle

Intraventricular septum

Tumor mass

Mitral valve

Left ventricle

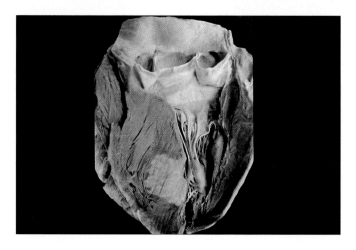

9   Secondary pericardial tumor. The pericardial cavity is opened to show the wide dissemination of tumor on the visceral pericardium of the right ventricle.

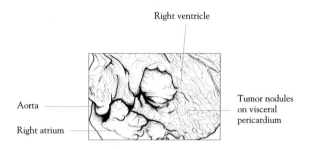

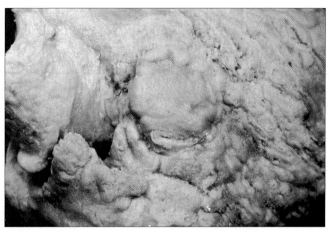

10   Schematic illustration of the auscultatory findings of left atrial myxoma. The tumor ejection sound occurs prior to the carotid pulse upstroke. The tumor 'plop' sound usually occurs later than that of the opening snap. Note that the absence of these sounds does not preclude the diagnosis.

CP=Carotid pulse; TE=tumor ejection sound; SM=systolic murmur; DM=diastolic murmur; HS=heart sounds; S_1=first heart sound; S_2=second heart sound; TP=tumor 'plop' sound.

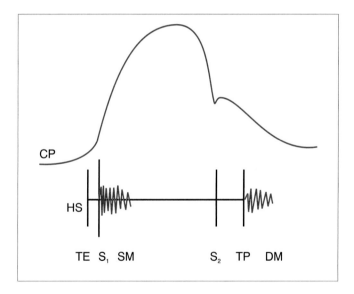

11

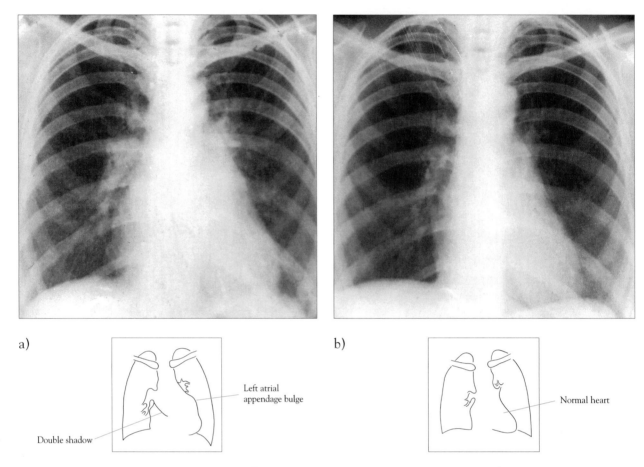

a) Double shadow

Left atrial appendage bulge

b) Normal heart

Left atrial myxoma. (a) The frontal chest X-ray in left atrial myxoma may show the features of left atrial enlargement, as in this case, with straightening of the left heart border, a left atrial appendage bulge, and a double shadow through the heart. There is haziness of the vessels, indicating pulmonary edema. The X-ray appearances may be very similar to those of mitral valve disease. (b) After removal of the myxoma, the X-ray appearances revert largely to normal.

12 Chest X-ray in right atrial myxoma showing pulmonary infarcts in the left lung field.

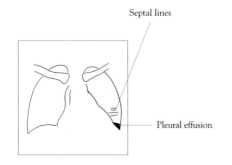

Septal lines

Pleural effusion

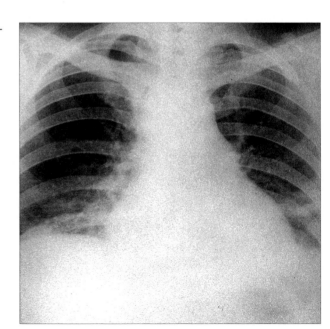

13

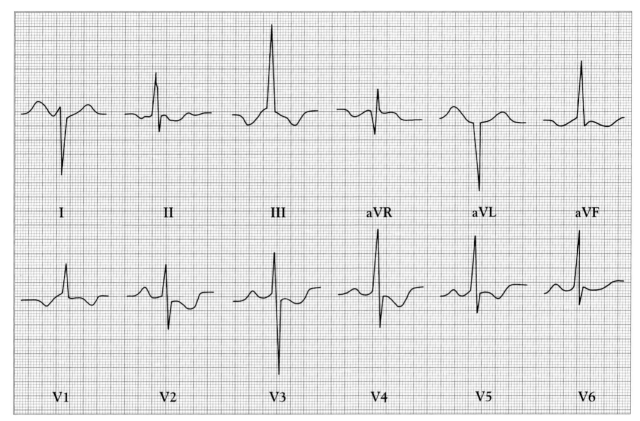

The electrocardiogram of a patient with left atrial myxoma. It shows low atrial (coronary sinus) rhythm with evidence of left atrial enlargement, with widespread T-wave inversion, dominant R-wave in V1, with deep S-wave in V5, indicating right ventricular hypertrophy.

14

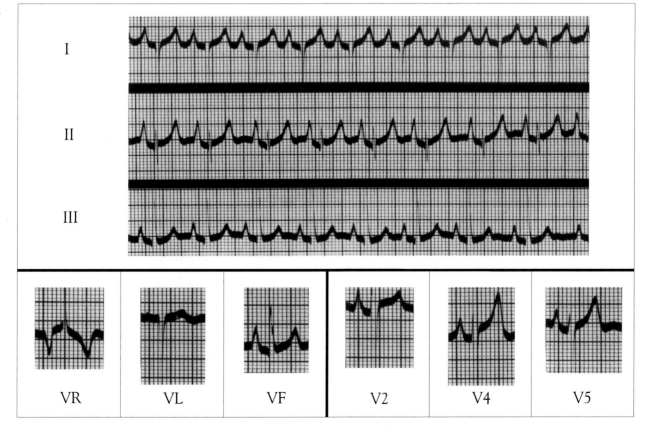

Electrocardiogram with tall P-waves in lead II indicating right atrial enlargement.

15

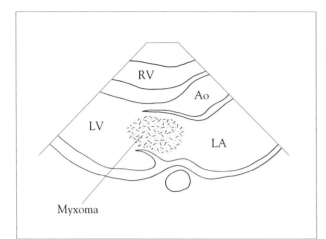
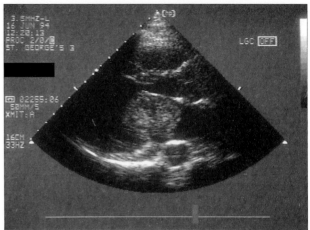

Parasternal long-axis view showing a large mass blocking the mitral valve orifice. Its location, attachment by a narrow pedicle to the atrial septum, and the absence of pericardial fluid make it almost certainly an atrial myxoma.

16 M-mode recording from the same patient as in [15], showing the echogenic mass within the mitral valve orifice. Since the blood flow into the left ventricle carries the tumor into the valve orifice, there is a brief interval between the opening of the mitral valve and appearance of the echoes.

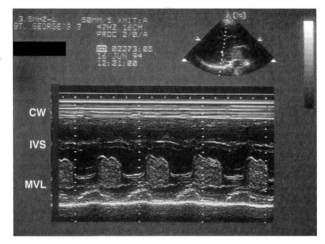

17

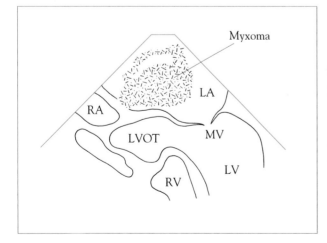
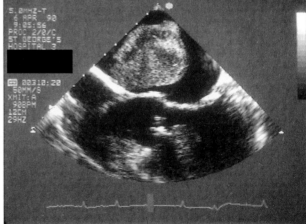

Transesophageal study showing the classical attachment of an atrial myxoma to the interatrial septum by a narrow pedicle; this allows the tumor to pivot freely, and move in and out of the mitral orifice.

18

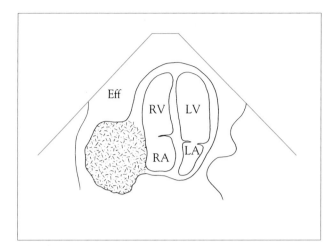 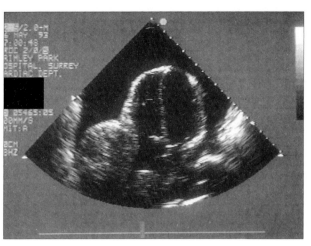

Apical four-chamber view showing a large, spherical mass attached to and invading the right atrial wall. In contrast to the typical myxoma, this is not in the left atrium, has a broad attachment point, and is associated with a very large pericardial effusion. This mass was later shown to be a hemangiosarcoma.

19

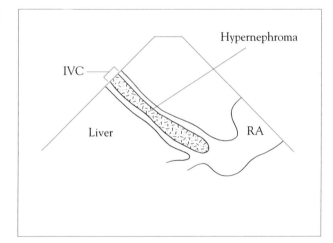 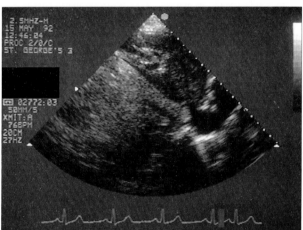

Subcostal view showing the inferior vena cava entering the right atrium. The lumen of the vena cava is largely filled with a sausage-like mass, the tip of which almost protrudes into the right atrium. This mass was later shown to be a hypernephroma.

20 Magnetic resonance image showing a left atrial mass attached to the interatrial septum.

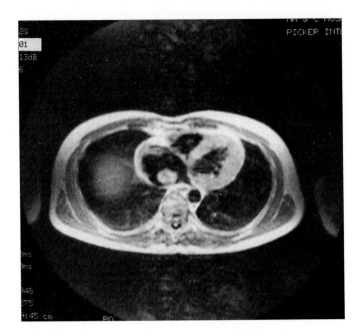

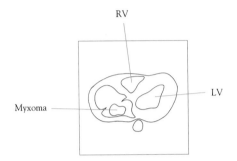

21 Magnetic resonance images in four contiguous transaxial planes showing a fibrosarcoma of the left ventricle.

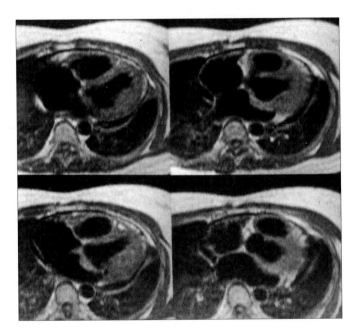

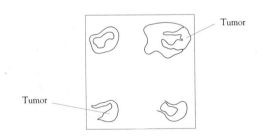

22 Magnetic resonance images of rhabdomyosarcoma. The upper spin echo image in the transaxial plane shows the tumor anteriorly around the right ventricle and atrium. The lower frame shows the same tumor in the coronal plane.

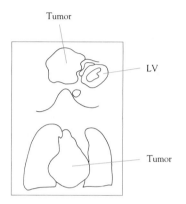

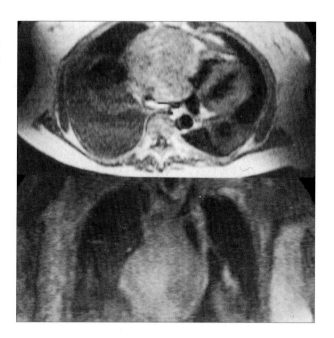

23

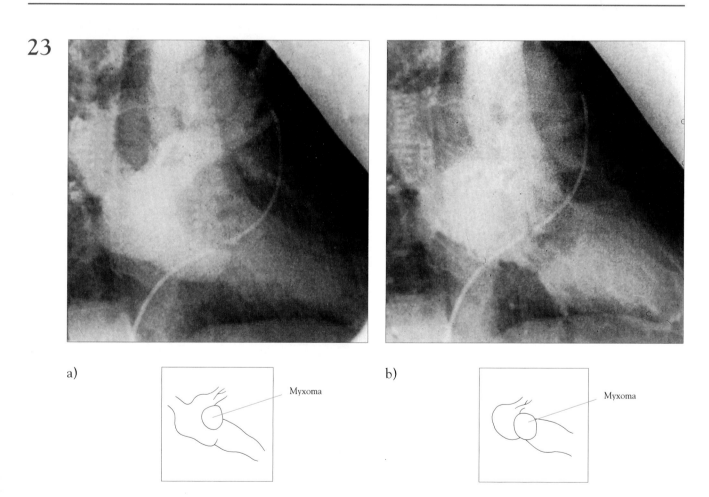

a)

b)

Angiography in left atrial myxoma. The majority of myxomata are mobile and can be visualized moving through the mitral valve during angiography. The myxoma has moved back into the left atrium in ventricular systole (a) and dropped down through the mitral valve, partially in the left ventricle, in ventricular diastole (b).

24   Right ventricular sarcoma. Right ventriculogram in the frontal view. This shows a large mass in the floor of the right ventricle with a small amount of contrast filling of the body of the right ventricle just above it.

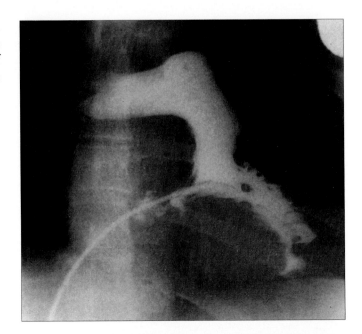

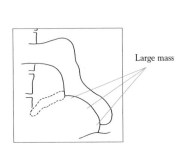

Large mass

25   Coronary arteriography showing a cardiac tumor in the same patient as [24]. The right coronary injection shows a pathologic circulation of the tumor in the floor of the right ventricle.

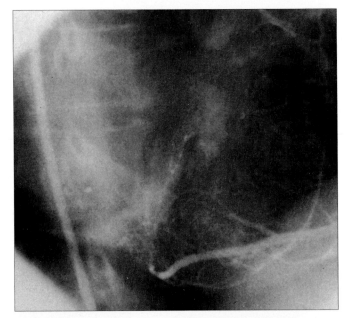

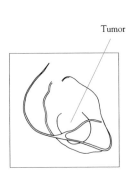

Tumor

26   Right atrial angiogram showing gross distortion of the normal cavity due to infiltration of the right atrial wall by tumor.

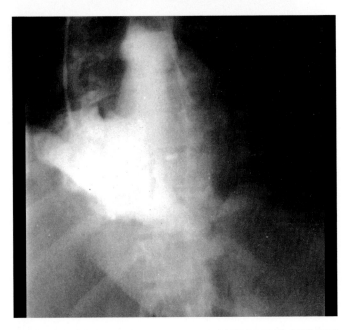

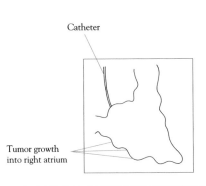

Catheter

Tumor growth into right atrium

27   Principles of management of cardiac tumors.

1. Echocardiographic evaluation as soon as the diagnosis is suspected

2. Surgical removal of atrial myxomata as soon as the diagnosis is established

3. Recurrence of myxomata is less than 5%

4. Partial or complete resection of fibromata and rhabdomyomata in symptomatic patients

PULMONARY EMBOLIC AND PULMONARY VASCULAR DISEASE

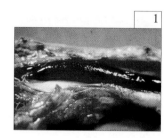

Pulmonary hypertension may occur in patients with:
1) an elevated pulmonary venous pressure due to abnormalities in the left heart, such as mitral stenosis, left atrial myxoma, cor triatriatum, and left ventricular disease of any etiology (post-capillary pulmonary hypertension);
2) increased pulmonary blood flow from a left-to-right intra- or extracardiac shunt, such as ventricular septal defect, atrial septal defect, or persistent ductus arteriosus;
3) intra- or extracardiac shunts with pulmonary vascular disease (Eisenmenger syndrome).

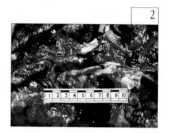

These conditions will be dealt with in their relevant sections. This section will include other causes:
4) pulmonary embolic disease;
5) chronic hypoxic conditions, including diseases of lung parenchyma and high altitude;
6) idiopathic (primary) pulmonary hypertension.

Pathology

Pulmonary embolism may be massive or minor, acute or chronic. Acute pulmonary embolism usually results from the passage of thrombus originating in a systemic vein [1] through the right side of the heart and lodging in the pulmonary arteries [2]. If the embolism is massive, the right ventricle becomes acutely dilated. If the embolism is minor, a pulmonary infarct may develop [3,4].

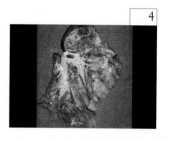

Chronic thromboembolic disease results in severe pulmonary hypertension due to long-standing obstruction to right ventricular outflow [5]. Histologically, the pulmonary arteries show mild medial hypertrophy, eccentric intimal fibrosis, and intraluminal fibrous septa, an appearance which distinguishes this condition from primary pulmonary hypertension [6]. Chronic hypoxia due to parenchymal lung disease or living at high altitude (high altitude precapillary pulmonary hypertension) may also cause changes in pulmonary arterioles with secondary pulmonary hypertension. The histologic changes include eccentric intimal fibrosis with longitudinal muscle bundles in the intima.

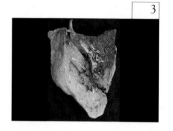

Some cases of pulmonary hypertension are due to primary disease of the small pulmonary arterioles, the cause of which is unknown. Histologically, there is medial hypertrophy, concentric and laminary intimal fibrosis with medial fibrinoid necrosis with or without arteritis, and the so-called 'plexiform' lesion [7,8]. Similar histologic appearances may be seen in patients with the Eisenmenger syndrome. There is an overall decrease in the number of pulmonary arteries, with a reduction in the caliber of the peripheral vessels [9,10]. In pulmonary hypertension, endothelial dysfunction (evident

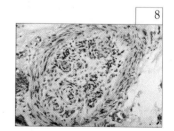

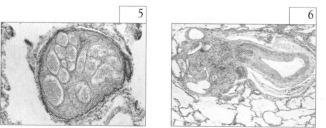

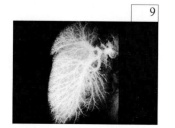

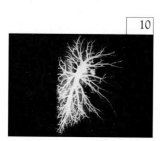

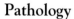

from lack of acetylcholine-induced pulmonary vasodilatation) and decreased tissue concentration of nitric oxide synthase required for the production of nitric oxide (lack of which may cause pulmonary vasoconstriction) have been documented. Increased vasoconstrictive substances, such as endothelins and thromboxanes, and compensatory vasodilatory agents, such as adrenomodulin and atrial and brain natriuretic peptides, also suggest a pathophysiologic role of pulmonary vascular endothelial dysfunction in the genesis of pulmonary hypertension. Endothelial dysfunction, in addition to pulmonary vasoconstriction, may promote proliferation and migration of smooth muscle cells in the pulmonary vessels and activate prothrombotic mechanisms, which increase the risk of thrombosis *in situ*.

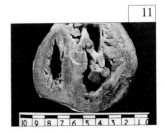

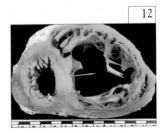

All cases of long-standing severe pulmonary hypertension will result in right ventricular hypertrophy [11]. With onset of right heart failure, right ventricular dilatation occurs [12]. In unexplained or primary pulmonary hypertension, pulmonary vascular and endothelial dysfunction (pulmonary vasoconstriction in response to acetylcholine) and abnormal endogenous endocrine metabolism (e.g. decreased endothelium-derived relaxing factors, increased endothelins, increased thromboxane A_2, and decreased prostacyclin) have been observed.

Presentation

Symptoms
Acute massive pulmonary embolism presents with the features of a sudden reduction in cardiac output (collapse and circulatory arrest). Sudden severe breathlessness is another common presentation. Pleuritic chest pain is usually not a feature of acute massive embolism, but there may have been prior episodes of pleurisy due to minor pulmonary embolism. Acute minor embolism usually results in pulmonary infarction, with pleurisy and/or hemoptysis being the main features. There is usually a clear predisposing factor for the development of thromboembolism, such as surgery, trauma, bed rest, neoplastic disease, severe generalized disease, or the taking of estrogens. Chronic pulmonary thromboembolic disease presents with the features of severe pulmonary hypertension (exertional dyspnea or syncope, sometimes with repetitive episodes of pleurisy and hemoptysis).

If pulmonary hypertension is due to chronic parenchymal lung disease, the symptomatology will be dominated by the respiratory abnormality.

Idiopathic (primary) pulmonary hypertension is most frequently seen in young women. The presentation is insidious, with increasing breathlessness, occasional exertional syncope, and sometimes hemoptysis. Angina-like chest pain sometimes occurs.

Signs
Massive pulmonary embolism will result in the physical signs of low cardiac output (peripheral vasoconstriction, hypotension, sinus tachycardia, oliguria, and cerebral confusion) and right ventricular failure (elevation of jugular venous pressure and a gallop rhythm at the left sternal edge). Minor pulmonary embolism causing pulmonary infarction has physical signs confined to the respiratory system, such as a pleural rub, lobar collapse or consolidation, or a pleural effusion.

Severe pulmonary hypertension, as occurs in long-standing hypoxic lung disease, chronic thromboembolic disease, or of idiopathic etiology gives rise to a loud pulmonary component of the second heart sound usually with normal respiratory variation in the width of splitting. There may be palpable right ventricular hypertrophy. The jugular venous pulse may show either abnormal dominance of the 'a' wave or a frank rise in venous pressure with or without obvious tricuspid regurgitation if there is additional right ventricular failure. Hepatic engorgement and fluid retention characterized by peripheral edema and ascites may be present. Respiratory failure is often present when the cause is long-standing parenchymal lung disease.

Investigations

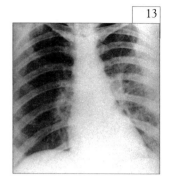

Radiology

In acute massive pulmonary embolism, the chest X-ray shows areas of oligemia due to patchy reduction in blood flow, interspersed with areas of compensatory hyperemia [13,14]. The central pulmonary arteries are not enlarged. In minor pulmonary embolism, the chest X-ray may be normal or show features consistent with pulmonary infarction (lobar collapse/consolidation with or without pleural effusion) [15].

In primary pulmonary hypertension, the heart and central pulmonary arteries are characteristically enlarged in a non-specific way and the peripheral vessels diffusely reduced in size [16].

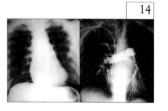

Thromboembolic pulmonary hypertension is distinguished from primary pulmonary hypertension by an irregular distribution of the vascular obliteration in the lungs [17]. In parenchymatous lung disease causing chronic pulmonary hypertension, the nature of the lung disease may be identified by specific appearances, but the cardiovascular changes are similar to those seen in pulmonary hypertension from other causes [18].

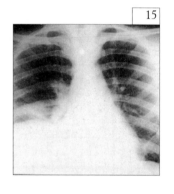

Electrocardiography

In acute massive pulmonary embolism, the electrocardiogram may show an $S_1 Q_3 T_3$ pattern [19], right bundle branch block [20], or right ventricular 'strain' with T-wave inversion over the anterior precordial leads [19]. Occasionally, staircase ST-segment changes are recognized. In minor pulmonary embolism, the electrocardiogram is normal unless there is additional significant cardiorespiratory disease. In chronic pulmonary hypertension from any cause, the electrocardiogram usually reflects the right ventricular hypertrophy with right axis deviation, right atrial enlargement, and T-wave inversion over the right ventricle (anterior precordial leads). The R-wave is dominant in lead V1 and the S-wave is dominant in V5 [21]. A qR pattern in V1 suggests severe right ventricular hypertrophy with pulmonary artery pressure almost equal to that of systemic arterial pressure.

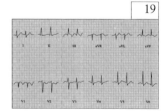

Arterial Blood Gases

Blood gases in massive pulmonary embolism usually show hypoxia and hypocapnia; in minor pulmonary embolism without additional cardiorespiratory disease, the gases will be normal. In chronic pulmonary hypertension due to lung disease, it is likely that there will be hypoxia and hypercapnia; in idiopathic and chronic thromboembolic pulmonary hypertension, there will be hypoxia.

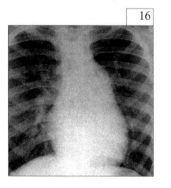

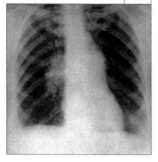

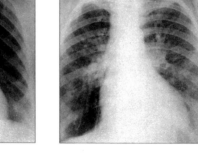

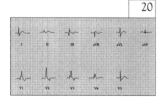

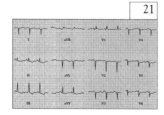

Nuclear Techniques

Simultaneous ventilation (using krypton-81m or xenon) and perfusion scans (using technetium-99m labeled macroaggregated albumin) will permit distinction between primary lung pathology, e.g. emphysema (matched ventilation-perfusion defects), and pulmonary vascular disease due to pulmonary embolism (where the ventilation scan is normal but there are variable defects of perfusion) [22–24].

The pulmonary angiogram demonstrates filling defects in the areas of perfusion defects detected by isotope scanning [25].

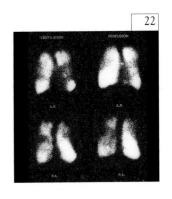

Echocardiography

Severe, chronic pulmonary hypertension leads to right ventricular hypertrophy and right atrial dilatation, features which can be recognized by echocardiography. In particular, the short-axis view shows flattening of the interventricular septum [26] and the abnormal pattern of contraction causes reversed or paradoxical motion of the septum on an M-mode recording [27].

Echocardiography is also able to identify causes of pulmonary hypertension secondary to left heart abnormalities such as mitral valve disease, atrial myxoma, or left ventricular disease. Transesophageal echocardiography usually provides visualization of the bifurcation of the main pulmonary artery and the proximal right pulmonary artery, which might show the presence of thrombus [28].

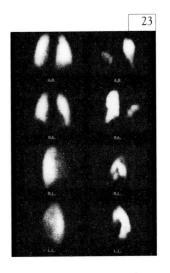

As long as there is detectable tricuspid or pulmonary regurgitation (usually the case in patients with valve or myocardial disease), continuous-wave Doppler allows right heart pressures to be measured. Tricuspid regurgitation allows assessment of systolic pulmonary artery pressure, while pulmonary regurgitation allows assessment of diastolic pressure in the main pulmonary artery [29,30].

Magnetic Resonance Imaging (MRI)

MRI has been used to detect proximal pulmonary emboli and has been shown to be highly sensitive compared with a pulmonary angiogram.

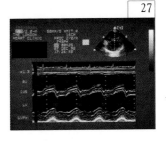

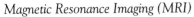

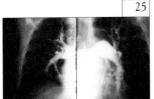

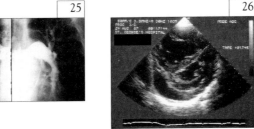

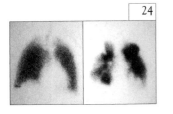

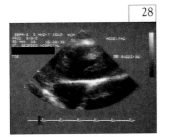

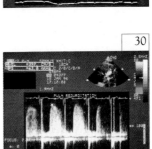

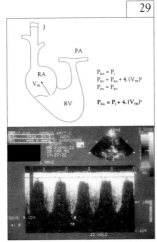

Cardiac Catheterization and Angiography

In acute massive pulmonary embolism, there is only moderate elevation of pulmonary artery pressure, distinguishing this condition from chronic thromboembolic disease, where the pulmonary artery pressures are usually much higher. In minor pulmonary embolism without additional significant cardiorespiratory disease, the pulmonary artery pressure is normal.

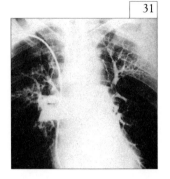

In massive pulmonary embolism, the angiogram shows obstruction to a major portion of the total pulmonary arterial bed [31]. In chronic thromboembolic pulmonary hypertension, the pulmonary trunk is enlarged and there is an asymmetric obliteration of pulmonary vessels, those unaffected by thrombus being tortuous and dilated [32]. There is a convex leading edge to contrast-filled vessels obstructed by thrombus, unlike the concave leading edge in acute embolism [33]. In primary (idiopathic) pulmonary hypertension, the pulmonary vasculature shows symmetric peripheral pruning [34].

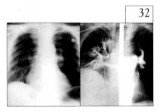

Principles of Management

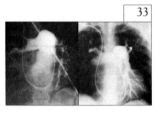

Anticoagulation with continuous intravenous infusion of heparin and subsequently with oral anticoagulation is the treatment of choice in minor pulmonary embolism to prevent extension and recurrence. In patients with massive pulmonary embolism who are critically ill with hemodynamic instability, intravenous or intrapulmonary administration of thrombolytic agents (streptokinase, urokinase, or recombinant tissue plasminogen activator) may help to restore normal hemodynamics more rapidly than can be achieved by heparin. In selected patients who are critically ill, and for whom thrombolysis is contraindicated or who are deteriorating on thrombolysis, catheter or surgical pulmonary embolectomy is life-saving. Long-term anticoagulation is required in patients with thromboembolic disease until the predisposing factors no longer apply. In patients with chronic thromboembolic disease, chronic pulmonary embolectomy has been performed, but the results are variable [35].

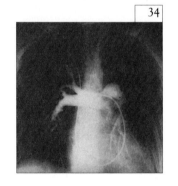

In primary pulmonary hypertension [36], pulmonary vasodilators such as calcium channel blocking drugs, prostacyclins, and inhaled nitric oxide may decrease pulmonary artery pressure and pulmonary vascular resistance in some patients. In selected patients, infusion of atrial natriuretic peptides or use of neutral endopeptidase inhibitors may decrease pulmonary artery pressure and pulmonary vascular resistance. Right atrial decompression with blade-balloon atrial septostomy may cause clinical improvement in selected patients. However, single- or double lung- or heart–lung transplants are the only effective treatment for severe pulmonary hypertension.

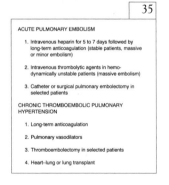

ACUTE PULMONARY EMBOLISM

1. Intravenous heparin for 5 to 7 days followed by long-term anticoagulation (stable patients, massive or minor embolism)

2. Intravenous thrombolytic agents in hemo-dynamically unstable patients (massive embolism)

3. Catheter or surgical pulmonary embolectomy in selected patients

CHRONIC THROMBOEMBOLIC PULMONARY HYPERTENSION

1. Long-term anticoagulation

2. Pulmonary vasodilators

3. Thromboembolectomy in selected patients

4. Heart–lung or lung transplant

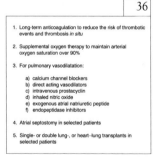

1. Long-term anticoagulation to reduce the risk of thrombotic events and thrombosis *in situ*

2. Supplemental oxygen therapy to maintain arterial oxygen saturation over 90%

3. For pulmonary vasodilatation:

   a) calcium channel blockers
   b) direct acting vasodilators
   c) intravenous prostacyclin
   d) inhaled nitric oxide
   e) exogenous atrial natriuretic peptide
   f) endopeptidase inhibitors

4. Atrial septostomy in selected patients

5. Single- or double lung-, or heart–lung transplants in selected patients

1 Thrombus in the femoral vein.

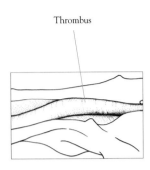

Thrombus

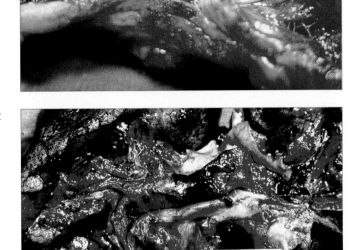

2 Large saddle embolus is seen astride both right and left pulmonary arteries.

Right pulmonary artery   Left pulmonary artery

Embolus

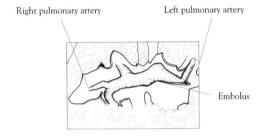

3 Pulmonary embolism in the lower lobe pulmonary artery branch resulting in infarction of the lung.

Lung infarction

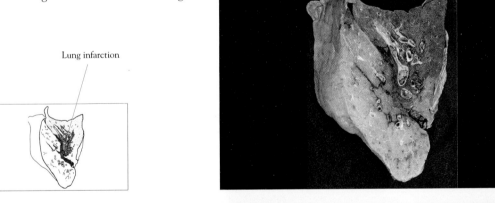

4 Minor pulmonary embolism in the upper lobe arteries resulting in infarction of the lung.

Pulmonary embolus   Infarction

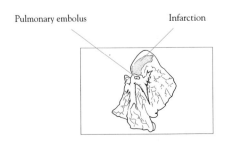

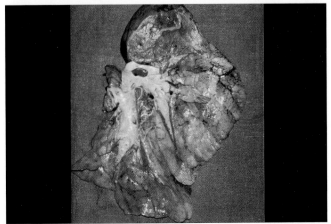

5 Cross-section through a pulmonary artery with a fibrous web-like structure within the lumen, due to organization of a thromboembolus.

Organized thromboembolus

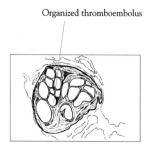

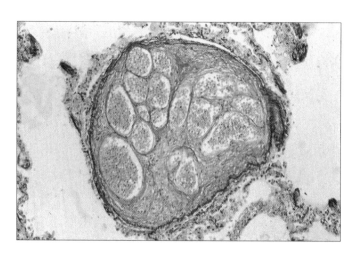

6 Histologic findings in chronic thromboembolic pulmonary hypertension showing mild medial hypertrophy, eccentric intimal fibrosis, and intraluminal fibrous septa.

Fibrous septa

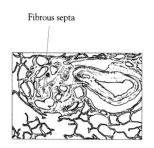

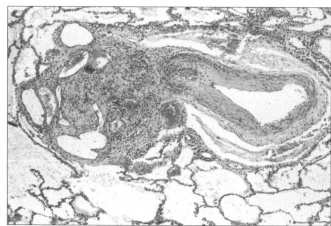

7 Normal pulmonary arteries (left panel) compared with small pulmonary artery affected by intimal fibrosis as a consequence of severe primary pulmonary hypertension (right panel).

Normal small pulmonary arteries   Lumen

Internal elastic lamina

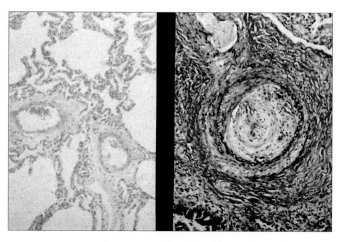

8 Complex angiomatoid lesions in small pulmonary arteries in primary pulmonary hypertension.

Small vascular spaces

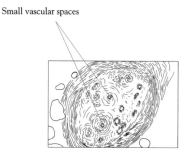

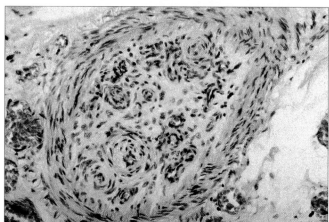

9   Normal post-mortem pulmonary arteriogram.

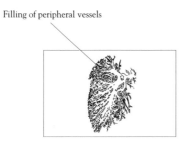

Filling of peripheral vessels

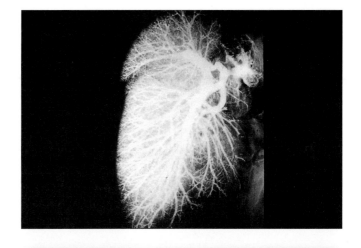

10   Post-mortem pulmonary arteriogram in primary pulmonary hypertension.

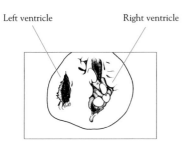

Peripheral 'pruning'

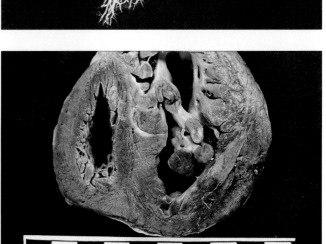

11   Gross right ventricular hypertrophy secondary to primary pulmonary hypertension. The right ventricular wall thickness and size greatly exceed those of the left ventricle.

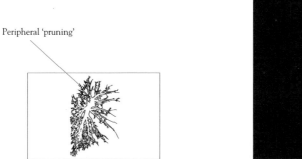

Left ventricle   Right ventricle

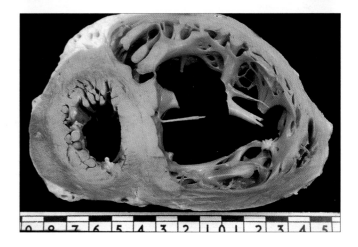

12   Right ventricular hypertrophy and dilatation secondary to pulmonary hypertension. Left ventricular cavity size remains normal or decreases.

Hypertrophic and dilated right ventricle

Normal left ventricle

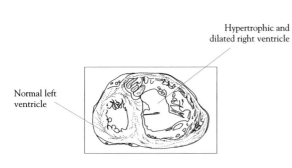

13   Chest X-ray of acute massive pulmonary embolism showing oligemia in the right lung with compensatory hyperemia in the left lung.

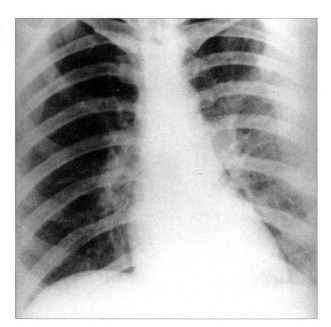

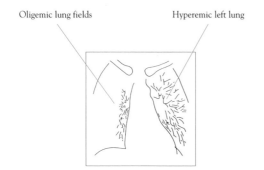

14

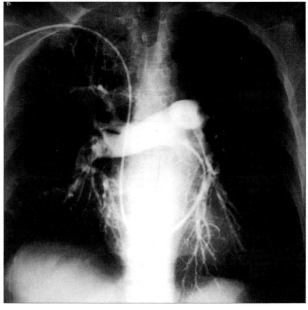

a)

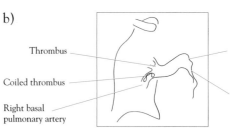

b)

The frontal chest X-ray (a) and pulmonary angiogram (b) in a patient with massive pulmonary embolism. The chest X-ray shows normal heart size and the lungs appearing generally oligemic. The pulmonary arteriogram shows massive pulmonary emboli, seen as intravascular filling defects and causing extensive obstruction of the main branch pulmonary arteries.

15   Chest X-ray of pulmonary infarction. Note the shadow at right lung base and elevated right hemidiaphragm.

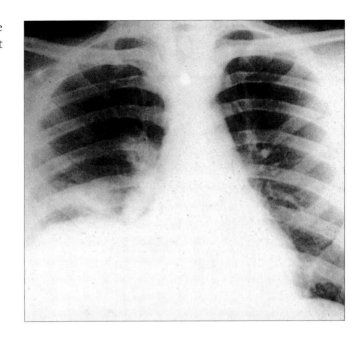

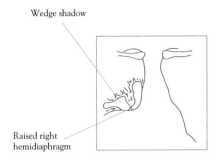

16   Chest X-ray of primary pulmonary hypertension showing large central pulmonary arteries and symmetric reduction in peripheral vessel size.

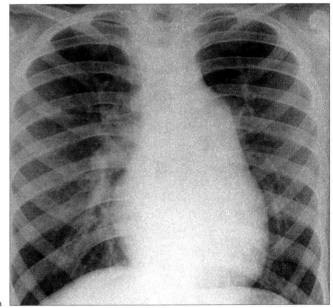

17   Chest X-ray in thromboembolic pulmonary hypertension showing large pulmonary trunk and right hilar artery. The left lung is oligemic.

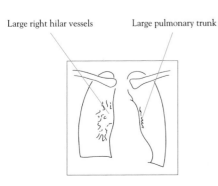

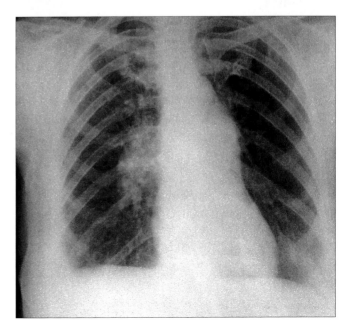

18 Chest X-ray in obstructive airways disease with cor pulmonale, showing large heart and hilar arteries with irregular pulmonary vascular obliteration.

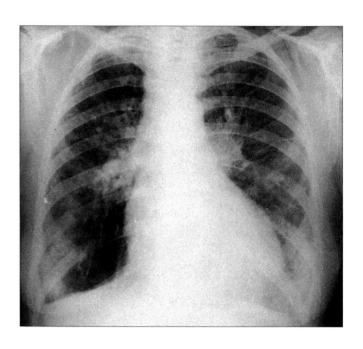

Large right hilar vessels

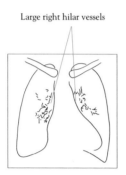

19

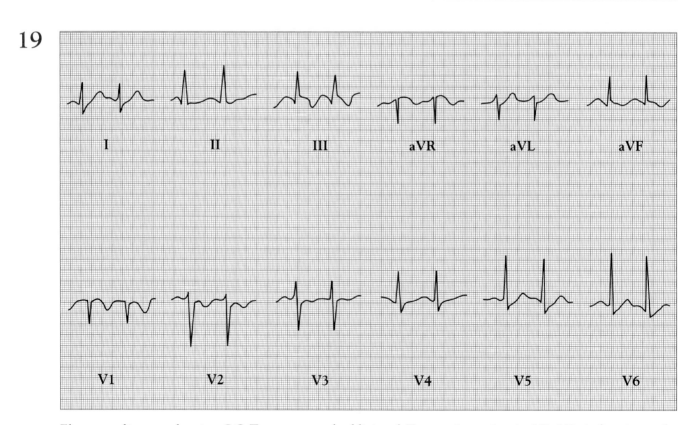

Electrocardiogram showing $S_1Q_3T_3$ pattern and additional T-wave inversion in V1–V3, indicating right ventricular strain.

20

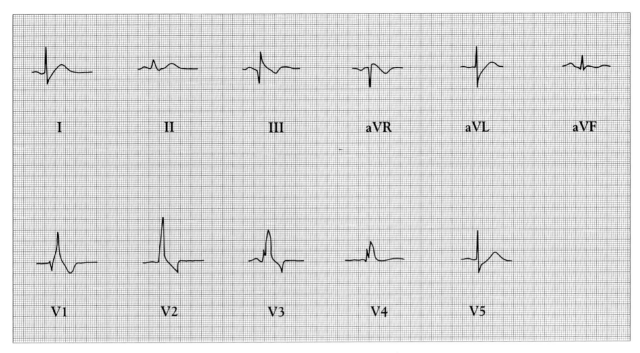

Electrocardiogram showing right bundle branch block.

21

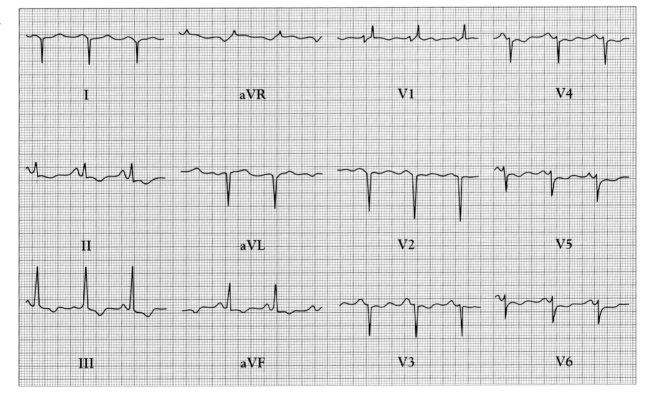

Electrocardiogram showing 'P' pulmonale, right axis deviation, and right ventricular hypertrophy.

22   Ventilation (left panel) and perfusion (right panel) lung scans in chronic obstructive airways disease, showing matched defects.

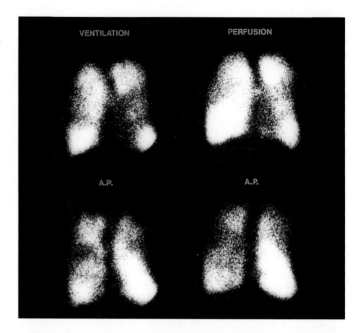

23   Ventilation (left panel) and perfusion (right panel) lung scans in pulmonary embolic disease, showing normal ventilation but multiple perfusion defects.

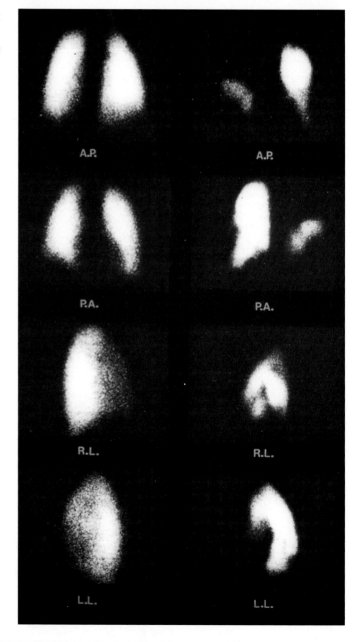

24

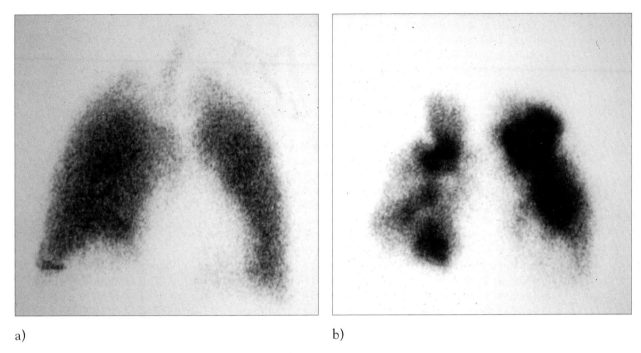

a) b)

Isotope scanning in pulmonary embolism. (a) The frontal ventilation scan, using krypton-81m, is normal in this patient. (b) Frontal perfusion scan, using intravenous technetium-99m, shows extensive perfusion defects, unaccompanied by ventilation defects, in both lungs, more marked on the right. These appearances are very suggestive of pulmonary embolic disease.

25

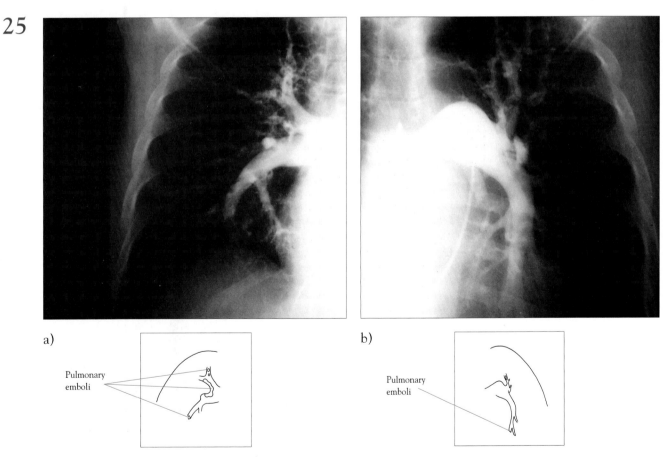

a) b)

Pulmonary angiogram to match the isotope scan shown in [24]. (a) Selective right pulmonary artery injection. (b) Selective left pulmonary artery injection. The pulmonary emboli appear as filling defects within the contrast-filled pulmonary arteries, their positions corresponding to the perfusion defects.

26

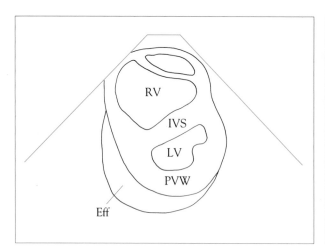
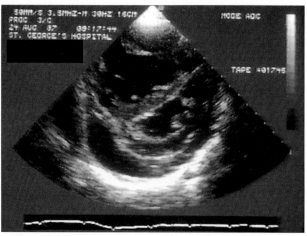

Parasternal short-axis view of a patient with right ventricular hypertrophy secondary to severe pulmonary hypertension. The right ventricle is enlarged and its walls abnormally thickened. High pressure in the right ventricle has distorted the shape of the interventricular septum, giving the left ventricle a D-shaped section. There is a small amount of fluid in the pericardial sac.

27 M-mode recording showing an enlarged right ventricle and characteristic septal motion of pulmonary hypertension. This has a reversed ('paradoxical') motion pattern, which may in part be due to concomitant tricuspid or pulmonary regurgitation.

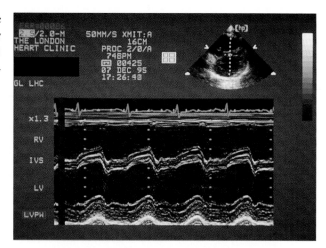

28

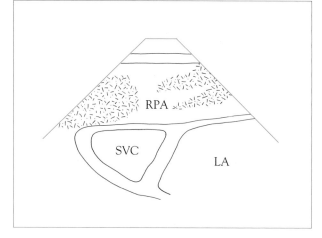
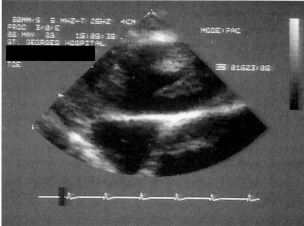

Transesophageal study in a patient with a massive pulmonary embolism. Multiple echogenic masses are seen in the proximal right pulmonary artery.

29

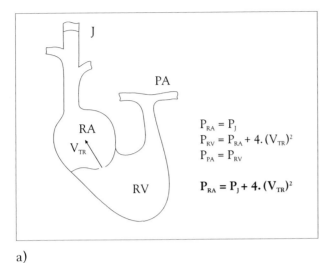

$$P_{RA} = P_J$$
$$P_{RV} = P_{RA} + 4.(V_{TR})^2$$
$$P_{PA} = P_{RV}$$

$$\mathbf{P_{RA} = P_J + 4.(V_{TR})^2}$$

a)

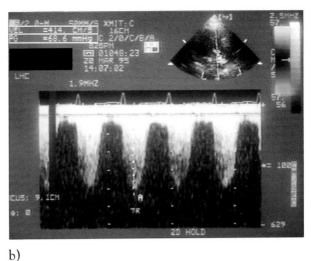

b)

(a) Diagram showing how pulmonary artery pressure can be determined from the velocity of a tricuspid regurgitation jet. Pressure in the right atrium can be determined from inspection of the jugular venous pulse. If any tricuspid regurgitation is present, the Bernoulli equation ($\Delta P = 4 \times V^2$) allows the (RV-RA) pressure gradient to be calculated from the velocity of the jet. Systolic pressure in the right ventricle equals that in the pulmonary arteries as long as there is no right ventricular outflow obstruction. (b) Continuous-wave spectral Doppler of tricuspid regurgitation. The peak jet velocity is 4 m/s, corresponding to a (RV-RA) gradient of 64 mmHg. Pulmonary artery pressure is thus equal to (RA pressure + 64) mmHg.

30 Continuous-wave spectral Doppler of pulmonary regurgitation in a patient with Eisenmenger's syndrome secondary to a large ventricular septal defect. The velocity of the regurgitant jet is almost 4 m/s showing that pulmonary diastolic pressure is about 60 mmHg.

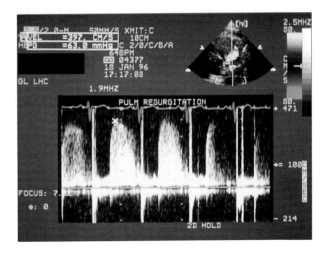

31 Pulmonary arteriogram in acute massive pulmonary embolism showing involvement of more than 50% of the major pulmonary arteries.

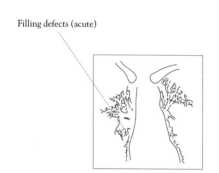

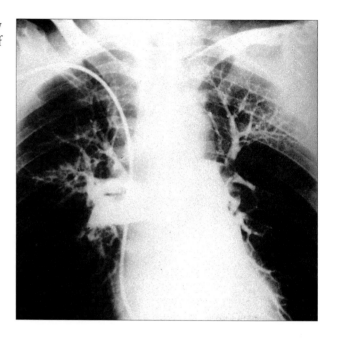

32

a)

b)

(a) Chest X-ray in a patient with chronic thromboembolic pulmonary hypertension, showing asymmetry of perfusion. The pulmonary vessels terminate beyond the hilum. (b) The pulmonary angiogram confirms that there is virtually no perfusion of the left lung and irregular perfusion of the right lung from long-standing pulmonary thromboembolic disease.

33

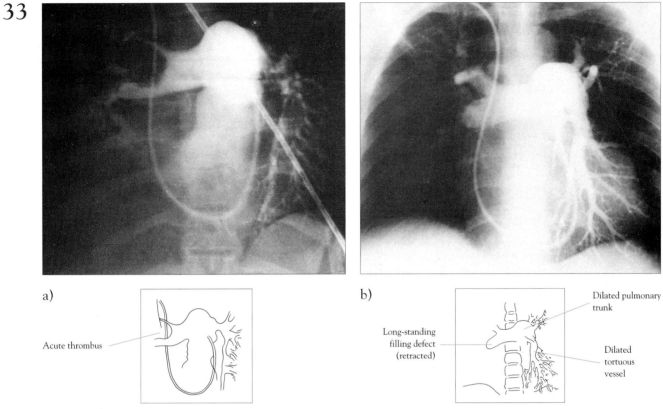

a)   Acute thrombus

b)   Long-standing filling defect (retracted)   Dilated pulmonary trunk   Dilated tortuous vessel

Pulmonary arteriogram in acute massive pulmonary embolism, showing (a) acute thrombus in the right pulmonary artery, causing a concave leading edge, contrasting with appearances in chronic thromboembolism (b) with a convex leading edge.

34 Pulmonary arteriogram in primary pulmonary hypertension, showing peripheral arterial pruning.

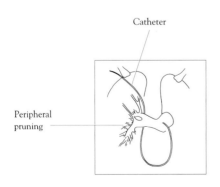

Catheter

Peripheral pruning

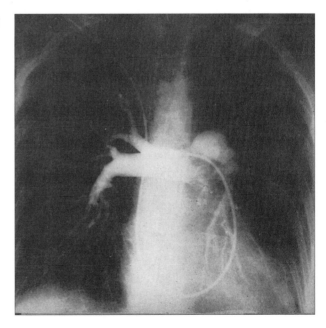

35 Principles of management of acute pulmonary embolism and chronic thromboembolic pulmonary hypertension.

ACUTE PULMONARY EMBOLISM

1. Intravenous heparin for 5 to 7 days followed by long-term anticoagulation (stable patients, massive or minor embolism)

2. Intravenous thrombolytic agents in hemodynamically unstable patients (massive embolism)

3. Catheter or surgical pulmonary embolectomy in selected patients

CHRONIC THROMBOEMBOLIC PULMONARY HYPERTENSION

1. Long-term anticoagulation

2. Pulmonary vasodilators

3. Thromboembolectomy in selected patients

4. Heart–lung or lung transplant

---

36 Principles of management of primary pulmonary hypertension.

---

1. Long-term anticoagulation to reduce the risk of thrombotic events and thrombosis *in situ*

2. Supplemental oxygen therapy to maintain arterial oxygen saturation over 90%

3. For pulmonary vasodilatation:

    a) calcium channel blockers
    b) direct acting vasodilators
    c) intravenous prostacyclin
    d) inhaled nitric oxide
    e) exogenous atrial natriuretic peptide
    f) endopeptidase inhibitors

4. Atrial septostomy in selected patients

5. Single- or double lung-, or heart–lung transplants in selected patients

---

PERICARDIAL DISEASE

Pathology

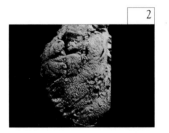

Disorders of the pericardium include acute and subacute inflammation, non-inflammatory effusion, chronic constriction, and congenital anomalies.

Pericardial thickening, internal and external adhesions, and pericardial calcification may be clinically silent and discovered incidentally. Acute and subacute inflammation of the pericardium can be caused by viral, bacterial, fungal, and other infectious agents. Inflammatory pericarditis may result from a vasculitis, immunopathies (e.g. drug reactions), myocardial infarction, dissecting aneurysm, pleural and pulmonary diseases, metabolic diseases (including uremia), neoplasms, trauma, and radiation. The most common causes of acute pericarditis, however, are viral infections [1]. In viral (Coxsackie) pericarditis, the myocardium may be involved by superficial extension of the inflammation (myopericarditis). Acute inflammatory pericarditis is characterized by a fibrinous exudate over the visceral and parietal pericardium [2], with varying amounts of turbid yellow fluid in the pericardial cavity. Histologic examination shows strands of fibrin deposited on the serosa with dilated blood vessels and acute inflammatory infiltrate.

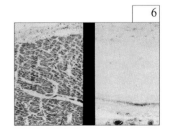

Acute myocardial infarction may be complicated by pericarditis. Episternopericarditis associated with transmural myocardial infarction is the most common form and is usually clinically silent. Dressler's or post-myocardial infarction syndrome occurs in approximately 3% of patients with acute myocardial infarction. Hemopericardium resulting from cardiac rupture is a catastrophic complication of acute myocardial infarction.

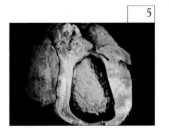

Pericardial effusion appears when fluid is produced too fast to be absorbed. Exudative effusion may result from inflammation, trauma, and malignancy [3]. Exudative effusion almost always contains large amounts of fibrin and a significant protein content. Transudative effusion has much less protein and no fibrin or blood. It occurs in salt and water retention, as in heart failure. Hemorrhagic pericarditis can occur in any type of pericarditis but most frequently with tuberculous infection and malignancies. Hemopericardium (which should be distinguished from hemorrhagic pericarditis) results from trauma, dissecting aneurysm, and cardiac rupture. Suppurative exudative effusions are mainly due to pyogenic infection and contain cellular debris and leukocytes [4].

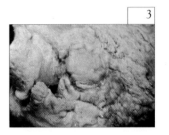

Chronic fibrosing pericarditis usually follows a clinically evident or silent episode of acute pericarditis due to any cause. Tuberculosis, which used to be the most frequent cause, is now relatively uncommon as a cause of constrictive pericarditis in developed countries [5]. Following an acute episode, constriction may be evident within three months (acute) or between three and twelve months (subacute). Occasionally, a clotted hemopericardium causes acute constriction or effusive constrictive pericarditis. Usually, the parietal and the visceral pericardium over most of the cardiac surfaces become adherent to each other. The usual cases of chronic constrictive pericarditis are due to a single sheet of fibrous tissue, in which a few lymphocytic foci are seen, with microscopic to gross calcium deposits. However, the pericardium may be grossly thickened in constrictive pericarditis [6]. Depending on the etiology, granulomas and giant cells may be seen.

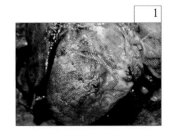

Secondary carcinoma commonly involves the pericardium. The tumor may appear as white nodules over the visceral pericardium or as a more diffuse sheet of tumor.

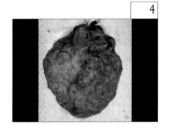

Presentation

Symptoms

The presenting symptom of acute pericarditis is sharp, usually severe, superficial central chest pain. The pain is worse with movement, breathing, and exertion, and reduced on sitting up. The pain may be over the trapezius, usually on the left side, but may be bilateral. Trapezius ridge pain is almost pathognomonic of pericarditis. Painful swallowing (odynophagia) is a rare presenting symptom. 'Flu'-like symptoms, with fever, malaise, myalgia, and cough may precede or accompany pericarditis.

Patients with a non-compressing pericardial effusion are usually asymptomatic. However, a very large effusion may cause compression of the adjacent structures and cause symptoms such as dysphagia, dyspnea, hoarseness, cough, hiccups, and abdominal fullness.

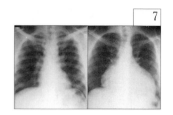

Patients with cardiac tamponade may present with non-specific symptoms or with dyspnea and fatigue. Air hunger is a manifestation of severe tamponade. Occasionally, patients present with presyncope or syncope.

Patients with constrictive pericarditis may complain of exertional fatigue, dyspnea, cough, and, occasionally, orthopnea, but more frequently ascites, edema, and abdominal discomfort are the presenting symptoms.

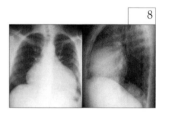

Signs
The hallmark of acute pericarditis is a pericardial rub, which may come and go. Pericardial rubs usually have a peculiar shuffling, creaking, scratching, or grating quality and consist of three (atrial systolic, ventricular systolic, and diastolic) components. However, rubs may be faint and simulate a murmur, and may consist of only one or two components. Occasionally, rubs may be palpable, like a thrill.

Non-compressing pericardial effusion may not be associated with any abnormal physical findings. Rarely, massive pericardial effusion may cause compression of the left bronchus, and dullness and tubular breathing between the angle of the left scapula and the spine (Ewart's sign). The heart sounds may appear distant.

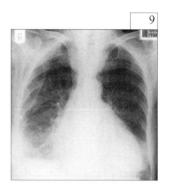

The crucial physical signs of cardiac tamponade are an elevated venous pressure, tachycardia, and pulsus paradoxus (a fall in systolic blood pressure of more than 10 mmHg during inspiration). The jugular venous pulse may show a dominant systolic descent. A third heart sound is not present. Heart sounds may be distant and, rarely, auscultatory alternans may be appreciated. Even when a large pericardial effusion is present, a pericardial rub may still be heard.

In chronic constrictive pericarditis, an elevated jugular venous pressure with inspiratory increase (Kussmaul's sign) may be present. In tamponade, Kussmaul's sign is absent, whereas in constriction, pulsus paradoxus is absent. A third heart sound usually indicates myocardial involvement. Ascites, hepatic enlargement, and edema are also present in many patients.

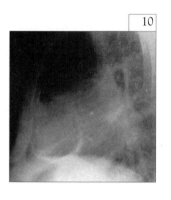

Investigations

Radiology
In acute pericarditis without effusion, the chest X-ray is normal. In the presence of a pericardial effusion, cardiomegaly without radiologic findings of pulmonary venous hypertension is present [7]. Inward displacement of the epicardial fat pad, along with cardiomegaly on plain film, also suggest pericardial effusion [8]. In constrictive pericarditis, cardiac size is normal or only slightly enlarged due to pericardial thickening or residual effusion [9]. In one-third of patients, pericardial calcification is recognized [10]. The calcification is mostly confined to the atrioventricular groove. The chest X-ray may be entirely normal in constrictive pericarditis.

Electrocardiography
During the acute phase of inflammatory pericarditis, elevation of the ST junction in almost all leads with ST-segment depression in leads aVR and V1 is characteristic [11]. PR-segment depression may also be present. In some patients, only non-specific ST-T changes are seen. During the recovery phase, T-wave inversion only with isoelectric ST-segments is present [12]. In significant pericardial effusion with or without tamponade,

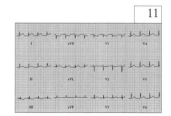

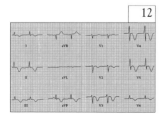

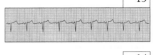

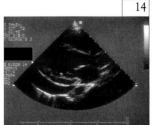

sinus tachycardia may be the only abnormal finding. Occasionally, partial or total electrical alternans is present [13]. Total (PQRST) electrical alternans is pathognomonic of cardiac tamponade with a large pericardial effusion.

Echocardiography

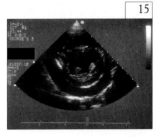

In acute fibrinous pericarditis, the echocardiogram can be completely normal. As soon as there is significant fluid within the pericardial sac, the visceral and parietal layers separate. This can readily be seen on a two-dimensional echocardiogram, which is the most sensitive means available for detecting the development of pericardial effusion. Normally, the two layers form a single echo (although slight separation can often be seen in systole). With the patient lying supine, a small effusion collects behind the left ventricle, resulting in the parietal pericardium showing as a bright, immobile echo separated from the moving myocardium by an echo-free space [14–16]. The fluid is never seen behind the left atrium; in this region, the pericardial sac forms a blind alley (the oblique sinus) around the pulmonary veins, which cannot easily distend. An important diagnostic sign in differentiating a pericardial from a pleural effusion is that the former forms a pointed wedge anterior to the thoracic aorta at the level of the atrioventricular groove, whereas the latter has a blunted edge up against the aorta [17].

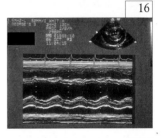

Qualitative assessment of the size of an effusion can be made. As the amount of fluid increases, it is seen anteriorly as well as posteriorly and the apical four-chamber view shows only the region adjacent to the left atrium remaining spared. Further fluid volume increases the separation of the layers [18]. Very large effusions allow the heart to move to and fro within the fluid-filled pericardium.

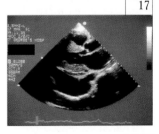

The rapid development of pericardial fluid may restrict cardiac filling, resulting in hemodynamic compromise. The first echocardiographic sign of this is usually collapse of the right atrial wall, although this is not usually of clinical significance [19]. Further increase of pressure within the pericardium causes diastolic collapse of the right ventricular wall and this is normally associated with a detectable degree of paradox in the arterial pulse [20]. Pulsed Doppler shows increased tricuspid filling velocities with a reciprocal decrease in left ventricular filling velocity (features of cardiac tamponade). Additional signs are engorgement of the inferior vena cava and large hepatic veins, and failure of these structures to change size with respiration.

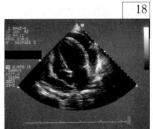

Chronic effusions, particularly those where the fluid contains blood or other protein-rich material, often contain seaweed-like fibrous strands, and these are likely to proceed to cause pericardial constriction [21]. When constriction is present, the tight pericardium surrounding the right ventricle prevents normal filling of the right ventricle leading to exaggerated tricuspid systolic ring motion associated with a dominant 'x' descent in the jugular venous pulse.

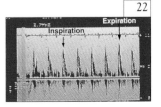

Pericardial constriction can be difficult to detect by echocardiography. The inability of the heart to accommodate any increase in right-sided volume during inspiration, except by reducing left-heart volume, can be demonstrated by Doppler. Using pulsed-wave Doppler, recordings are made of diastolic flow across the mitral and tricuspid valves: normally, there is obvious respiratory variation in tricuspid flow, and little or none in mitral flow, but in the presence of constriction, mitral flow velocities are seen to diminish during inspiration [22].

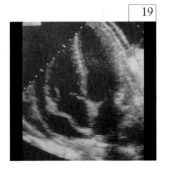

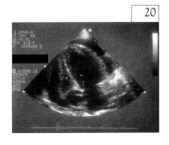

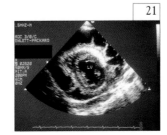

Magnetic Resonance Imaging (MRI) and Computed Tomography (CT)
Both MRI and CT are useful in demonstrating anatomic abnormalities in a patient with the hemodynamic abnormalities of constriction. Both MRI and CT are very sensitive for the detection of pericardial thickening [23,24]. CT is good for detecting calcification in the pericardium; in constriction, MRI demonstrates impaired diastolic filling from the superior vena caval flow.

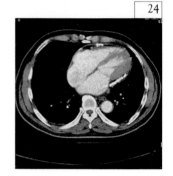

Laboratory Studies
Routine blood tests, including ESR, are carried out for diagnosing the etiology of pericarditis but these tests are rarely revealing. Specific tests, including pericardial biopsy, are sometimes necessary for diagnosing the etiology of pericardial effusion.

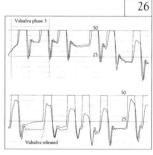

Cardiac Catheterization and Angiography
Cardiac catheterization and angiography play little part in the diagnosis or management of patients with acute pericarditis or pericardial effusion. In rare patients with suspected cardiac tamponade, determination of the hemodynamics may confirm the diagnosis. In tamponade, mean right atrial, right ventricular, and mean capillary wedge pressures are equal. The right atrial pressure confirms the dominance of the systolic descent. In low-pressure tamponade, which occurs in the presence of hypovolemia, the right atrial pressure may be as low as 5–6 mmHg but increases rapidly to a high level during volume expansion, and equalization of the pressures becomes apparent.

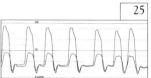

In patients with suspected constrictive pericarditis, it may be desirable to confirm the hemodynamic abnormalities of constriction by cardiac catheterization. The characteristic findings are equalization of the right and left ventricular end-diastolic pressures (by contrast with restrictive cardiomyopathy), and a 'dip and plateau' pattern of ventricular diastolic pressure wave forms [25]. The difference between the left and right ventricular end-diastolic pressures in constriction is less than 5 mmHg and this difference does not increase during volume expansion, Valsalva, or Müller maneuvers [26]. The right ventricular end-diastolic pressure exceeds one-third of its systolic pressure, and right ventricular systolic pressure is not usually higher than 45 mmHg. The wave form of the right atrial pressure may show a dominant 'y' descent if there is important myocardial involvement.

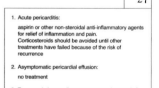

Principles of Management

Acute pericarditis should be treated with aspirin or other non-steroidal anti-inflammatory agents [27]. Corticosteroids should not be used until other treatments have failed because of the risk of recurrence. Specific therapy of the etiology of pericardial disease should be given if such therapy exists.

Asymptomatic pericardial effusion does not require any treatment. Pericardiocentesis, with or without pericardial biopsy, may be required for diagnosis in rare patients.

Tamponade is usually a cardiac emergency and removal of pericardial fluid by paracentesis or surgical drainage is mandatory. Pericardiectomy is the only effective treatment of symptomatic constrictive pericarditis, although significant myocardial involvement may make the procedure less effective.

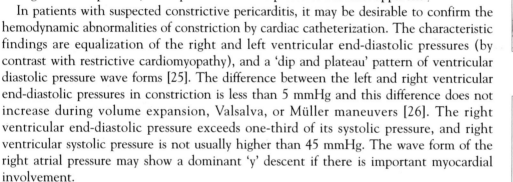

1. Acute pericarditis:
   aspirin or other non-steroidal anti-inflammatory agents for relief of inflammation and pain. Corticosteroids should be avoided until other treatments have failed because of the risk of recurrence

2. Asymptomatic pericardial effusion:
   no treatment

3. Tamponade is a cardiac emergency and removal of pericardial fluid by paracentesis or surgical drainage is mandatory

4. Symptomatic constrictive pericarditis:
   surgical decortication

1 Viral pericarditis. The visceral pericardium is red and inflamed, with a roughened surface due to deposition of fibrin.

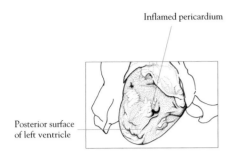

Inflamed pericardium

Posterior surface of left ventricle

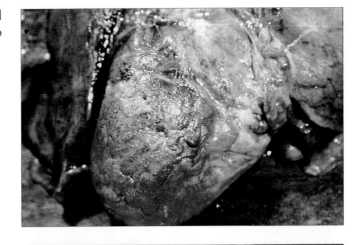

2 Acute pericarditis. A thick fibrinous exudate covers the surface of the heart.

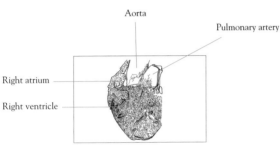

Aorta

Pulmonary artery

Right atrium

Right ventricle

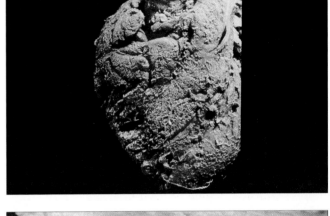

3 Secondary pericardial tumor. The pericardial cavity is opened to show the wide dissemination of tumor on the visceral pericardium of the right ventricle.

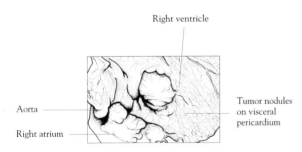

Right ventricle

Aorta

Tumor nodules on visceral pericardium

Right atrium

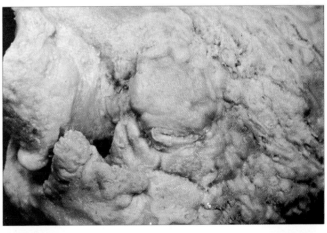

4 Bacterial pericarditis. Purulent exudate on visceral pericardium.

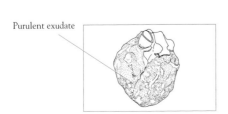

Purulent exudate

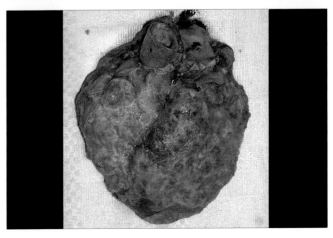

5 Chronic constrictive pericarditis. A window has been cut through the thickened parietal pericardium which forms a rough constrictive membrane. Note also the shaggy exudate on the visceral pericardium.

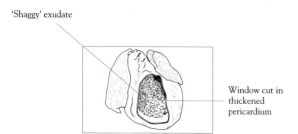

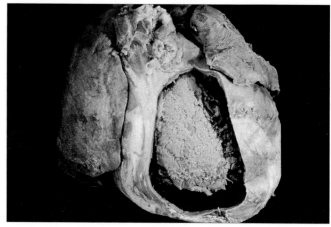

6 Histologic section of normal pericardium (left panel). The pericardium forms a thin layer on the myocardium. Histologic section of grossly thickened pericardium (right panel) in chronic constrictive pericarditis. (Both sections are taken at the same magnification.)

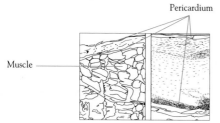

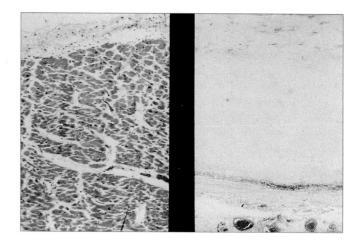

7

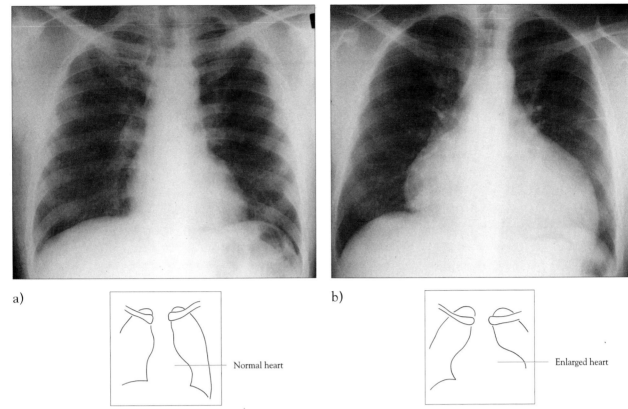

Pericardial effusion. (a) This patient's chest X-ray was initially normal. (b) Three months later, the heart shadow is markedly enlarged, with a rather globular appearance. In spite of this, the lung vessels appear entirely normal. Rapid increase in the size of the heart shadow, and the association of what appears to be a large heart shadow with lungs showing no evidence of pulmonary edema, are very suggestive of a pericardial effusion.

8

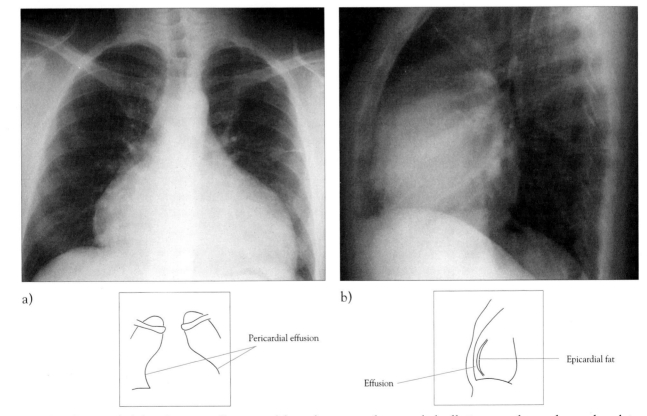

Displaced epicardial fat. Occasionally, a confident diagnosis of pericardial effusion may be made on the plain film. (a) The frontal view (same patient as in [7]) shows the large heart and clear lungs. (b) The lateral view shows the displacement inwards of the double edge of the epicardial fat line by the effusion and can be identified when the effusion separates it from the sternum.

9 Constrictive pericarditis. The heart shadow may be normal or enlarged as in this example.

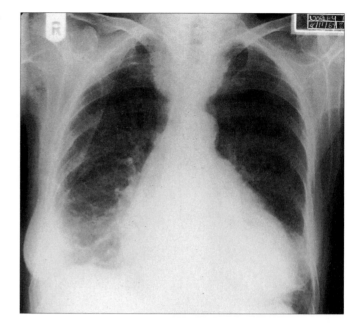

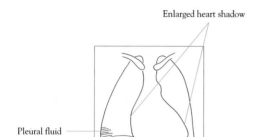

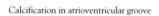

10 Lateral chest X-ray showing calcification in the atrioventricular groove in a patient with chronic constrictive pericarditis.

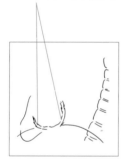

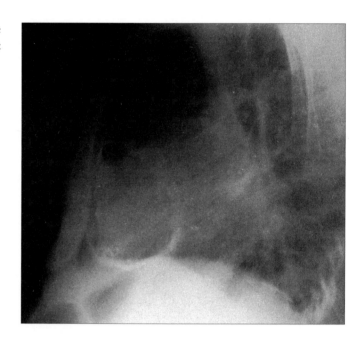

11

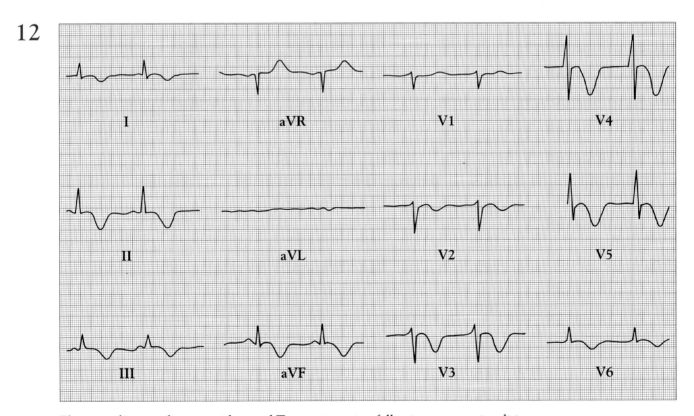

Electrocardiogram showing widespread concave ST-segment elevation in a patient with acute pericarditis. Note the ST-segment depression in leads aVR and V1, and widespread PR-segment depression.

12

Electrocardiogram showing widespread T-wave inversion following acute pericarditis.

13

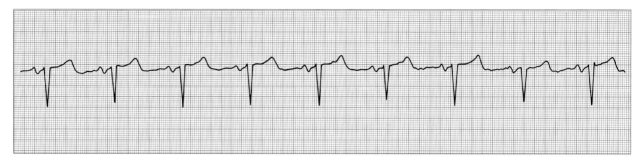

Low-voltage QRS complexes with smaller and larger amplitudes of the QRS complexes (partial electrical alternans) may be seen in cardiac tamponade.

14

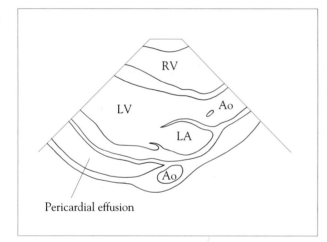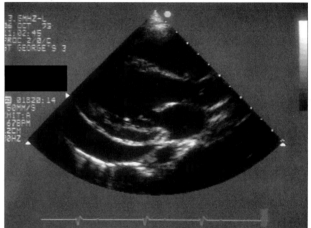

Parasternal long-axis view from a patient with a moderate sized pericardial effusion. The fluid is seen as an echo-free space behind the heart when the patient is lying down. It is not present behind the left atrium, where the oblique sinus effectively prevents accumulation of fluid in this region of the pericardium.

15

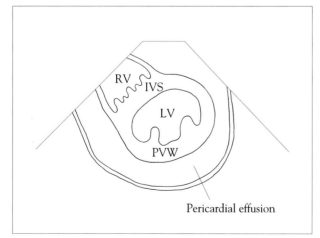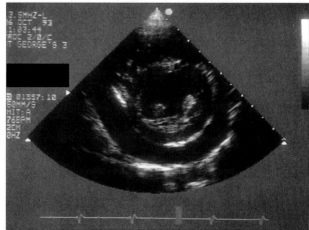

Parasternal short-axis view of the same patient as in [14].

16   M-mode recording from the same case as in [14] and [15], showing the echo-free space behind the left ventricle.

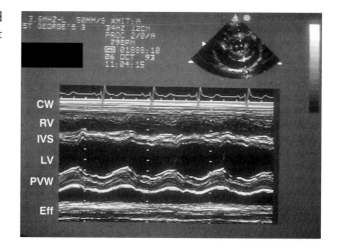

17

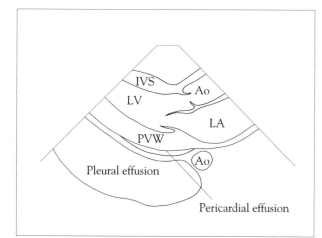

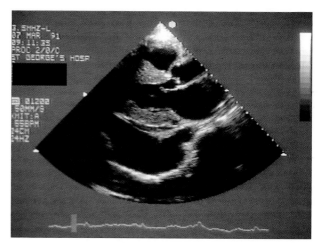

Parasternal long-axis view showing a small pericardial effusion with a large left pleural effusion. The pericardial fluid tapers off before reaching the descending thoracic aorta, whereas the pleural effusion abuts and is seen posterior to the aorta.

18

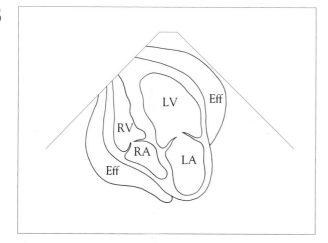

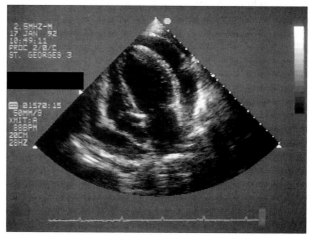

Apical four-chamber view of a large pericardial effusion. This allows the heart to move within the pericardium and may manifest as marked variations in the amplitude of the ECG complexes. Note that the region adjacent to the left atrium is spared.

19

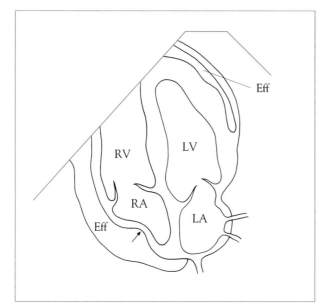 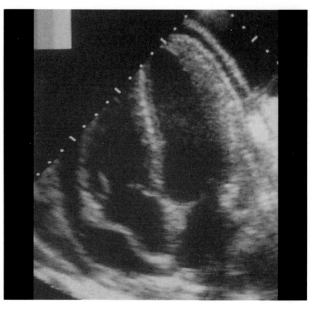

Moderate or large effusions cause partial collapse of the right atrial wall (arrow), seen in this apical four-chamber view. This is not associated with hemodynamic dysfunction.

20

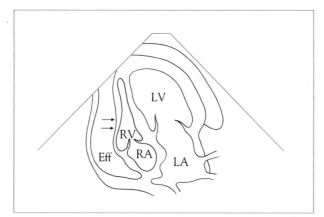 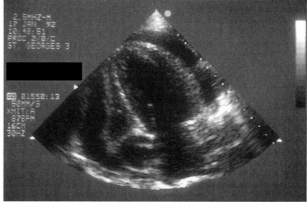

Diastolic collapse (arrows) of the right ventricular wall, seen in this apical four-chamber view, is a sign of hemodynamic compromise and manifests clinically as an exaggerated reduction in pulse pressure on inspiration ('pulsus paradoxus').

21

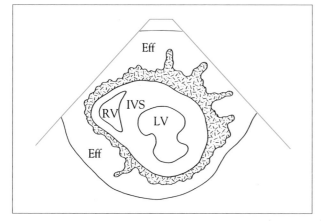 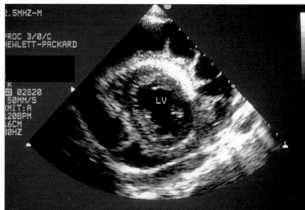

Parasternal short-axis view of a case of tuberculous pericarditis with chronic pericardial effusion. There are multiple seaweed-like strands of protein material within the fluid.

22   Changes in transmitral Doppler flow in constrictive pericarditis, illustrating diminished transmitral flow during inspiration.

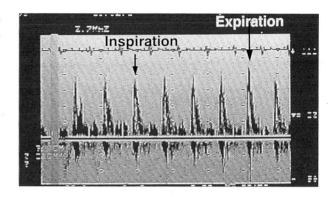

23

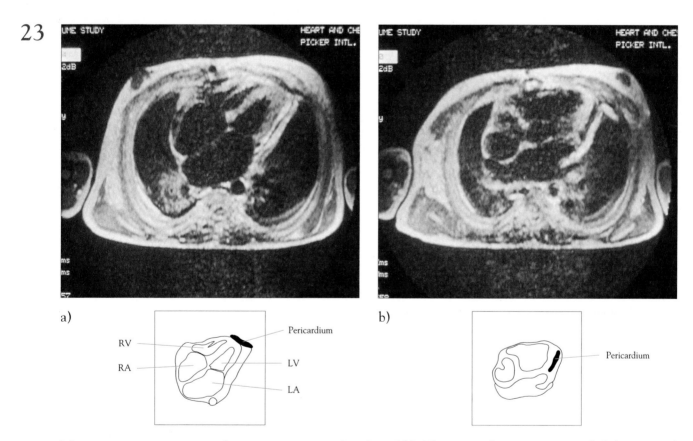

a)

b)

Magnetic resonance images of constrictive pericarditis (a and b). The pericardium appears as a dark line around the heart and in this case it is grossly thickened, which is highly suggestive of a diagnosis of constrictive pericarditis.

24 Ultrafast cine CT of constrictive pericarditis. There are obvious calcium deposits in the pericardium, particularly around the lateral wall and anteriorly around the right ventricle.

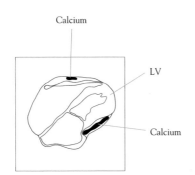

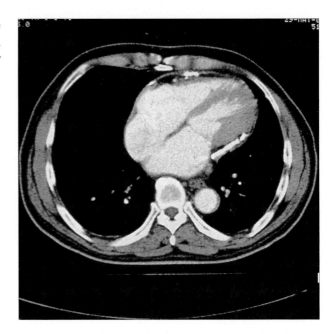

25

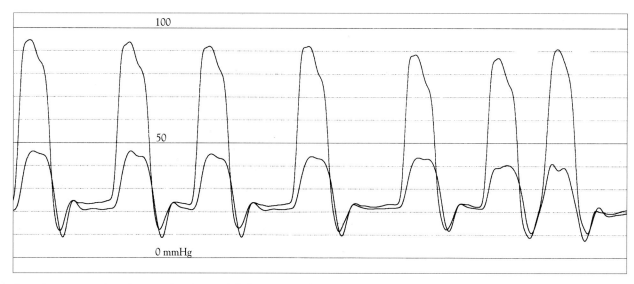

Simultaneous recordings of right and left ventricular pressures showing 'dip and plateau' wave forms and equalization of right and left ventricular diastolic pressures.

26

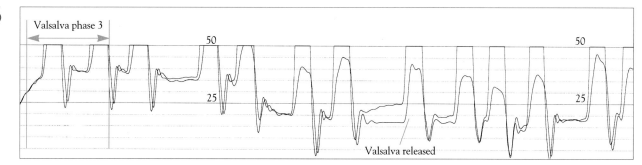

Right and left ventricular diastolic pressures remain equal during the Valsalva maneuver.

27   Principles of management of pericardial disease.

1. Acute pericarditis:

   aspirin or other non-steroidal anti-inflammatory agents for relief of inflammation and pain.
   Corticosteroids should be avoided until other treatments have failed because of the risk of recurrence

2. Asymptomatic pericardial effusion:

   no treatment

3. Tamponade is a cardiac emergency and removal of pericardial fluid by paracentesis or surgical drainage is mandatory

4. Symptomatic constrictive pericarditis:

   surgical decortication

A

'a' wave
Fallots's tetralogy 314
heart failure 97, 121
hypertension 138, 163
mitral stenosis 170, 171
mitral regurgitation 189
persistent ductus arteriosus 296
pulmonary embolic and pulmonary
vascular disease 387
pulmonary stenosis 306, 307, 312
restrictive cardiomyopathy 360
tricuspid valve disease 252, 256
ventricular septal defect 283
accelerated hypertension, *see*
malignant hypertension
ACE inhibitors
AMI 53, 82, 83
dilated cardiomyopathy 333,
341
adenosine-induced stress in stable
angina, thallium imaging 6, 20
adrenal disease causing hypertension
134, 150-1
isotope scanning 137, 160
IV urography 137, 159
age and blood pressure 129, 140
airway disease, *see* lung
aldosteronism, primary 134, 151
ambulatory BP monitoring 136,
155-6
ambulatory ECG
angina (stable) 5, 15
hypertrophic cardiomyopathy
343, 351
ammonia (^{13}N) for PET scan in
stable angina 7, 25
amyloid heart disease
ECG 360, 364
echocardiography 360, 365
myocardial infiltration 359,
362, 365
analgesic nephropathy 137, 158
aneurysms, aortic
aortic regurgitation with 231,
238
imaging 233, 242, 247
in hypertension 143
aneurysms, cerebral, in hypertension
132, 145, 146
aneurysms, LV
in angina (stable) 7, 28
in heart failure 93, 100, 107
echocardiography 97, 114
MRI 125
X-ray 95, 106

in MI (acute) 47, 52, 59, 74
echocardiography 52, 74
false aneurysms 77
MRI 52, 76
ventriculography 51, 69
in MI (old) 107
angina
effort, diagnostic features 4, 11
post-MI 54
stable 3-33
definition 3
investigations 4-8, 12-31
management (principles)
8-9, 31-7
pathophysiology and pathology
3, 10-11
presenting symptoms/signs 3,
11-12
unstable 40-6
definition 40
investigations 40-1, 44-6
management (principles) 42,
46
pathophysiology and pathology
40, 43
presenting symptoms/signs 40
variant (Prinzmetal's; vasospastic)
34-9
definition 3
investigations 34-5, 38-9
management (principles) 36,
39
pathophysiology and pathology
34, 36
presenting symptoms/signs 34,
36
angiography (cardiac)
pericardial disease 408, 419
tumors 373-4, 383-4
ventricular, *see* ventriculography
see also catheterization
angiography (vascular)
aortic, *see* aortography
coronary (coronary arteriography)
angina (stable) 8, 29-30
angina (unstable) 41, 45-6
angina (variant) 35, 39
heart failure 98, 123
MI 53, 79-80, 81
tumor 384
pulmonary vasculature, normal
post-mortem 393
pulmonary vasculature in disease
390, 402-3
embolus 389, 390, 399, 402
renal 137, 157, 159

angioplasty, coronary, in stable
angina 9, 32
perfusion imaging in assessment
of 6, 22
angiotensin-converting enzyme
inhibitors, *see* ACE inhibitors
ankylosing spondylitis, aortic
regurgitation 230, 236
aorta (including aortic root)
aneurysms, *see* aneurysms
aortic regurgitation with
abnormalities of 230, 235-6
aortic enlargement 231
radiology 231
in aortic stenosis 207, 214
coarctation, *see* aortic coarctation
dissection, *see* aortic dissection
override (of ventricular septum)
in Fallot's tetralogy 314, 315,
316, 319, 320
in PDA 296, 300
aortic arch
knuckle of, abnormalities 321,
324, 325
right-sided, in Fallot's tetralogy
314, 317
aortic coarctation 321-7
hypertension with 135, 139, 152,
155, 165
investigations 321-2, 323-4
management (principles) 322
pathophysiology and pathology
314, 316
presentation 321
aortic dissection
aortic regurgitation due to 230
imaging 233, 243, 248
in hypertension 166
aortic regurgitation 230-50
definition 230
in hypertension 163
investigations 231-4, 237-50
Doppler 163, 232-3, 245-6
management (principles) 234,
250
pathology 230, 235-6
presenting symptoms/signs 230-1,
237
aortic stenosis 206-29
investigations 207-10, 213-28
management (principles) 210,
228-9
pathophysiology and pathology
206-7, 211-12
presenting symptoms/signs 207,
213

subvalvar, *see* subvalvar aortic
  stenosis
supravalvar, *see* supravalvar aortic
  stenosis
valvar 206
aortic valve
  premature closure in hypertrophic
    cardiomyopathy 344, 352
  regurgitation due to, *see* aortic
    regurgitation
  stenosis, pathology 206
    see also aortic stenosis
aortography
  aortic coarctation 322, 327
  aortic regurgitation 233-4, 249-50
  aortic stenosis 225
  PDA 298, 304-5
arrhythmias
  in angina (stable) in exercise
    stress testing 4-5, 14
  in heart failure 96, 109, 110, 111
  in hypertrophic cardiomyopathy
    343, 351
  in MI 54, 84-8
  in mitral regurgitation 189
  see also specific arrhythmias
arterial blood gases in pulmonary
  vascular disease 388
arterial disease in hypertension
  large arteries 131, 142-3
  small arteries 131, 143-4
arteriography, *see* angiography
  (vascular)
arteriolar disease in hypertension 131
atheroma in hypertension 131, 143
  coronary 132, 145
  renal 147
atheromatous plaque, *see* plaque
atherosclerosis, coronary 3, 10
  angiogram 30
atherosclerotic plaque, *see* plaque
atrial enlargement, left
  with atrial myxoma 372, 379
  in heart failure
    echocardiography 95, 96, 103,
      113
    in restrictive cardiomyopathy
      360, 364
    X-ray 95, 103
  in mitral stenosis 170, 176, 177
    X-ray 171, 179
atrial enlargement, right, with atrial
  myxoma 372, 379
atrial fibrillation
  in heart failure 109
  in MI 54, 88
  in mitral regurgitation 189, 196

atrial septum
  defect 269-82
    investigations 270-2, 274-83
    management (principles) 272
    ostium primum, *see* ostium
      primum ASD
    ostium secundum, *see* ostium
      secundum ASD
    pathophysiology and pathology
      269, 273-4
    presenting symptoms/signs 269,
      274
  myxoma attached to 380, 382
atrial thrombus, *see* thrombus
atrial tumors, *see* tumors *and specific
  types*
atrioventricular block in AMI 54, 87
auscultation (sounds and murmurs)
  aortic coarctation 321
  aortic regurgitation 231, 237
  aortic stenosis 207, 213
  atrial myxoma 372, 377
  atrial septal defect 269, 274
  hypertrophic cardiomyopathy 343,
    347
  mitral prolapse 189, 194
  mitral stenosis 170, 175
  pulmonary stenosis 306, 309
  tricuspid disease 251, 252, 256
  VSD 283, 287
Austin–Flint murmur, aortic
  regurgitation 231, 237

B

bacterial pericarditis 405, 409
balloon angioplasty, *see* angioplasty
balloon-tipped thermodilution
  catheter 98, 120
balloon valvuloplasty, *see*
  valvuloplasty
bat's wing appearance of pulmonary
  vessels 136, 155
beta-blockers, heart failure 99
bicuspid aortic valve, congenitally
  206, 211
  aortic coarctation and 321, 323
  echocardiography 208, 217, 218,
    241
  regurgitation 230, 235
bifascicular block in AMI 54, 88
block, heart
  in aortic stenosis 208, 217
  bundle branch, *see* bundle branch
    block
  in cardiomyopathy (dilated) 331,
    332, 336
  in Ebstein's anomaly 252, 259

in heart failure 96, 108
in MI
  atrioventricular 54, 87
  bifascicular 54, 88
in mitral regurgitation 189, 197
in pulmonary vascular disease 388,
  397
blood flow
  Doppler studies, *see* Doppler
    studies
  myocardial, *see* myocardial
    ischemia; myocardial perfusion
blood gases, arterial, in pulmonary
  vascular disease 388
blood pool imaging
  aortic regurgitation 232, 246
  aortic stenosis 209
  cardiomyopathy
    dilated 332, 339
    hypertrophic cardiomyopathy
      344
    restrictive 360
  heart failure 97-8, 117-18
  mitral regurgitation 191, 203
  tricuspid disease 254
blood pressure
  ambulatory monitoring 136,
    155-6
  high, *see* hypertension
  oral contraceptives and 147
  population/age/gender distribution
    129, 140
brain, vascular disease in
  hypertension 129, 132, 145-6
bundle branch block
  left
    aortic stenosis and 208, 217
    dilated cardiomyopathy and
      331, 332, 336
    heart failure and 96, 108
    mitral regurgitation and 189,
      197
  right
    in Ebstein's anomaly 252, 259
    in pulmonary vascular disease
      388, 397

C

calcification
  aorta
    aortic regurgitation with 231,
      238
    in PDA 296, 300
  aortic (valve) 207, 215
    bicuspid 206, 211
    echocardiography 208, 219

senile aortic stenosis and 206, 212
X-ray 215
coronary, CT imaging 7, 22
LA in mitral stenosis 171, 179
mitral valve, in chronic mitral stenosis 170, 178
mitral valve ring/annular 189, 195
pericardial, X-ray 359, 363, 406, 412
cancers, *see* malignancies
captopril renogram 137, 161
carcinoid disease, tricuspid valve in 251, 253, 255
carcinoma, secondary, pathology 371, 376, 405
cardiac disease/procedures, *see* heart *and references below*
cardiomegaly, *see* heart
cardiomyopathy 329-58
dilated (in heart failure etc.) 331-41
angiography 98, 122, 333
definition 331
ECG 108, 109, 110, 331, 336-7
echocardiography 96, 112, 332, 337-8
management (principles) 333, 341
MRI 124, 332, 339
other investigations 93, 101, 332-4, 335-40
pathophysiology and pathology 331, 334
presentation 331
hypertrophic 342-58
definition 342
investigations 343-5, 348-57
management (principles) 345, 358
pathophysiology and pathology 342, 346-7
presenting signs and symptoms 342-3, 347
ischemic 93, 123
restrictive 359-69
definition 359
investigations 359-60, 363-8
management (principles) 361, 368
pathophysiology and pathology 359, 362
presentation 359
RV 111

carotid disease in hypertension 142, 143
catheter valvuloplasty, *see* valvuloplasty
catheterization, cardiac
angina
stable 8, 29
unstable 41, 45
variant 35, 39
aortic coarctation 322
aortic regurgitation 232, 249
aortic stenosis 209, 222-4
ASD 271
cardiomyopathy
dilated 333
hypertrophic 345, 356
restrictive 361
Fallot's tetralogy 315
heart failure 98, 120-1
MI 52, 78-9
mitral regurgitation 191, 204
mitral stenosis 172, 184
PDA 297, 304-5
pericardial disease 408
pulmonary stenosis 307
pulmonary vascular disease 390, 402-3
tricuspid disease 254, 264
tumors 373
VSD 285
see also angiography
cerebrovascular disease, blood pressure and 129, 132, 145-6
Charcot–Bouchard aneurysm 132, 145
chordal rupture, mitral (and consequent regurgitation) 188, 192
echocardiography 190, 199
signs 189, 194
X-ray 189, 194
circle of Willis aneurysm 132, 146
coarctation of aorta, *see* aortic coarctation
computed tomography (conventional)
angina
stable 7, 27
unstable 41
variant 35
aortic regurgitation 232, 247
aortic stenosis 209
cardiomyopathy
dilated 332, 340
hypertrophic 345, 355
restrictive 360, 366
heart failure 99

MI 52, 78
mitral regurgitation 191
mitral stenosis 172
pericardial disease 408, 418
tumors 373
computed tomography (single photon emission), *see* single photon emission CT
computed tomography in stable angina, single photon emission 5, 18
congenital heart disorders 267-327
aortic regurgitation with 230
bicuspid aortic valve, *see* bicuspid aortic valve
contraction band necrosis in AMI 47, 57
cor pulmonale 396
coronary artery (disease)
atheroma, in hypertension 132, 145
atherosclerosis, *see* atherosclerosis
calcification, CT imaging 7, 22
in Kawasaki disease 3, 10
thallium scanning in severe disease 6, 21
thrombus, thrombolytic therapy, *see* thrombolysis
vasospasm, *see* spasm
coronary artery (techniques)
angiography, *see* angiography (vascular)
angioplasty, *see* angioplasty
bypass graft in stable angina 9, 31
stents in stable angina 9, 33
creatine kinase (MB fraction), AMI 50, 65
Cushing's syndrome 134, 150

D
diabetes 134, 152
diastolic blood flow in mitral stenosis 172, 183
diastolic blood pressure
age and 129, 140
in constrictive pericarditis 408, 419
in mitral stenosis (LV) 172, 184
see also end-diastolic pressure
diastolic filling in restrictive cardiomyopathy 360
diastolic function (of ventricle)
in aortic stenosis 208, 220
in hypertension 138
diastolic pulmonary artery pressure measurement, pulmonary regurgitation allowing 389, 401

digital subtraction angiography, renal 137, 159

dipyridamole-induced stress in stable angina, thallium imaging 6, 19

dobutamine-induced stress in stable angina
  echocardiography 7, 28
  thallium imaging 6, 20

Doppler studies
  aortic coarctation 322, 326
  aortic regurgitation 163, 232-3, 245-6
  aortic stenosis 208-9, 221
  ASD 270-1, 278, 279, 280
  cardiomyopathy
    dilated 332, 338
    hypertrophic 344, 354
    restrictive 360, 366
  Fallot's tetralogy 315, 319
  heart failure 97, 115-16
  MI 51, 73-4
  mitral regurgitation, see mitral regurgitation
  mitral stenosis 172, 183-4
  PDA 297, 302, 303
  pericardial disease 407, 417
  pulmonary stenosis 307, 311
  tricuspid disease, see tricuspid valve disease
  VSD 284, 285, 290, 291, 292

drugs see specific (types of) drugs and entries under pharmacologic

ductus arteriosus, persistent 296-305
  investigations 296, 299-305
  management (principles) 298
  pathophysiology and pathology 296, 299
  presenting symptoms/signs 296, 299

dysrhythmias, see arrhythmias

E

'e' wave
  heart failure 97, 116
  hypertension 138, 163, 164
  restrictive cardiomyopathy 360

Ebstein's anomaly
  investigations 252, 253, 254, 257, 259, 263, 264
  management 254, 266
  pathology 251, 255
  presenting symptoms/signs 251, 256

ECG, see electrocardiography

echocardiography

angina
  stable 7-8, 27-8
  unstable 41
  variant 35, 38

aortic coarctation 322, 326

aortic regurgitation 163, 232-3, 241-6

aortic stenosis 208-9, 217-21

ASD 270-1, 278-81

cardiomyopathy
  dilated 96, 112, 332, 337-8
  hypertrophic 343-4, 351-4
  restrictive 360, 364-6

Doppler, see Doppler studies

Fallot's tetralogy 315, 318-19

heart failure 96-7, 112-17

hypertension 138, 161-4

MI 51, 71-5

mitral regurgitation 189-90, 198-202

mitral stenosis 171-2, 181-3

PDA 297, 302-3

pericardial disease 407, 414-17

pulmonary stenosis 307, 310-12

pulmonary vascular disease 389, 400-2

tricuspid disease 184, 253, 260-3
  in heart failure 97, 116

tumors 372-3, 380-1

ventricular hypertrophy (left) 161-2, 208, 220, 344, 352, 353

ventricular septal defect 284-5, 290-3

eclampsia 135, 153

ectopic beats in AMI 54, 84

edema, pulmonary
  in AMI 54-5, 89, 145
    management 54-5, 89
    X-ray 49, 60
  in aortic regurgitation 231, 239
  in aortic stenosis 214
  in heart failure 95, 102, 103, 104, 105
  in hypertension 131, 145
  in mitral regurgitation due to chordal rupture 189, 194

effort angina, diagnostic features 4, 11

effusions
  pericardial 366
    echocardiography 407, 414-16
    management 408, 419
    presentation 406
    X-ray 406, 411
  pleural
    in heart failure 95, 102, 104

in mitral stenosis 170, 177

Eisenmenger's syndrome
  ASD and 269
    imaging 270, 275
  PDA and 296, 300
  pulmonary regurgitation in 401
  VSD and 283
    auscultation 283, 287
    investigations 284, 288, 289, 401

ejection fraction, LV
  in dilated cardiomyopathy 331, 334
  stable angina and 6, 24

electrocardiography
  angina
    stable 4-5, 13-15
    unstable 41, 44
    variant 34-5, 36-7
  aortic coarctation 322
  aortic regurgitation 232, 240
  aortic stenosis 208, 216-17
  ASD 270, 277
  cardiomyopathy
    dilated 108, 109, 110, 331, 336-7
    hypertrophic 343, 349-51
    restrictive 360, 364
  exercise, see exercise stress testing
  Fallot's tetralogy 314, 318
  heart failure 96, 106-11
  hypertension 135-6, 154
  MI
    acute 49-50, 61-5, 96, 106, 197
    old 96, 107
  mitral regurgitation 189, 196-7
  mitral stenosis 171, 180
  papillary muscle rupture 197
  PDA 297, 310
  pericardial disease 406-7, 413-14
  pulmonary stenosis 307, 310
  pulmonary vascular disease 388, 396-7
  tricuspid disease 252, 259
  tumors 372, 379
  ventricular hypertrophy, see hypertrophy
  ventricular septal defect 284, 289

electrophysiologic studies, hypertrophic cardiomyopathy 343

embolism/embolic thrombus, pulmonary
  arteriogram 390, 403
  cardiac catheterization and angiography 390
  ECG 388, 396, 397

echocardiography 389, 400
heart failure with 94, 102
management 390, 404
MRI 389
nuclear imaging 389, 398, 399
pathology 94, 102, 386, 391, 392
presentation 387
X-ray 388, 394
encephalopathy, hypertensive 132, 146
end-diastolic pressure (ventricles)
in constrictive pericarditis 408, 419
LV
in aortic regurgitation 233, 249
in heart failure 98, 121
in restrictive cardiomyopathy 361, 367
end-diastolic volumes in dilated cardiomyopathy 332, 339
end-systolic volumes in dilated cardiomyopathy 332, 339
endocarditis, infective
aortic regurgitation and 230, 235, 241
echocardiography and clinical signs of 190, 201, 241
endocrinopathies causing hypertension 134, 150-1
endomyocardial fibrosis 359, 362
angiography 361, 367
exercise angina (effort angina), diagnostic features 4, 11
exercise stress testing
ECG
AMI 50, 66
angina (stable) 4-5, 13, 14
oxygen consumption in heart failure 99, 124

F

Fallot's tetralogy 314-20
investigations 314, 317-20
management (principles) 315
pathophysiology and pathology 314, 316
pulmonary stenosis 313, 314, 316
presentation 314
fibrillation
atrial, see atrial fibrillation
ventricular, in AMI 54, 85
fibrinoid necrosis 131, 144
fibromuscular dysplasia 137, 159
fibrosarcoma, MRI 382

fibrosis
endomyocardial, see endomyocardial fibrosis
interstitial, in dilated cardiomyopathy 331, 334
foramen ovale, patent 269, 273
fundus in hypertension 130, 141, 142

G

gender and blood pressure 129, 140
Gerbode defect 283
glomerulonephritis 133-4, 149-50
IV urography 136, 158
red cell casts 153

H

heart
block, see block
catheterization, see catheterization
enlargement (cardiomegaly)
in aortic coarctation 321, 324
in ASD 270, 275
in dilated cardiomyopathy 331, 335
in heart failure 95, 105
in hypertrophic cardiomyopathy 343, 348
in mitral regurgitation 189, 195
in restrictive cardiomyopathy 359, 363
in hypertension 131-2, 144-5
sounds and murmurs, see auscultation
surgery in heart failure 99
tamponade, see tamponade
see also specific parts
heart failure 91-125
definition 93
dilated cardiomyopathy in, see cardiomyopathy
hypertensive, echocardiography 162
in pulmonary hypertension 97, 116, 117
investigations 95-9, 102-25
management (principles) 99, 125
MI and, see myocardial infarction
pathophysiology and pathology 93-4, 100-2
presenting symptoms/signs 94-5
hemangiosarcomas 381
hemodynamic abnormalities
angina (unstable) 41

cardiomyopathy
dilated 333, 340
restrictive 359, 363
heart failure 98, 120
MI 52-3, 78-9
pericardial constriction 408
tumors 373, 374
see also specific abnormalities and methods of investigation
hemosiderosis in mitral valve disease 170, 178
hepatic veins in tricuspid regurgitation, systolic reflux into 253, 262
hiatus hernia 12
hormonal disorders causing hypertension 134, 150-1
hyaline thickening 131, 144
hypernephroma 373, 381
hypertension 127-66
accelerated/malignant, see malignant hypertension
benign 129
classification 129, 130
by cause 129-30
investigation 135-9, 154-66
management (principles) 129, 139, 140, 166
pathology/disease risks 129, 131-2, 142-7
pathophysiology 140-2
prevalence 129-30, 140
primary/essential, definition 129-30
see also pulmonary hypertension (primary)
prognosis 130, 141
pulmonary, see pulmonary hypertension
secondary 133-5, 147-53
definition 129
see also specific causes
symptoms/signs 130
'white coat' 136, 156
hypertrophic cardiomyopathy, see cardiomyopathy
hypertrophy
LV
angiogram 226
in aortic regurgitation 232, 240
in aortic stenosis 206, 208, 211, 216, 226
ECG 96, 108, 135-6, 154, 189, 196, 208, 216, 232, 240, 284, 289

echocardiography 161-2, 208, 220, 344, 352, 353
in heart failure 96, 108
in hypertension 131, 135-6, 144, 154, 161-2, 164
in hypertrophic cardiomyopathy 342, 344, 346, 352, 353
in mitral regurgitation 189, 196
MRI 164
in VSD 284, 289
medial 131
RV
with atrial myxoma 372, 379
ECG 171, 180
in Fallot's tetralogy 314, 318
pulmonary stenosis due to 306, 308
in pulmonary vascular disease/hypertension 387, 388, 389, 393, 397, 400
with VSD 285, 293
septal (ventricular), see ventricular septum
hypokinesia, LV global 98, 122

I

infarction
acute myocardial, see myocardial infarction
pulmonary
atrial myxoma and 372, 378
emboli and 386, 388, 391, 394
X-ray 388, 394, 395
infections causing pericarditis 405, 409
infundibular pulmonary stenosis 306, 308
in Fallot's tetralogy 314, 316
intimal thickening 131, 142, 143
intravenous urography, see urography
ischemia
myocardial, see myocardial ischemia
renal 133
ischemic cardiomyopathy 93, 123
ischemic heart disease 1-90
general pathophysiology 3
heart failure in 93
mitral regurgitation in 190, 201
see also specific diseases
isotope scans, see nuclear imaging
isovolumic relaxation time
hypertension and 138, 163
restrictive cardiomyopathy and 360, 366

J

Joint National Committee, hypertension classification 129, 141

K

Kawasaki disease 3, 10
Kerley B-lines, see septal lines
kidney see entries under renal
krypton-81m ventilation–perfusion scans in pulmonary vascular disease 389, 399

L

laboratory studies
AMI 50
pericardial disease 408
tumors 373
lung
disease (causing pulmonary hypertension) 388
obstructive 396, 398
edema, see edema
infarcts, see infarction
vasculature see entries under pulmonary

M

magnetic resonance imaging
angina
stable 7, 26
unstable 41, 45
variant 35
aortic coarctation 322, 327
aortic regurgitation 232, 247, 248
aortic stenosis 209, 222
ASD 271, 281-2
cardiomyopathy
dilated 124, 332, 339
hypertrophic 345, 355
restrictive 360
Fallot's tetralogy 315, 319
heart failure 99, 124, 125
hypertension 138-9, 164-6
MI 52, 76-7
mitral regurgitation 191, 203
mitral stenosis 172
PDA 297, 304
pericardial disease 408, 417
pulmonary stenosis 307, 312
pulmonary vascular disease 389
tricuspid disease 254, 263
tumors 373, 382-3
ventricular hypertrophy (left) 164
ventricular septal defect 285, 293-4

malignancies, cardiac
investigations 372, 373, 381, 382, 383, 384
pathology 371, 376-7
pericardial, secondary 371, 376
malignant/accelerated hypertension
definition 130
fibrinoid necrosis in 131
kidney in 130, 147
retinopathy 142
mammary artery (internal) in aortic coarctation, dilatation 322, 323, 327
Marfan's syndrome
aortic regurgitation 230, 242, 248, 249
mitral regurgitation 188, 193
mechanical complications of AMI 55, 89
medial hypertrophy 131
melanoma, pathology 371, 376
metastases
echocardiography 373, 381
pathology 371, 376
pericardial 371
mitral regurgitation 188-205
definition 188
Doppler echocardiography 172, 184, 190, 202
in AMI 51, 73
in dilated cardiomyopathy 332, 338
in heart failure 97, 115
in hypertrophic cardiomyopathy 344
investigations (other than Doppler) 189-91, 194-204
in hypertrophic cardiomyopathy 344, 353
in restrictive cardiomyopathy 361, 364, 367
management (principles) 191, 205
in MI 53, 81, 188, 192, 193
imaging 51, 73
pathology 188, 192-3
presenting symptoms/signs 188-9, 194
primary 191
secondary 191
'v'-wave in 53, 81
mitral valve
calcification, see calcification
in hypertrophic cardiomyopathy, abnormalities 344, 352, 353

leaflets
    in hypertrophic
        cardiomyopathy 342, 346
    myxomatous appearance 190,
        198, 199
    premature closure in aortic
        regurgitation 232, 243, 244
    prolapse (and consequent
        regurgitation)
        echocardiography 190, 198,
            199, 200
        symptoms 188
    regurgitation, see mitral
        regurgitation
    stenosis 169-87
        definition 169
        investigations 170-2, 176-85
        management (principles)
            172-3, 185-6
        pathology 169, 174-5
        presenting symptoms/signs
            169-70, 175
        tumor movement involving
            372-3, 380
        vegetations 169, 174, 190, 200
mitral valvuloplasty 172-3, 185, 186
Mobitz type I and II second-degree
    AV block in AMI 87
Monckeberg's aortic stenosis 206,
    212
murmurs, see auscultation
muscle fibers, vacuolated, in dilated
    cardiomyopathy 331, 334
myocardial infarction, acute 47-90
    definition 47
    heart failure and 93, 100, 104,
        106
    in hypertension 132
    investigations 49-53, 60-82
        ECG, see electrocardiography
    management (principles) 53-5,
        82-90
    mitral regurgitation, see mitral
        regurgitation
    non-Q-wave (subendocardial) 55
    pathophysiology and pathology
        47-8, 56-9
        papillary muscle, see papillary
            muscle damage
    pericarditis in 55, 405
    presenting symptoms/signs 48
    pulmonary edema in, see edema
myocardial infarction, old
    ECG 96, 107
    heart failure and 96, 107
myocardial ischemia

non-cardiac conditions with
    discomfort similar to 4, 12
    silent 5, 15
    in stable angina, mechanism 3,
        11
myocardial metabolism, PET scans,
    see positron emission tomography
myocardial perfusion/blood flow in
    stable angina
    nuclear imaging 5-7, 12-25, 119
    PET scans, see positron emission
        tomography
    see also reperfusion
myocarditis, rheumatic 169
myocardium
    amyloid infiltration, see amyloid
    hibernating 7, 25, 98, 119, 120
    in hypertrophic cardiomyopathy,
        histology 342, 347
    stunned 51, 70
myxoma, atrial
    investigations 372-4, 378, 379,
        380
    management (principles) 374,
        385
    pathology 371, 375
    presentation 371, 372, 377
myxomatous appearance, mitral
    leaflets 190, 198, 199

N

neoplasms, see tumors
nephroblastoma (Wilms' tumor)
    148
nephrosclerosis 132, 146
nitrogen-13 ammonia for PET scan
    in stable angina 7, 25
nuclear imaging (myocardial
    perfusion)
    angina
        stable 5-7, 17-25, 119
        unstable 41
        variant 35, 38
    aortic regurgitation 233, 246
    aortic stenosis 209
    ASD 271
    cardiomyopathy
        dilated 332
        hypertrophic 344, 355
        restrictive 360
    heart failure 97-8, 117-19
    MI 50
    mitral regurgitation 191, 203
    pulmonary vascular disease 389,
        398-9
    tricuspid disease 254

tumors 373
nuclear imaging (renal/adrenal)
    137-8, 160-1

oral contraceptives and blood
    pressure 147
ostium primum ASD 269, 273
    angiography 271-2, 282
    ECG 270, 277
    echocardiography 270, 278, 279
    X-ray 270, 276
ostium secundum ASD 269, 273
    ECG 270, 277
echocardiography 270, 278, 280,
    281
oxygen consumption in heart failure,
exercise testing 99, 124

P

P-waves
    atrial myxoma 379
    mitral stenosis 171, 180
pacing, prophylactic, AMI patients
    54, 88
papillary muscle damage/infarction
    47, 51, 57, 58, 73, 188, 192
    ECG 197
    pulmonary artery and capillary
        wedge pressure recording 53, 81
perfusion, see myocardial perfusion;
    ventilation–perfusion scans
pericarditis
    acute/subacute
        ECG 406, 413
        management 408, 419
        pathology 405, 409
        presentation 405
    in AMI 55, 405
    constrictive/chronic constrictive
        catheterization studies 408
        CT 409, 418
        diagnostic investigations 359,
            360, 361, 363, 366
        echocardiography 407, 417
        MRI 409, 417
        pathology 10, 405
        X-ray 406, 412
pericardium 405-19
    calcification, X-ray 359, 363, 406,
        412
    effusions, see effusions
    thickening 360, 366, 405
    tumors
        pathology 371, 376, 405
        secondary 371, 376
        signs 372

pharmacologic causes of
  hypertension 135, 137, 158
pharmacologic management
  angina
    stable 8-9
    unstable 42, 46
  dilated cardiomyopathy 333, 341
  heart failure 99
  MI 53-5, 82, 83
  mitral regurgitation 205
  see also specific (types of) drugs
pharmacologic stress testing in
stable angina
  echocardiography 7, 28
  thallium imaging 6, 19-20
phase imaging in radionuclide
ventriculography 6, 23
  LV aneurysm 51, 69
pheochromocytoma 134, 151, 159
plaque, atheromatous and
  atherosclerotic 3
  angina and
    stable 10, 30
    unstable 40, 43
  hypertension and 143
  MI and 47, 53
pleural effusions, *see* effusions
polycystic kidney disease
  IV urography 136-7, 158
  ultrasound 137, 160
positron emission tomography
  (myocardial blood flow and
  metabolism)
  angina (stable) 7, 25
  heart failure 98, 120
PR interval
  Ebstein's anomaly and pre-
    excitation syndrome 252, 259
  hypertrophic cardiomyopathy
    343, 350
pre-excitation, in hypertrophic
  cardiomyopathy 350
pre-excitation syndrome 252, 259
pregnancy, hypertension of 135, 153
pressure–volume relation, restrictive
  cardiomyopathy 359, 363
Prinzmetal's angina, *see* angina
pseudoaneurysm, LV, in AMI 52, 75
pulmonary artery/trunk
  in ASD 270, 275
  in Fallot's tetralogy 314, 317
  in mitral stenosis 171, 179
  in papillary muscle infarction,
    pressure 53, 81
  in PDA 296, 300, 313

in pulmonary stenosis 306, 307,
  309, 310
stenosis of, *see* pulmonary stenosis
  in VSD 284, 288
pulmonary capillary wedge pressure
  in dilated cardiomyopathy 333,
    340
  in heart failure 98, 121
  in mitral regurgitation 191, 204
  in mitral stenosis 172, 184
  in papillary muscle infarction 53,
    81
pulmonary edema, *see* edema
pulmonary embolism, heart failure
  with 94, 102
pulmonary hypertension
  (primary/idiopathic/essential)
  arteriogram 390, 403
  management 390, 404
  pathology 386-7, 392, 393
  X-ray 388, 395
pulmonary hypertension (secondary
  and in general/unspecified)
  386-403
  ASD and 270, 275
  heart failure in 97, 116, 117
  investigations 388-90, 394-403
  management (principles) 390,
    404
  pathology 386, 391-3
  presentation 387
  thromboembolic, *see*
    thromboembolic pulmonary
    hypertension
  tricuspid regurgitation and 262
  venous, *see* pulmonary veins
  VSD and 285, 288, 293
pulmonary infarcts, *see* infarction
pulmonary non-vascular tissue,
  see lung
pulmonary regurgitation allowing
  diastolic pulmonary artery pressure
  measurement 389, 401
pulmonary stenosis (including
  pulmonary valve) 306-13
  in Fallot's tetralogy 313, 314, 316
  investigations 306-7, 309-13
    angiographic 209-10, 226, 307,
      313
  management (principles) 307
  pathophysiology and pathology
    306, 308
  presenting symptoms/signs 306-9
pulmonary–systemic flow ratio, *see*
  Qp/Qs ratio
pulmonary valve stenosis, *see*

pulmonary stenosis
pulmonary vascular disease and
  abnormalities (in general) 386-403
  in Fallot's tetralogy 317
  investigations 388-90, 394-403
  management (principles) 390,
    404
  pathology 386, 391-3
  presentation 387
  with VSD 283, 284, 287, 288
pulmonary veins
  anomalous, ASD and 270, 276
  hypertension
    in dilated cardiomyopathy 331
    in hypertrophic
      cardiomyopathy 343, 348
    in restrictive cardiomyopathy
      359
  in mitral stenosis 170, 177
pyelonephritis, chronic 133
  IV urography 136, 148

Q

Q-waves
  cardiomyopathy
    dilated 331, 337
    hypertrophic 343, 349
  MI
    acute 49, 61, 62, 63, 65
    old 107
  see also $S_1/Q_3/T_3$ pattern
Qp/Qs (pulmonary/systemic flow
  ratio), ASD
  Doppler 271
  MRI 271, 282
QR pattern, mitral stenosis 171, 180
QRS complexes
  AMI 84, 85, 86, 87, 88
  amyloid heart disease 360, 364
  hypertrophic cardiomyopathy 343,
    350

R

R-wave
  atrial myxoma 379
  PDA 297, 310
  ventricular hypertrophy (left)
    135-6, 154
  ventricular septal defect 284, 289
radiology (X-ray)
  angina
    stable 4
    unstable 40
  aortic coarctation 321-2, 324-5
  aortic regurgitation 231, 237-9
  aortic stenosis 207-8, 213-16

ASD 270, 274-6
cardiomyopathy
  dilated 331, 335
    hypertrophic 343, 348
    restrictive 359, 363
catheter for pulmonary capillary
  wedge pressure measurement 121
Fallot's tetralogy 314
heart failure 95, 102-5
hypertension 136, 154-5
MI 49, 60
mitral regurgitation 189, 194-5
mitral stenosis 170-1, 176-9
PDA 296, 299-300
pericardial disease 406, 411-12
pulmonary stenosis 306, 309
pulmonary vascular disease 388,
  394-6, 402
tricuspid disease 252, 257-8
tumors 372, 378
VSD 284, 288
radionuclide imaging, see nuclear
  imaging
Reavan's syndrome (syndrome X) 3,
  11, 134
red cell casts 135, 153
remodeling
  arterial/arteriolar 131
  ventricular 93, 101
renal disease (caused by
  hypertension) 132, 146-7
  malignant hypertension 130, 147
  red cell casts 135, 153
renal disease (causing hypertension)
  133-5, 147-50
  parenchymal 133-4, 136-7,
    148-50, 158
  radiologic investigations 136-7,
    137-8, 139, 160-1, 165
  vascular (e.g. renal artery stenosis)
    133, 136, 137, 139, 143-4,
    147-8, 157, 159, 165
renal tumors, metastatic
  echocardiography 373, 381
  pathology 376
reperfusion in AMI
  injury 47, 57
  stunned myocardium following
    51, 70
retinopathy, hypertensive 130, 141,
  142
revascularization procedures,
  perfusion imaging in assessment of
  6, 22
rhabdomyoma, pathology 371, 376

rhabdomyosarcoma
  MRI 383
  pathology 371, 376
rheumatic fever
  aortic valve in
    calcification 219
    regurgitation 230, 235, 239
    stenosis 206, 212
  mitral disease 169, 174, 175
    angiography 204
  tricuspid disease 251, 255
    echocardiography 253
    X-ray 252, 258
  see also endocarditis
rib notching in aortic coarctation
  321, 324
Roger's VSD 283

S
S-wave
  atrial myxoma 379
  LV hypertrophy 136, 154
  PDA 297, 310
  see also $S_1/Q_3/T_3$ pattern; ST-
    segment changes; ST-T
    abnormalities
sarcomas
  echocardiography 381
  MRI 382, 383
  pathology 371, 376
scintigraphy, see nuclear imaging
scleroderma 133, 149
septa, heart, see atrial septum;
  ventricular septum
septal lines (including Kerley
  B-lines)
  in heart failure 95, 104
  in hypertension 136, 155
  in mitral stenosis 170, 177
sex and blood pressure 129, 140
shock, cardiogenic 55, 89
shunts
  ASD 269
    echocardiography 271, 280
  Fallot's tetralogy 315, 320
  PDA 297, 303
  VSD 283
    angiography 285, 295
    echocardiography 285, 291,
      292
single photon emission CT
  angina (stable) 5, 18
  MI 66
sinus venosus defect 269, 273
  echocardiography 270-1, 279
sonography, see ultrasound

sounds, see auscultation
spasm, coronary artery
  in MI etiology 48, 59
  in variant angina
    mechanism 34, 36
    provocation tests 35, 39
spondylitis, ankylosing, aortic
  regurgitation in 230, 236
$S_1/Q_3/T_3$ pattern, pulmonary
  embolism 388, 396
ST-segment changes
  angina
    stable 4-5, 13, 14, 15
    unstable 41, 44
    variant 34-5, 36-7
  heart failure 106, 107
  MI 49, 50, 61, 62, 63, 65, 66, 86,
    87, 106
  pericarditis 406, 413
ST-T abnormalities
  aortic coarctation 322, 325
  aortic regurgitation 232, 240
  aortic stenosis 208, 216
  cardiomyopathy (dilated) 331,
    336
  heart failure 96, 108, 109
  mitral regurgitation 189, 196
  see also T-wave abnormalities
Starling function in dilated
  cardiomyopathy 331, 334
stents, coronary, in stable angina 33
stress testing
  angina (stable)
    ECG 4-5, 13, 14
    echocardiography 7, 28
    thallium scanning 6, 19-20, 21
    ventriculography 6, 24
  by exercise, see exercise stress
    testing
  heart failure 99
  MI 50, 66
  pharmacologic, see
    pharmacologic stress testing
  stroke and blood pressure 129
subendocardial MI 55
subvalvar aortic stenosis 206-7, 212
  angiography 227, 228
  withdrawal pressure tracing 209,
    223
  X-ray 208
supravalvar aortic stenosis 206
  angiography 225, 226
  withdrawal pressure tracing 209,
    223
  X-ray 208, 215, 216

surgery, cardiac
    in heart failure 99
    tumors 374, 385
    see also specific procedures
syndrome X 3, 11, 134
syphilitic disease
    aorta 231, 238
    aortic valve 236
systolic blood pressure
    age and 129, 140
    oral contraceptives and 147
systolic function (LV), reduced
    93-4, 101
    in aortic stenosis 208, 220
    echocardiography 7, 27, 138, 208,
        220
    in hypertension 138
    in restrictive cardiomyopathy 360,
        365
systolic pulmonary artery pressure
    measurement, tricuspid valve
    regurgitation allowing 389, 401

T

T-wave abnormalities (inversion
    etc.)
    angina
        stable 4, 14
        unstable 41, 44
    aortic stenosis 216
    heart failure 96, 111
    hypertrophic cardiomyopathy 343,
        349, 350
    hypertrophy of LV 136, 154
    MI 49, 61, 64
    PDA 297, 310
    pericarditis 406, 413
    pulmonary vascular disease 388,
        396
    tumors 372, 379
    see also $S_1/Q_3/T_3$ pattern; ST-
        segment changes; ST-T
        abnormalities
tachycardias, ventricular
    in angina (stable) 14
    in heart failure 110, 111
    in hypertrophic cardiomyopathy
        343, 351
    in MI 54, 85, 86
tamponade, cardiac
    in AMI 47, 58
    ECG 406-7, 414
    management 408
    presentation 407
technetium-99m imaging
    angina (stable) 5, 6, 18

heart failure 97-8
    MI 50, 67-8
    renovascular disease 137, 160
tetralogy of Fallot, *see* Fallot's
    tetralogy
thallium-201 imaging
    angina (stable) 5-6, 7, 16-22, 26
    heart failure 98, 119
    MI 66
thermodilution catheter,
    balloon-tipped 98, 120
thromboembolic pulmonary
    hypertension, chronic
    angiography 402
    management 390, 404
    pathology 386, 392
    X-ray 388, 395, 402
thrombolysis
    coronary (in AMI) 53
        arteriography 53, 79
    pulmonary embolus 390, 404
thrombus
    coronary artery 47, 56
        thrombolytic therapy, *see*
            thrombolysis
    embolic, *see* embolism
    LA
        in dilated cardiomyopathy 332,
            338
        in mitral stenosis 169, 171,
            175, 182
    LV
        in AMI 52, 75, 77, 78
        in heart failure 97, 114
    LV/RV in restrictive
        cardiomyopathy 360, 365
tomography, *see* computed
    tomography; positron emission
    tomography; thallium-201 imaging
tricuspid valve disease (acquired -
    stenosis/regurgitation etc.) 251-66
    Doppler studies 184, 253, 260-3
        in dilated cardiomyopathy 332,
            338
        in heart failure 97, 116
    investigations (other than
        Doppler) 252-4, 257-65
        in restrictive cardiomyopathy
            361, 368
    pathology 251, 255
    presenting symptoms/signs 251-2,
        256
    in pulmonary hypertension
        allowing systolic pulmonary
        artery pressure measurement 389,
        401

tricuspid valve disease (congenital),
    see Ebstein's anomaly
tumors 371-85
    adrenal 134, 150, 151
        imaging 137, 159, 160
    cardiac 371-85
        investigations 372-4, 378-84
        management (principles) 374,
            385
        pathology 371, 375-7
        presentation 371-2, 377
    malignant, *see* malignancies
    renal 148

U

ultrasound
    cardiac, *see* echocardiography
    renal 137, 160
urography, intravenous 136-7, 157-8
    chronic pyelonephritis 136, 148

V

'v' wave and mitral regurgitation 53,
    81, 191, 204
vacuolated muscle fibers in dilated
    cardiomyopathy 331, 334
valve disease 167-266
    see also specific valves
valvuloplasty
    aortic 210, 228, 229
    mitral 172-3, 185, 186
vasodilators, pulmonary 390, 404
vasospasm, coronary, *see* spasm
vasospastic angina, *see* angina
vegetations
    aortic 241
    mitral 169, 174, 190, 200
vein bypass graft surgery, coronary
    disease 9, 31
ventilation–perfusion scans,
    pulmonary vascular disease 389,
    398-9
ventricles
    aneurysm, *see* aneurysm
    arrhythmias
        in angina (stable) 14
        in heart failure 110, 111
        in hypertrophic
            cardiomyopathy 343, 351
        in MI 54, 85, 86
    cardiomyopathy of right 111
    diastolic blood in left, in mitral
        stenosis 172, 184
    dilated/enlarged left
        in aortic regurgitation 232,
            244

in dilated cardiomyopathy 332, 333, 339, 340
dilated/enlarged right, in pulmonary hypertension 387, 393
ejection fraction (left), see ejection fraction
end-diastolic pressure, see end-diastolic pressure
function
    diastolic, see diastolic function
    in dilated cardiomyopathy 331, 334
    in restrictive cardiomyopathy 360, 363, 365, 366
    systolic, see systolic function
hypertrophy, see hypertrophy
hypokinesia (global) of left 98, 122
infarction, right 55, 89
    nuclear imaging 50, 67
mitral annular dilatation with disease of left 190, 202
pseudoaneurysm in left, in AMI 52, 75
remodeling 93, 101
septum, see ventricular septum
thrombus, see thrombus
tumors
    angiography 384
    pathology 376
walls, thinning in dilated cardiomyopathy 331, 332, 334, 337
ventricular septum
    aorta overriding, in Fallot's tetralogy 314, 315, 316, 319, 320

damage in AMI 47, 58
    echocardiography 51, 74
    X-ray 49, 60
defect 283-95
    in Fallot's tetralogy 315, 318, 319
    investigations 284-5, 288-95
    management (principles) 285
    pathophysiology and pathology 283, 286-9
    presenting symptoms/signs 283, 287
Eisenmenger's syndrome and, see Eisenmenger's syndrome
flattening and motion in pulmonary hypertension 389, 400
hypertrophy and thickening 342, 346
    angiography 357
    echocardiography 343, 351, 352
    MRI/CT 345, 355
    X-ray 343, 348
ventriculography
    contrast left
        angina (unstable) 41
        aortic stenosis 209, 210, 224, 226, 227, 228
        ASD 271-2, 282
        dilated cardiomyopathy 98, 122, 333, 340
        heart failure 98, 122
        hypertrophic cardiomyopathy 345, 356-7

MI 53, 82
mitral regurgitation 191, 204-5
mitral stenosis 172, 185
restrictive cardiomyopathy 361, 367
VSD 285, 294-6
contrast right
    aortic stenosis 209-10, 226
    Fallot's tetralogy 315, 320
    hypertrophic cardiomyopathy 345, 357
    pulmonary stenosis 209-10, 226, 307, 313
    restrictive cardiomyopathy 361, 368
    sarcoma 384
    tricuspid disease 254, 264-5
radionuclide
    angina (stable) 6, 23, 24
    MI 51, 69-70
    tumors 373
Venturi effect 344, 353
viral pericarditis 405, 409

W

'white coat' hypertension 136, 156
Wilms' tumor 148
Wolff–Parkinson–White (pre-excitation) syndrome, ECG 252, 259

X

X-ray, see radiology